ASSESSMENT in Speech-Language Pathology

Pathology

A Resource Manual

ASSESSMENT in Speech-Language Pathology

A Resource Manual

5th Edition

Kenneth G. Shipley

Julie G. McAfee

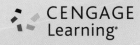
CENGAGE
Learning®

Australia • Brazil • Japan • Korea • Mexico • Singapore • Spain • United Kingdom • United States

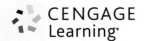

Assessment in Speech-Language Pathology: A Resource Manual, Fifth Edition
Author(s): Kenneth G. Shipley, Julie G. McAfee

SVP, GM Skills & Global Product Management: **Dawn Gerrain**

Product Director: **Matt Seeley**

Product Manager: **Laura Stewart**

Senior Director, Development: **Marah Bellegarde**

Product Development Manager: **Juliet Steiner**

Content Developer: **Deborah Bordeaux**

Product Assistant: **Deb Handy**

Vice President, Marketing Services: **Jennifer Ann Baker**

Marketing Manager: **Jon Sheehan**

Senior Production Director: **Wendy Troeger**

Production Director: **Andrew Crouth**

Senior Content Project Manager: **Kenneth McGrath**

Managing Art Director: **Jack Pendleton**

For product information and technology assistance, contact us at **Cengage Learning Customer & Sales Support, 1-800-354-9706**

For permission to use material from this text or product, submit all requests online at **www.cengage.com/permissions**.
Further permissions questions can be e-mailed to **permissionrequest@cengage.com**

Library of Congress Control Number: 2014959400

Book Only ISBN: 978-1-2851-9807-1

Package ISBN: 978-1-2851-9805-7

Cengage Learning
20 Channel Center Street
Boston, MA 02210
USA

Cengage Learning is a leading provider of customized learning solutions with office locations around the globe, including Singapore, the United Kingdom, Australia, Mexico, Brazil, and Japan. Locate your local office at: **www.cengage.com/global**

Cengage Learning products are represented in Canada by Nelson Education, Ltd.

To learn more about Cengage Learning, visit **www.cengage.com**

Purchase any of our products at your local college store or at our preferred online store **www.cengagebrain.com**

Notice to the Reader

Publisher does not warrant or guarantee any of the products described herein or perform any independent analysis in connection with any of the product information contained herein. Publisher does not assume, and expressly disclaims, any obligation to obtain and include information other than that provided to it by the manufacturer. The reader is expressly warned to consider and adopt all safety precautions that might be indicated by the activities described herein and to avoid all potential hazards. By following the instructions contained herein, the reader willingly assumes all risks in connection with such instructions. The publisher makes no representations or warranties of any kind, including but not limited to, the warranties of fitness for particular purpose or merchantability, nor are any such representations implied with respect to the material set forth herein, and the publisher takes no responsibility with respect to such material. The publisher shall not be liable for any special, consequential, or exemplary damages resulting, in whole or part, from the readers' use of, or reliance upon, this material.

Printed in China
Print Number: 03   Print Year: 2017

CONTENTS

PART II   OBTAINING, INTERPRETING, AND REPORTING ASSESSMENT INFORMATION   63

PART III   RESOURCES FOR ASSESSING COMMUNICATIVE DISORDERS   181

LIST OF TABLES

LIST OF FORMS

LIST OF FIGURES

The purpose of the *Assessment in Speech-Language Pathology: A Resource Manual* is to provide students and professionals with user-friendly information, materials, and procedures for use in the assessment of communicative disorders. The *Resource Manual* is a collection of resource materials applicable to a variety of assessment and diagnostic activities. The items included are practical and easy to use. Materials published previously, but unavailable in a single source, as well as materials developed specifically for this work are included.

New in this fifth edition:

- Expanded information on foundations of assessment, including HIPAA guidelines and instructions for determining chronological age

- New information and samples of individualized education plans (IEPs) and individualized family service plans (IFSPs)

- New content related to childhood apraxia of speech

- New content related to early intervention

- New content on autism that reflects current DSM-5 definition

- Dedicated chapters for autism and augmentative and alternative communication (AAC)

- New and updated chapter on voice disorders, with inclusion of laryngectomy and cleft lip and palate

- New content related to neurocognitive disorders that reflects current DSM-5 definitions

- Dedicated chapter for medical diagnoses associated with communicative disorders

- New chapter with quick reference materials and caregiver handouts

- Updated and new recommendations for published assessment tools, sources of additional information, online resources, and apps useful for assessment

- Digital version of the book, which is completely searchable for text, charts and tables, images, forms, and more

- Online access to downloadable forms

Assessment in Speech-Language Pathology: A Resource Manual contains many reproducible forms, sample reports, and quick-reference tables. Guidelines for interpreting assessment data for specific disorders are also included. The text is divided into four major sections. Part I highlights preparatory considerations. Psychometric principles are summarized, including standardization, validity, and reliability. Descriptions of norm-referenced testing, criterion-referenced testing, and authentic assessment are provided, including advantages and disadvantages of each approach. Preparatory considerations when working with multicultural clients are described as well.

Part II includes procedures and materials for obtaining assessment information, interpreting assessment data, and reporting assessment findings to clients, caregivers, and other professionals. It also includes case history forms and a wide range of interpretive information, interview questions for various and specific communicative disorders, and instructions and examples for reporting assessment information.

Part III provides a variety of materials and suggestions for assessing communicative disorders. Chapter 5 includes general assessment procedures, materials, and worksheets common to all disorders. The remaining chapters are dedicated to specific communicative disorders. Each chapter contains a variety of reference materials, worksheets, procedural guidelines, and interpretive assessment information specifically designed to address the unique characteristics of speech, fluency, language, voice, dysphagia, or neurologically based disorders.

Part IV is a quick-reference section covering hearing disabilities; medical conditions associated with communicative disorders; normal speech, language, and motor development; and tables, images, and caregiver handouts. Some tables and images from earlier chapters are duplicated in this section, but are presented in a caregiver-handout format to enhance the assessment process.

Each chapter includes a listing of "Sources of Additional Information." The Internet sites recommended were deemed appropriate and stable at the time of printing. Because the Internet is a dynamic environment, some sites may no longer exist or may have changed in content. We apologize for any frustration this may cause. New in this edition, apps appropriate for speech-language assessment are also recommended. Again, this is a burgeoning industry and continually changing. Consider those listed here a springboard into exploring apps for diagnostic purposes.

Prior editions contained a CD with supplemental material. We are pleased to now offer this content online. Forms found throughout the text are available in downloadable format to meet individual clinical needs. Many of the stimulus materials used for assessment are also available, including storyboard art, illustrations, and reading passages. These can be used in their digital form or downloaded and printed. Clinicians are encouraged to download content onto a flash drive or other portable storage device so that they have access to these files if they work in environments where Internet access is not readily available.

Assessment in Speech-Language Pathology: A Resource Manual can be a valuable resource for beginning or experienced clinicians. No other manual provides such a comprehensive package of reference materials, explanations of assessment procedures, practical stimulus suggestions, and hands-on worksheets and screening forms.

ABOUT THE AUTHORS

Kenneth G. Shipley is Professor of Communicative Disorders and Deaf Studies and Special Assistant to the Provost at California State University, Fresno. Previously, he served as Chair of the Department of Communicative Disorders and Deaf Studies, Associate Dean of the College of Health and Human Services, and the university's Associate Provost. During his career, he also taught at the medical school at the University of Nevada; served as a speech-language pathologist in the schools; taught in a classroom for children with severe oral language disorders; and practiced in various hospital, educational, and private-practice settings.

Dr. Shipley received his bachelor's and master's degrees from California State University, Los Angeles, and his doctoral degree from Wichita State University. He also completed the Management Development Program at Harvard University. Dr. Shipley has authored and co-authored a number of books, instructional programs, and assessment instruments in speech-language pathology; presented or co-presented more than 30 scientific papers at such conferences as Annual Conventions of the American Speech-Language-Hearing Association; and has had a number of articles published in various major journals in the field. He also coaches intermediate and senior high school girls' golf.

Julie G. McAfee received her bachelor's and master's degrees from California State University, Fresno. She has significant experience serving a variety of adult and child populations. Over the years, she has enjoyed working in acute care hospitals, rehabilitation hospitals, skilled nursing facilities, client homes, preschools, and elementary schools. She is currently in a private practice in the Bay Area of Northern California and serves clients of all ages and conditions. Mrs. McAfee is passionate about helping individuals obtain the highest possible level of communicative ability in order to improve their quality of life. She is grateful for the opportunity to stay abreast of changes in the field in all areas, and enjoys sharing her knowledge, research, and experience with other professionals and all who are affected by a communicative disorder.

Mrs. McAfee is also an accomplished flutist with a bachelor's degree in music performance. She has toured internationally and continues to perform in Northern California.

ACKNOWLEDGMENTS

Our grateful appreciation is extended to our colleagues, friends, and family members who offered support and help with this project. M. N. Hegde, Deborah Davis, Celeste Roseberry-McKibbin, Mary Lou Cancio, Henriette Langdon, Lisa Loud, Barbara Papamarcos, Maxine Rucker, Jennifer Lowe, and Linda Gabrielson reviewed or assisted with portions of this text at various stages of preparation and provided helpful suggestions and comments along the way.

We also thank Kenneth McGrath, Laura Stewart, Deborah Bordeaux and Jack Pendleton at Cengage Learning for their guidance during the review and production process, with special thanks extended to Patricia Gaworecki for her substantial contributions. Our appreciation is extended to the professional reviewers who provided helpful feedback during the draft stages of this project. We are grateful to the many publishers and authors who allowed us to include their works in this book. Our families were especially encouraging and supportive during the development of this Resource Manual. We extend our love and appreciation to Peggy, Jennifer, Adam, Mathias, Janelle, and Timothy. This book could not have been written without your support.

Reviewers

Cengage Learning would like to thank the following reviewers for their valuable feedback throughout the revision process:

Paula S. Currie, Ph.D., CCC-SLP
Southeastern Louisiana University
Hammond, LA

Julie Fuller-Boiling, Ed.D.
Eastern Kentucky University
Richmond, KY

Lennette J. Ivy, Ph.D., CCC-SLP
The University of Mississippi
University, MS

Frank Kersting
Western Kentucky University
Bowling Green, KY

Carney Sotto, Ph.D., CCC-SLP
University of Cincinnati
Cincinnati, OH

Deborah Rainer, M.S., CCC-SLP
Baylor University
Waco, TX

Stacy Wagovich, Ph.D.
University of Missouri
Columbia, MO

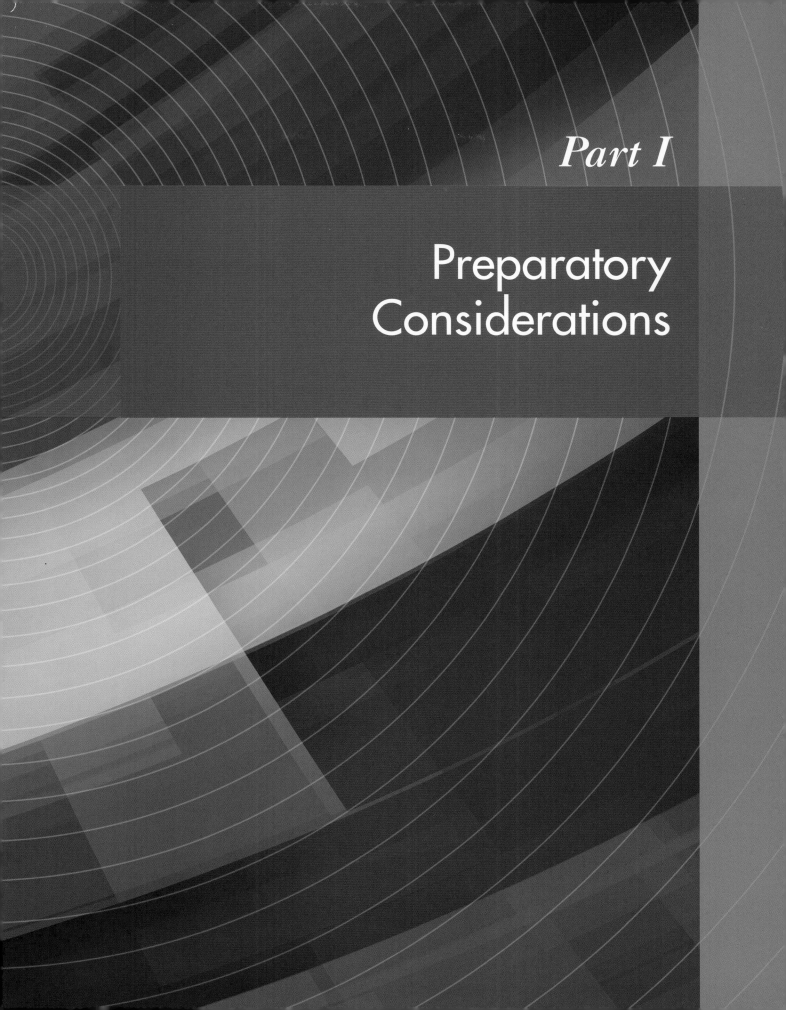

Part I

Preparatory Considerations

FOUNDATIONS OF ASSESSMENT

Before venturing into the assessment process, it is important to gain an understanding of the underlying principles and philosophies of assessment in speech-language pathology. The foundations of assessment provide the framework for all clinical activities. This chapter will define assessment and describe the foundations of assessment that cause it to be meaningful and useful.

OVERVIEW OF ASSESSMENT

Assessment is the process of collecting valid and reliable information, integrating it, and interpreting it to make a judgment or a decision about something. It is the process of measuring communicative behaviors of interest. Assessment is synonymous with evaluation. The outcome of an assessment is usually a diagnosis, which is the clinical decision regarding the presence or absence of a disorder and, often, the assignment of a diagnostic label. Speech-language pathologists use assessment information to make professional diagnoses and conclusions, identify the need for referral to other professionals, identify the need for treatment, determine the focus of treatment, determine the frequency and length of treatment, and make decisions about the structure of treatment (e.g., individual versus group sessions, treatment with or without caregiver involvement). Ultimately, all initial clinical decisions are based on information derived from an assessment process.

For an assessment to be meaningful and useful, it must have foundational integrity. This integrity may be assured if each assessment adheres to these five principles:

1. *A good assessment is thorough.* It should incorporate as much relevant information as possible so that an accurate diagnosis and appropriate recommendations can be made.

2. *A good assessment uses a variety of assessment modalities.* It should include a combination of interview and case history information, formal and informal testing, and client observations.

3. *A good assessment is valid.* It should truly evaluate the intended skills.

4. *A good assessment is reliable.* It should accurately reflect the client's communicative abilities and disabilities. Repeated evaluations of the same client should yield similar findings, provided there has been no change in the client's status.

5. *A good assessment is tailored to the individual client.* Assessment materials that are appropriate for the client's age, gender, skill levels, and ethnocultural background should be used.

Completing an assessment involves gathering relevant information, assimilating it, drawing conclusions, and then sharing the findings and recommendations. We have summarized the process by providing this overview of seven steps the clinician should take in completing an assessment:

1. Obtain historical information about the client, the client's family or caregivers, and the nature of the disorder.

2. Interview the client, the client's family or caregivers, or both.

3. Evaluate the structural and functional integrity of the oralfacial mechanism.

4. Sample and evaluate the client's speech and language use and abilities in the areas of articulation and speech, language, fluency, voice, and resonance. In the case of a dysphagia assessment, assess the client's chewing and swallowing abilities.

5. Screen the client's hearing or obtain evaluative information about hearing abilities.

6. Evaluate assessment information to determine impressions, diagnosis or conclusions, prognosis, and recommendations.

7. Share clinical findings through an interview with the client or caregiver, formal written records (such as a report), and informal verbal contacts (such as a telephone contact with a physician).

The overall emphasis of each assessment differs depending on the client, the type of disorder, the setting, the client's history, the involvement of the caregivers, and other factors. For example:

- Some disorders have extensive histories; others do not.
- Clients have different primary communicative problems. Some exhibit problems of articulation, others of voice, still others of fluency, and so forth.
- Some cases involve extensive interviewing; others do not.
- Some cases require detailed written reports, whereas others do not.

Even though assessment emphases differ across clients, some consideration of each of the seven general areas listed above is necessary with most clients.

ASSESSMENT METHODS

The end purpose of an assessment in speech-language pathology is to draw a conclusion about an individual's communicative abilities. The paths to that end are varied. There are several methods and approaches that are appropriate for validly and reliably collecting assessment data. Regardless of the approach used, it is always important to use the most recent edition of a published test. This is required by insurance and law agencies, and it is also a best practice to not use outdated or obsolete materials. The following sections describe norm-referenced assessment, criterion-referenced assessment, and authentic assessment approaches. Each method has advantages and disadvantages. Although they are differentiated here, they sometimes overlap. Most clinicians use a combination of these methods to obtain the most complete assessment data.

Norm-Referenced Tests

Most of the commercially available tests used by speech-language pathologists are norm-referenced tests. They are most commonly used for evaluating clients for articulation or language disorders. Norm-referenced tests are always standardized. They allow a comparison of an individual's performance to the performance of a larger group, called a normative group. Norm-referenced tests help answer the question, "How does my client compare to the average?" It is the responsibility of test developers to determine normative standards that will identify what *average* is for a given test. Test developers accomplish this by administering the

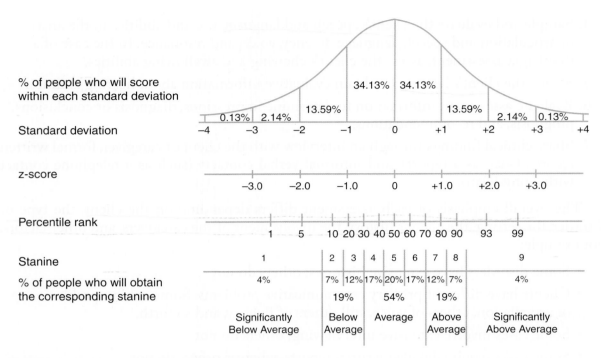

FIGURE 1-1.   Depiction of the Normal Distribution

test to a representative sample group. The results of this sample are analyzed to establish the *normal distribution*. This normal distribution then provides a range of scores by which others are judged when they take the same test.

The normal distribution is often depicted using a bell-shaped curve, as shown in Figure 1-1. The normal distribution is symmetrical. The height and width of the bell are dependent upon two quantities: the *mean* and the *standard deviation*. The mean determines the peak, and it represents the average performance. (In a perfect distribution, the peak also depicts the *median*, which is the middle of the distribution, and the *mode*, which is the most frequently occurring score.) The standard deviation determines the width, or spread, and it represents the distribution away from the group average. The *Empirical Rule* for a normal curve states that:

- 68% of all outcomes will fall within one standard deviation of the mean (34% on each side).
- 95% of all outcomes will fall within two standard deviations of the mean (47.5% on each side).
- 99.7% of all outcomes will fall within three standard deviations of the mean (49.85% on each side).

There are advantages and disadvantages of using norm-referenced tests. Some of the advantages include the following:

- The tests are objective.
- The skills of an individual can be compared to those of a large group of similar individuals.

- Test administration is usually efficient.
- Many norm-referenced tests are widely recognized, allowing for a common ground of discussion when other professionals are involved with the same client.
- Clinicians are not required to have a high level of clinical experience and skill to administer and score tests (administration and interpretation guidelines are clearly specified in the accompanying manual).
- Insurance companies and school districts prefer known test entities for third-party payment and qualification for services.

Some of the disadvantages include the following:

- Norm-referenced tests do not allow for individualization.
- Tests are generally static; they tell what a person knows, not how a person learns.
- The testing situation may be unnatural and not representative of real life.
- The approach evaluates isolated skills without considering other contributing factors.
- Norm-referenced tests must be administered exactly as instructed for the results to be considered valid and reliable.
- Test materials may not be appropriate for certain populations, such as culturally and linguistically diverse clients.

Criterion-Referenced Tests

Criterion-referenced tests do not attempt to compare an individual's performance to any-one else's (as opposed to norm-referenced tests); rather they identify what a client can and cannot do compared to a predefined criterion. These tests help answer the question, "How does my client's performance compare to an expected level of performance?" Criterion-referenced tests assume that there is a level of performance that must be met for a behavior to be acceptable. Any performance below that level is considered deviant. For example, when evaluating an aphasic client, it is not helpful to compare the client's speech and language skills to a normative group. It is much more meaningful to compare the client's abilities to a clinical expectation—in this example, intelligible and functional speech and language.

Criterion-referenced tests are used most often when assessing clients for neurogenic disorders, fluency disorders, and voice disorders. They may also be used for evaluating some aspects of articulation or language. Criterion-referenced tests may or may not be standardized.

There are advantages and disadvantages of using criterion-referenced tests. Some of the advantages include the following:

- The tests are usually objective.
- Test administration is usually efficient.
- Many criterion-referenced tests are widely recognized, allowing for a common ground of discussion when other professionals are involved with the same client.
- Insurance companies and school districts prefer known test entities for third-party payment and for qualification for services.
- With nonstandardized criterion-referenced tests, there is some opportunity for individualization.

Some of the disadvantages include the following:

- The testing situation may be unnatural and not representative of real life.
- The approach evaluates isolated skills without considering other contributing factors.
- Standardized criterion-referenced tests do not allow for individualization.
- Standardized criterion-referenced tests must be administered exactly as instructed for the results to be considered valid and reliable.

Authentic Assessment Approach

Authentic assessment is also known as *alternative assessment* or *nontraditional assessment*. Like criterion-referenced assessment, authentic assessment identifies what a client can and cannot do. The differentiating aspect of authentic assessment is its emphasis on contextualized test stimuli. The test environment is more realistic and natural. For example, when assessing a client with a fluency disorder, it may not be meaningful to use contrived repeat-after-me test materials. It may be more valid to observe the client in real-life situations, such as talking on the phone to a friend or talking with family members during a meal at home.

Another feature of authentic assessment is that it is ongoing. The authentic assessment approach evaluates the client's performance during diagnostic and treatment phases. Assessment information is maintained in a *client portfolio*, which offers a broad portrait of the client's skills across time and in different settings. When appropriate, the client actively participates in reviewing the portfolio and adding new materials. This provides an opportunity for the client to practice self-monitoring and self-evaluation. Artifacts of the client's performance on standardized tests, nonstandardized tests, and treatment tasks are items that are included in the client's portfolio.

Using an authentic assessment approach requires more clinical skill, experience, and creativity than does formal assessment because skills are assessed qualitatively. Testing environments are manipulated to the point of eliciting desired behavior, yet not so much that the authentic aspect of the client's responses is negated. There are several strategies recommended for evaluating clients using an authentic assessment approach, which can be modified for different clinical situations. They are:

- Systematic observations
- Real-life simulations
- Language sampling
- Structured symbolic play
- Short-answer and extended-answer responses
- Self-monitoring and self-assessment
- Use of anecdotal notes and checklists
- Videotaping
- Audiotaping
- Involvement of caregivers and other professionals

There are advantages and disadvantages to using an authentic assessment approach. Advantages include the following:

- The approach is natural and similar to the real world.
- Clients participate in self-evaluation and self-monitoring.
- The approach allows for individualization. This is particularly beneficial with culturally diverse clients or special needs clients, such as those who use Augmentative or Alternate Communication (AAC) systems.
- The approach offers flexibility.

Disadvantages include the following:

- The approach may lack objectivity.
- Procedures are not usually standardized, thus reliability and validity are less assured.
- Implementation requires a high level of clinical experience and skill.
- The approach is not efficient, requiring a lot of planning time.
- Authentic assessment may be impractical in some situations.
- Insurance companies and school districts prefer known test entities for third-party payment and qualification for services.

Dynamic assessment (DA) is a form of authentic assessment. The purpose of dynamic assessment is to evaluate a client's learning potential based on his or her ability to modify responses after the clinician provides teaching or other assistance. It is an especially appropriate strategy when assessing clients with cognitive communication disorders or those from culturally and linguistically diverse backgrounds (enabling clinicians to distinguish between a language disorder and language difference).

The dynamic assessment approach follows a test-teach-retest method. Specifically:

1. A test is administered without prompts or cues to determine current performance.
2. The clinician teaches strategies specific to the skills being evaluated, observing the client's response to instruction and adjusting teaching accordingly. (This is referred to as a *mediated learning experience*, or *MLE*.)
3. The test is re-administered and results from the pre- and post-test are compared.

The clinician pays particular attention to teaching strategies that were effective at improving the client's success. These may include use of cuing (e.g., verbal, visual, tactile, or auditory), graduated prompting, making environmental adjustments, conversational teaching (e.g., asking questions such as "Why did you . . .?" and then instructing "Ah, I see . . . ."), or other strategies.

Dynamic assessment allows the clinician, as part of the diagnostic process, to determine baseline ability and identify appropriate goals and strategies for intervention. If one of the clinician's purposes is to discern a language difference versus a language impairment, it is helpful to note that clients who do not demonstrate improvement following teaching likely have a language impairment, whereas clients who are able to make positive changes following brief teaching experiences are likely to have a language difference.

PSYCHOMETRIC PRINCIPLES

Psychometrics refers to the measurement of human traits, abilities, and certain processes. It is what speech-language pathologists do when evaluating a client's communication. The basic principles of psychometrics are described in the following sections. Read one of the texts on research methodology and evaluation listed in the "Sources of Additional Information" at the end of this chapter for more detailed information on these principles.

Validity

Test validity means that a test truly measures what it claims to measure. There are several types of validity:

- *Face validity* means that a test looks like it assesses the skill it claims to assess. A layperson can make this judgment. Face validity alone is not a valuable measure of validity because it is based merely on appearance, not on content or outcomes.

- *Content validity* means that a test's contents are representative of the content domain of the skill being assessed. For example, a valid articulation test should elicit all phonemes, thereby assessing the spectrum of articulation. Content validity is related to face validity; content validity, though, judges the actual content of the test (rather than superficial appearance) and is judged by individuals with expert knowledge.

- *Construct validity* means a test measures a predetermined theoretical construct, which is an explanation of a behavior or attribute based on empirical observation. For example, the theoretical construct that preschool children's language skills improve with age is based on language development studies. Therefore, a valid test of early language development will show improved language skills when administered to normally developing preschool children of progressively increasing ages.

- *Criterion validity* refers to validity that is established by use of an external criterion. There are two types of criterion validity:
  - *Concurrent validity* refers to a test's validity in comparison to a widely accepted standard. For example, the Stanford-Binet Intelligence Scale is already accepted as a valid assessment of intelligence. Newer intelligence tests are compared to the Stanford-Binet, which serves as the criterion measure.
  - *Predictive validity* refers to a test's ability to predict performance (the criterion measure) in another situation or at a later time. It implies that there is a known relationship between the behaviors the test measures and the behaviors or skills exhibited at some future time. College entrance exams, such as the Graduate Record Examination (GRE), are used because of their predictive validity. The GRE scores are expected to predict future academic performance.

Reliability

Reliability means results are replicable. When administered properly, a test gives consistent results on repeated administrations or with different interpreters judging the same administration. There are several types of reliability:

- *Test-retest reliability* refers to a test's stability over time. It is determined by administering the same test multiple times to the same group and then comparing the scores.

If the scores from the different administrations are the same or very similar, the test is considered stable and reliable.

- *Split-half reliability* refers to a test's internal consistency. Scores from one half of the test correlate with results from the other half of the test. The halves must be comparable in style and scope and all items should assess the same skill. This is often achieved by dividing the test into odd-numbered questions and even-numbered questions.

- *Rater reliability* refers to the level of agreement among individuals rating a test. It is determined by administering a single test and audio- or videotaping it so it can be scored multiple times. There are two types of rater reliability:
  - *Intra-rater reliability* is established if results are consistent when the same person rates the test on more than one occasion.
  - *Inter-rater reliability* is established if results are consistent when more than one person rates the test.

- *Alternate form reliability*, also called *parallel form reliability*, refers to a test's correlation coefficient with a similar test. It is determined by administering a test (Test A) to a group of people and then administering a parallel form of the test (Test B) to the same group of people. The two sets of test results are compared to determine the test's alternate form reliability.

Standardization

There are many commercially available speech and language assessment tools that are standardized. Standardized tests, also called *formal* tests, are those that provide standard procedures for the administration and scoring of the test. Standardization is accomplished so that test-giver bias and other extraneous influences do not affect the client's performance and so that results from different people are comparable. Most of the standardized tests clinicians use are norm-referenced. But *standardized* is not synonymous with *norm-referenced*. Any type of test can be standardized as long as uniform test administration and scoring are used.

Test developers are responsible for clearly outlining the standardization and psychometric aspects of a test. Each test's manual should include information about:

- The purpose(s) of the test
- The age range for which the test is designed and standardized
- Test construction and development
- Administration and scoring procedures
- The normative sample group and statistical information derived from it
- Test reliability
- Test validity

It is important to become familiar with this information before using any standardized test for assessment purposes. Lack of familiarity with this information or inappropriate application of it could render results useless or false.

Form 1-1, "Test Evaluation Form," is a worksheet that may be helpful for evaluating test manuals to determine whether they are worthwhile assessment tools. It is also helpful to read test reviews in professional journals or to consult analyses published by the Buros Institute of Mental Measurements, an organization dedicated to monitoring the quality of commercially published tests.

STANDARDIZED TEST ADMINISTRATION

Read the accompanying manual before administering any standardized test. Each is unique in administration protocols and scoring. There are some foundational principles that apply to most tests, and these are described in the following sections.

Determining Chronological Age

Chronological age is the exact age of a person in years, months, and days. It is important for analyzing findings from standardized tests, as it allows the clinician to convert raw data into meaningful scores.

To calculate chronological age:

1. Record the test administration date as year, month, day.
2. Record the client's birth date as year, month, day.
3. Subtract the birth date from the test date. If necessary, borrow 12 months from the year column and add to the month column, reducing the year by one, and/or borrow 30 or 31 days (based on number of days in month borrowed from) from the months column and add to the days column, reducing the month by one.

Two examples are presented here. The first is a complicated example, requiring two instances of borrowing—12 months were borrowed from the year column, and 31 days were borrowed from the month column (which became May, not April, after the first borrow, so 31 days borrowed):

Test date is April 2, 2015. Client's birth date is December 12, 2008.

$$
\begin{array}{rrr}
2015 & 4 & 2 \\
-2008 & 12 & 12 \\
\hline
\end{array}
$$

Adjusted after borrowing from month and year columns:

$$
\begin{array}{rrr}
2014 & 15 & 33 \\
-2008 & 12 & 12 \\
\hline
6 & 3 & 21 \\
\end{array}
$$

Chronological age is 6 years, 3 months, 21 days.

The second is a simpler example, requiring no borrowing of months or days:

Test date is July 25, 2015. Client's birth date is May 10, 2005.

$$
\begin{array}{rrr}
2015 & 7 & 25 \\
-2005 & 5 & 10 \\
\hline
10 & 2 & 15
\end{array}
$$

Chronological age is 10 years, 2 months, 15 days.

Easy-to-use chronological age calculators are available online and as apps that can be downloaded onto smartphones or tablets. The user plugs in the test date and birth date and chronological age is automatically calculated. A few of the free chronological age calculators available include:

- Chronological Age Calculator App, by Smarty Ears Apps
- Pearson Assessments, Chronological Age Calculator: http://www.pearsonassess ments.com/hai/Images/ageCalculator/ageCalculator.htm
- Super Duper Publications, Chronological Age Calculator: available as an app or online at http://www.superduperinc.com/AgeCalculator/

For preemie infants and toddlers, it is important to consider *adjusted age*, also referred to as *corrected age*. Adjusted age takes into account the gestational development that was missed due to premature delivery. For example, a normal 10-month old baby born 8 weeks premature would be more similar, developmentally, to a normal 8-month old. This is important when considering milestones that have or have not been achieved and when applying standardized norms. Adjusted age is determined by using the child's due date, rather than actual birth date, when calculating chronological age. Adjusted age becomes less relevant as a child grows, and is generally not a consideration for children over age 3.

Basals and Ceilings

Basal refers to the starting point for test administration and scoring. *Ceiling* refers to the ending point. Basals and ceilings allow the tester to hone in on only the most relevant testing material. It would not be worthwhile or efficient, for example, to spend time assessing pre-speech babbling skills in a client who speaks in sentences, or vice versa.

It is important to read test manuals to determine basals and ceilings. Typically, a starting point is suggested according to a client's age. The basal is then established by eliciting a certain number of consecutively correct responses. If the basal cannot be established from the recommended starting point, test items before the suggested starting point are administered until the predetermined number of consecutively correct responses is elicited. For example, if a test's basal is three consecutively correct responses, and the recommended starting point is test item #20, the tester will start test administration on item #20. If, however, the client does not answer three consecutive prompts correctly, the tester will work backwards from test item #20 until the basal is established (i.e., administer test items #19, #18, #17, etc.).

The test ceiling is also predetermined and stated in the test manual. A ceiling is typically determined by a requisite number of consecutively incorrect responses. It is imperative to review the manual before administering a test. Basals and ceilings vary with every test. Many tests do not have a basal or ceiling and are designed to be administered in their entirety. And in some cases, certain subsets of an individual test require a basal and ceiling, whereas other subtests of the same test do not.

Standardized Administration, Modification, and Accommodation

Standardized tests are designed to be administered in a formulaic manner. That makes them, by definition, standardized. It is important to administer test items according to the protocol outlined in the test manual. For example, if the test is to be administered without repeating prompts or cuing, then do not repeat or cue. If the test is to be administered within a specified period of time, do not allow extra time. It is also important to understand the population for which the test was designed. Normative scores are not valid for a client who is not reflected in the normative sample, even when standardized administration is applied. That said, our clients do not always match a test's profile, and special considerations sometimes need to be made when administering a test.

Accommodations are minor adjustments to a testing situation that do not compromise a test's standardized procedure. For example, large-print versions of visual stimuli may be used, or an aide may assist with recorded responses. As long as the content is not altered, the findings are still considered valid and norm-referenced scores can still be applied.

In contrast, *modifications* are changes to the test's standardized administration protocol. For example, a test giver might re-word or simplify instructions, allow extra time on timed tests, repeat prompts, offer verbal or visual cues, skip test items, allow the test taker to explain or correct responses, and so forth. Any such instance of altering the standardized manner of administration invalidates the norm-referenced scores.

Understanding Standardized Test Scores

Once a test is administered, scores can be calculated and findings can be interpreted. A *raw score* is the initial score obtained based on number of correct responses. Read the test manual to determine how to calculate raw scores (and other scores) for a given test. Some tests award more than one point for a correct response. Incorrect calculation of raw score will skew all findings and make test results inaccurate. Raw scores are not meaningful until converted to scaled scores, which include z-scores, percentiles, and stanines. Scaled scores allow the tester to compare the abilities of the test taker to the appropriate normative sample (as defined by the test designer in terms of age, gender, ethnicity, etc.).

A *z-score*, also called *standard score*, allows the clinician to compare the client's score to the normative sample. The z-score tells how many standard deviations the raw score is from the mean. The z-score is useful because it shows where an individual score lies along the continuum of the bell-shaped curve, and thus tells how different the test taker's score is from the average.

Percentile rank is another expression of individual standing in comparison to the normal distribution. The percentile rank tells the percentage of people scoring at or below a particular score. For example, scoring in the 75th percentile indicates that the individual scored higher than 75% of the people taking the same test. The 50th percentile is the median; 50% of the test takers obtained the median score.

Stanine (standard nine) is an additional method of ranking an individual's test performance. A stanine is a score based on a 9-unit scale, where a score of 5 describes average performance. Each stanine unit (except for 1 and 9) is equally distributed across the curve. Most people (54%) score stanines of 4, 5, or 6; few people (8%) score a stanine of 1 or 9.

Test manuals provide specific instructions for interpreting raw scores. It is always important to read the statistical data in each test manual before drawing conclusions about a client's performance. As a general guideline, though, there is cause for concern if a client performs near the bottom 5% of the normal distribution, or approximately -1.5 to -2 standard deviations below the mean (Haynes & Pindzola, 2012).

The *confidence interval* represents the degree of certainty on the part of the test developer that the statistical values obtained are true. Confidence intervals allow for natural human variability to be taken into consideration. Many test manuals provide statistical data for a confidence interval of 95% (some lower, but the higher the better when considering test reliability). This allows the clinician to obtain a range of possible scores in which the true value of the score exists 95% of the time. In other words, a 95% confidence interval provides a range of reliable scores, not just a single reliable score.

Many test manuals provide scores for *age equivalence* (or sometimes *grade equivalence*). Be aware that these scores are the least useful and most misleading scores obtained from a standardized test. An age-equivalent score is the average raw score for a particular age. For example, if 30 is the average raw score for 8-year olds, then all test takers who obtain a raw score of 30 obtain an age-equivalent score of 8 years. Although it seems logical that raw scores transfer easily to age equivalence, age-equivalent scores do not take into account the normal distribution of scores within a population. It would be incorrect to conclude that a 10-year-old child with an age-equivalent score of 8 years is performing below expectations based on age equivalence alone. It could very well be true that the 10-year-old's score is within the range of normal variation. Age-equivalent and grade-equivalent scores are not considered a reliable measure and should generally not be used.

HEALTH INSURANCE PORTABILITY AND ACCOUNTABILITY ACT (HIPAA)

The *Health Insurance Portability and Accountability Act (HIPAA)* is a federal law designed to improve the health care system by:

- Allowing consumers to continue and transfer health insurance coverage after a job change or job loss,
- Reducing health care fraud,
- Mandating industry-wide standards for electronic transmission of health care information and billing, and
- Protecting the privacy and confidentiality of health information.

The law affects all consumers of health services. It also affects all health care practitioners who transmit any information in electronic form for which a national standard has been established. Many speech-language pathologists, particularly those working in a private practice, are required to comply with the law. Clinicians who are uncertain if they are a "covered entity" (required participant) should certainly do their homework to find out. And, if they are covered entities, they should follow the letter of the law, as there are significant fines for noncompliance. HIPAA is regulated by the U.S. Department of Health and Human Services (DHHS). Detailed information about HIPAA, including what constitutes a covered entity, electronic submission standards, privacy policies, and more, can be found on the DHHS website at www.hhs.gov.

Some of the major requirements of HIPAA that affect speech-language pathologists include the following:

- Health care providers must obtain a National Provider Identifier (NPI) number.
- All clients must be given a copy of the clinician's privacy policies. Clients must sign an acknowledgement that they received a copy. The privacy policy must also be posted in a prominent location in the clinician's place of business.
- All protected health information must be handled confidentially. Clinicians may transmit only the minimum information about a client that is necessary to conduct business. This applies to oral, paper, and electronic information.
- National standards for electronic health care transactions must be followed.
- Clinicians must maintain an "accounting of disclosures," which is a record of all instances when a client's information is shared.
- Business associates who manage health care information on behalf of a provider must also comply with HIPAA regulations.

These points are for general knowledge only. The need for clinicians who are covered entities to do further research and become informed providers cannot be overemphasized.

CODE OF FAIR TESTING PRACTICES IN EDUCATION

The *Code of Fair Testing Practices in Education*, presented in Figure 1-2, was developed by the Joint Committee on Testing Practices, which is sponsored by professional associations such as the American Psychological Association, the National Council on Measurement in Education, the American Association for Counseling and Development, and the American Speech-Language-Hearing Association. The guidelines in the *Code* were developed primarily for use with commercially available and standardized tests, although many of the principles also apply to informal testing situations.

There are two parts to the *Code*: one is for test developers and publishers, the other is for those who administer and use the tests. Only the sections for test users are presented in Figure 1-2.

A. *Selecting Appropriate Tests.* Test users should select tests that meet the intended purpose and that are appropriate for the intended test takers.

1. Define the purpose for testing, the content and skills to be tested, and the intended test takers. Select and use the most appropriate test based on a thorough review of available information.

2. Review and select tests based on the appropriateness of test content, skills tested, and content coverage for the intended purpose of testing.

3. Review materials provided by test developers and select tests for which clear, accurate, and complete information is provided.

4. Select tests through a process that includes persons with appropriate knowledge, skills, and training.

5. Evaluate evidence of the technical quality of the test provided by the test developer and any independent reviewers.

6. Evaluate representative samples of test questions or practice tests, directions, answer sheets, manuals, and score reports before selecting a test.

7. Evaluate procedures and materials used by test developers, as well as the resulting test, to ensure that potentially offensive content or language is avoided.

8. Select tests with appropriately modified forms or administration procedures for test takers with disabilities who need special accommodations.

9. Evaluate the available evidence on the performance of test takers of diverse subgroups. Determine, to the extent feasible, which performance differences may have been caused by factors unrelated to the skills being assessed.

B. *Administering and Scoring Tests.* Test users should administer and score tests correctly and fairly.

1. Follow established procedures for administering tests in a standardized manner.

2. Provide and document appropriate procedures for test takers with disabilities who need special accommodations or those with diverse linguistic backgrounds. Some accommodations may be required by law or regulation.

3. Provide test takers with an opportunity to become familiar with test question formats and any materials or equipment that may be used during testing.

4. Protect the security of test materials, including respecting copyrights and eliminating opportunities for test takers to obtain scores by fraudulent means.

5. If test scoring is the responsibility of the test user, provide adequate training to scorers and ensure and monitor the accuracy of the scoring process.

6. Correct errors that affect the interpretation of the scores and communicate the corrected results promptly.

7. Develop and implement procedures for ensuring the confidentiality of scores.

FIGURE 1-2. Code of Fair Testing Practices in Education

C. *Reporting and Interpreting Test Results.* Test users should report and interpret test results accurately and clearly.

1. Interpret the meaning of the test results, taking into account the nature of the content, norms or comparison groups, other technical evidence, and benefits and limitations of test results.

2. Interpret test results from modified test or test administration procedures in view of the impact those modifications may have had on test results.

3. Avoid using tests for purposes other than those recommended by the test developer unless there is evidence to support the intended use or interpretation.

4. Review the procedures for setting performance standards or passing scores. Avoid using stigmatizing labels.

5. Avoid using a single test score as the sole determinant of decisions about test takers. Interpret test scores in conjunction with other information about individuals.

6. State the intended interpretation and use of test results for groups of test takers. Avoid grouping test results for purposes not specifically recommended by the test developer unless evidence is obtained to support the intended use. Report procedures that were followed in determining who were and who were not included in the groups being compared, and describe factors that might influence the interpretation of results.

7. Communicate test results in a timely fashion and in a manner that is understood by the test taker.

8. Develop and implement procedures for monitoring test use, including consistency with the intended purposes of the test.

D. *Informing Test Takers.* Test users should inform test takers about the nature of the test, test taker rights and responsibilities, the appropriate use of scores, and procedures for resolving challenges to scores.

1. Inform test takers in advance of the test administration about the coverage of the test, the types of question formats, the directions, and appropriate test-taking strategies. Make such information available to all test takers.

2. When a test is optional, provide test takers or their parents/guardians with information to help them judge whether a test should be taken—including indications of any consequences that may result from not taking the test (e.g., not being eligible to compete for a particular scholarship)—and whether there is an available alternative to the test.

3. Provide test takers or their parents/guardians with information about rights test takers may have to obtain copies of tests and completed answer sheets, to retake tests, to have tests rescored, or to have scores declared invalid.

4. Provide test takers or their parents/guardians with information about responsibilities test takers have, such as being aware of the intended purpose and uses

FIGURE 1-2. Continued

of the test, performing at capacity, following directions, and not disclosing test items or interfering with other test takers.

5. Inform test takers or their parents/guardians how long scores will be kept on file and indicate to whom, under what circumstances, and in what manner test scores and related information will or will not be released. Protect test scores from unauthorized release and access.

6. Describe procedures for investigating and resolving circumstances that might result in canceling or withholding scores, such as failure to adhere to specified testing procedures.

7. Describe procedures that test takers, parents/guardians, and other interested parties may use to obtain more information about the test, register complaints, and have problems resolved.

Reprinted with permission. *Code of Fair Testing Practices in Education.* (2004). *Washington, DC: Joint Committee on Testing Practices.* (Mailing Address: Joint Committee on Testing Practices, Science Directorate, American Psychological Association, 750 First Street, NE, Washington, DC 20002-4242; http://www.apa.org/.)

FIGURE 1-2.   Continued

CODE OF ETHICS FOR SPEECH-LANGUAGE PATHOLOGISTS

Speech-language pathologists have an obligation to provide services with professional integrity, achieve the highest possible level of clinical competence, and serve the needs of the public. Clinicians need to be aware of biases and prejudices that may be personally held or prevalent in society. Such biases and prejudices should not hinder the assessment process. It is the clinician's responsibility to determine whether a communicative disorder exists, and if so, recommend a treatment plan that is in the best interests of the client. Negative feelings or attitudes should never affect clinical impressions or decisions.

Principles of professional ethics and conduct are outlined in the American Speech-Language-Hearing Association (ASHA) Code of Ethics. The ASHA Code of Ethics can be found online at http://www.asha.org/Code-of-Ethics/.

CONCLUDING COMMENTS

This chapter highlighted the foundational aspects of assessment. Assessment was defined and the overall assessment process was outlined. Psychometric principles were discussed. Information about norm-referenced, criterion-referenced, and authentic assessment was provided, including advantages and disadvantages of each approach. Although each aspect of assessment was differentiated from the others, in true clinical settings some of these concepts and approaches overlap.

SOURCES OF ADDITIONAL INFORMATION

Print Sources

Groth-Marnat, G. (2009). *Handbook of psychological assessment* (5th ed.). Hoboken, NJ: John Wiley & Sons.

Carlson, J. F., Geisinger, K. F., & Jonson J. L. (Eds.). (2014). *The nineteenth mental measurements yearbook.* Lincoln, NE: University of Nebraska Press.

Losardo, A., & Notari-Syverson, A. (2011). *Alternative approaches to assessing young children* (2nd ed.). Baltimore, MD: Brookes Publishing.

Maddox, T. (Ed.). (2008). *Tests: A comprehensive reference for assessments in psychology, education, and business* (6th ed.). Austin, TX: Pro-Ed.

Schiavetti, N., Metz, D. E., & Orlikaff, R. F. (2010). *Evaluating research in communicative disorders* (6th ed.). Upper Saddle River, NJ: Pearson.

Electronic Sources

Buros Institute of Mental Measurements:
http://www.buros.org

Educational Resource Information Center (ERIC):
http://www.ed.gov

Form 1-1.

Test Evaluation Form

Title of Test: _____

Author: _____

Publisher: _____

Date of Publication: _____

Age Range: _____

Instructions: Evaluate the test in each of the areas below using the following scoring system:

> G = Good
> F = Fair
> P = Poor
> NI = No Information
> NA = Not Applicable

Purposes of the Test

_____ A. The purposes of the test are described adequately in the test manual.

_____ B. The purposes of the test are appropriate for the intended local uses of the instrument.

Comments:

Construction of the Test

_____ A. Test was developed based on a contemporary theoretical model of speech-language development and reflects findings of recent research.

_____ B. Procedures used in developing test content (e.g., selection and field-testing of test items) were adequate.

Comments:

(continues)

Adapted from *Speech and Language Assessment for the Bilingual Handicapped*, 2nd ed. (pp. 175–177), by L. J. Mattes and D. R. Omark, 1991, Oceanside, CA: Academic Communication Associates.

Form 1-1. continued

Procedures

A. Procedures for test administration:

_____ 1. Described adequately in the test manual.

_____ 2. Appropriate for the local population.

B. Procedures for scoring the test:

_____ 1. Described adequately in the test manual.

_____ 2. Appropriate for the local population.

C. Procedures for test interpretation:

_____ 1. Described adequately in the test manual.

_____ 2. Appropriate for the local population.

Comments:

Linguistic Appropriateness of the Test

_____ A. Directions presented to the child are written in the dialect used by the local population.

_____ B. Test items are written in the dialect used by the local population.

Comments:

(continues)

Adapted from *Speech and Language Assessment for the Bilingual Handicapped*, 2nd ed. (pp. 175–177), by L. J. Mattes and D. R. Omark, 1991, Oceanside, CA: Academic Communication Associates.

Form 1-1. continued

Cultural Appropriateness of the Test

_____ A. Types of tasks that the child is asked to perform are culturally appropriate for the local population.

_____ B. Content of test items is culturally appropriate for the local population.

_____ C. Visual stimuli (e.g., stimulus pictures used with the test) are culturally appropriate for the local population.

Comments:

Adequacy of Norms

_____ A. Procedures for selection of the standardization sample are described in detail.

_____ B. Standardization sample is an appropriate comparison group for the local population in terms of:

_____ 1. Age

_____ 2. Ethnic background

_____ 3. Place of birth

_____ 4. Community of current residence

_____ 5. Length of residence in the United States

_____ 6. Socioeconomic level

_____ 7. Language classification (e.g., limited English proficient)

_____ 8. Language most often used by child at home

_____ 9. Language most often used by child at school

_____ 10. Type of language program provided in school setting

Comments:

(continues)

Adapted from *Speech and Language Assessment for the Bilingual Handicapped*, 2nd ed. (pp. 175–177), by L. J. Mattes and D. R. Omark, 1991, Oceanside, CA: Academic Communication Associates.

Form 1-1. continued

Adequacy of Test Reliability Data

_____ A. Test-retest reliability

_____ B. Alternate form reliability

_____ C. Split-half or internal consistency

Comments:

Adequacy of Test Validity Data

_____ A. Face validity

_____ B. Content validity

_____ C. Construct validity

_____ D. Concurrent validity

_____ E. Predictive validity

Comments:

Adapted from *Speech and Language Assessment for the Bilingual Handicapped*, 2nd ed. (pp. 175–177), by L. J. Mattes and D. R. Omark, 1991, Oceanside, CA: Academic Communication Associates.

Chapter 2

MULTICULTURAL CONSIDERATIONS

Culturally and linguistically diverse (CLD) clients present unique challenges to clinicians assessing communicative skills. These clients come from a wide range of socioeconomic circumstances, educational and cultural linguistic backgrounds, and personal experiences. They also demonstrate varying degrees of English proficiency. No single chapter or book can provide all of the information needed to effectively serve each individual. The materials presented in this chapter are intended to provide core information and serve as a springboard for becoming fully prepared to assess CLD clients.

PREASSESSMENT KNOWLEDGE

Evaluating a client with a multicultural linguistic background often requires some amount of preassessment research. Before evaluating a CLD client, a clinician needs to understand the client's culture, normal communication development associated with the culture, and the client's personal history. Without this knowledge, assessment procedures may be inappropriate, and diagnostic conclusions may be incorrect.

Know the Culture of the Client

Every culture has a set of pragmatic social rules that guide communicative behaviors. Knowledge of these rules enables clinicians to exchange information with clients and their caregivers in a culturally sensitive manner. A disregard for these rules may be offensive, could result in misunderstandings, and could lead to an inaccurate diagnosis. We have listed several social customs and beliefs that may be relevant when communicating with CLD clients and caregivers. Information about specific cultural groups was obtained from Goldstein (2000), Roseberry-McKibbin (2008), and Westby (2002). Be aware that within each culture, there is individual variation. What is true for a culture as a whole may not be true for an individual from that culture.

1. *Cultural groups have differing views of disability and intervention.* In some cultures (e.g., Asian), having a disability is considered the person's fate and any recommended intervention may be considered futile. In other cultures, parents may feel personally responsible for a child's disability (e.g., certain Hispanic groups). In certain religions (e.g., Hindu, Native American Spiritism), it is believed that a disability is a spiritual gift or punishment. In these cases, the client may be opposed to any intervention that would change the disability. Some cultures (e.g., Asian, Native American) rely on non-Western methods of treatment or healing, such as herbal remedies, massage, hot baths, and acupuncture, and may be skeptical of a clinician's ability to help.

2. *Cultural groups hold diverse views of a woman's role in society.* In some cultures (e.g., Arab), clients or their caregivers may not respect female professionals. It may be socially inappropriate for a female professional to make any physical contact with a man, such as a handshake, or to ask a man direct questions. Female caregivers may not respect suggestions offered by a female professional who is not also a mother. These cultural social rules can be particularly problematic because many speech-language pathologists are women. In some cultures (e.g., Asian), women and young girls are primarily care providers for the family, and school-aged girls may be frequently absent from or drop out of school to care for other family members at home.

3. *Cultural groups hold different views of familial authority.* In some cultures (e.g., Middle Eastern regions, Hispanic, Asian), the father is the spokesperson for the family and the highest authority. Addressing anyone other than the father may be considered disrespectful. In other cultures (e.g., Asian, Middle Eastern regions, Native American), it is the godparents, grandparents, aunts, uncles, or tribal elders who make familial decisions.

4. *Names and titles you will use during communicative exchanges may vary among different cultures.* In some cultures (e.g., Asian), it is more common to address certain family members by relationship rather than name (e.g., *Grandmother* rather than *Mrs. Chang*). When you are unsure, it is best to simply ask how an individual prefers to be addressed.

5. *Certain cultural groups may be uncomfortable with many of the case history and interview questions that are often asked in some settings in the United States.* In some cultures (e.g., African American), certain questions may be perceived as rude and highly personal. In these cases, it is wise to establish a rapport with the client and caregivers before asking personal questions. This may require that all of the salient information is gathered across multiple visits rather than during an initial interview.

6. *Certain cultural groups may be uncomfortable with some of the testing practices we traditionally use.* For example, not all cultural groups use pseudoquestions. These are questions that are asked not to gain new knowledge but to test the person being questioned. In our mainstream culture it is common to ask a child "Where is your nose?" even when we already know where the child's nose is. Some CLD clients (e.g., Native American) would probably not answer the question so as not to insult the person asking. In a diagnostic session, this cultural difference requires the clinician to be particularly creative in assessing a client's speech and language abilities. In some cultures (e.g., African American, Hispanic, Native American), children learn mostly by observation. These clients may be unwilling to attempt unfamiliar tasks or may expect a demonstration of assessment tasks. "Testing" itself may be a completely unfamiliar concept.

7. *Individual achievement is viewed differently among cultural groups.* In some cultural groups (e.g., Middle Eastern, African American) group performance is valued more highly than individual performance; showing individual achievement, as expected in many traditional testing situations, may be socially inappropriate. Some cultures (e.g., Asian) value humility and modesty very highly. Touting individual achievement may be frowned upon.

8. *Cultural groups hold differing views about a child's behavior in the company of adults.* In some cultural groups (e.g., Asian), children are expected to be seen and not heard. In other groups, children do not initiate conversations (e.g., Hispanic). In contrast, people from certain cultures (e.g., African American) expect a very high level of conversational participation from their children.

9. *Cultural groups maintain different views about the use of eye contact in communication.* In some cultures (e.g., African American, Hispanic), it is disrespectful for a child to make frequent or prolonged eye contact with adults because it is perceived as a challenge to authority. In Asian populations, adults also avoid prolonged eye contact with other adults. In contrast, in mainstream American culture, we expect children and adults to look us in the eyes when we speak to them.

10. *Cultural groups view time differently.* In some cultures (e.g., Hispanic, Native American, Middle Eastern), arriving on time for an appointment or answering questions within a proposed time frame is superfluous.

11. *Different cultural groups express disapproval in varying ways.* In some cultures (e.g., Asian), it can be considered inappropriate to contradict others. Caregivers may appear cooperative and agreeable during interview situations; however, they may be merely "saving face" or showing courteous respect while having no intention of following through with your recommendations or requests. They may also smile and appear agreeable, even when they are quite angry.

12. *Perceptions of personal space vary across cultures.* In some cultures (e.g., Middle Eastern, Hispanic, Asian), it may be common to have many people living in a relatively small home or apartment. Also, in some cultures (e.g., Hispanic), physical distance between people is rather close. They may be offended if you step away from them during conversation. In contrast, other cultures (e.g., Japanese) are more comfortable with a greater amount of personal space. In some cultures (African American), physical touch is used to express approval. In contrast, other cultures (Japanese) exhibit very limited physical contact during social interactions.

13. *Certain cultural groups expect varying amounts of small talk before engaging in the business at hand.* In some cultures (e.g., Hispanic, Arab), it is rude to jump right to business without engaging in a satisfactory level of preliminary small talk.

14. *Some cultural groups harbor generalized mistrust of other cultural groups.* These are typically politically driven hostilities. Whether justified or not, it is important to be aware of them.

The degree to which an individual has been acculturated into the mainstream American culture will shape the adherence to these social rules. Some individuals may not share most of the dispositions common to their cultural background. In such cases, stereotyping them would be offensive. For instance, it would be inappropriate to assume that an Asian woman is a full-time care provider when, in fact, she is a highly educated professional pursuing a full-time career.

Ethnography is one method of becoming more culturally knowledgeable. Ethnography is the scientific study of a culture. Ethnographic research is accomplished by observing and interviewing members of a culture. Its purpose is to understand a culture from an insider's perspective without interjecting personal judgments or biases.

The "Clinician's Cultural Competence Worksheet," Form 2-1, is helpful for collecting information about a client's cultural background. There are several potential strategies for obtaining this information:

- Interview members of the cultural community.
- Observe the members of the community in naturalistic situations.
- Ask the client to share about his or her culture.
- Consult with other professionals, particularly speech-language pathologists who are from the same cultural group or who have extensive experience working with individuals from that group.
- Read as much relevant professional literature as possible.
- Read some of the classical literature from the client's culture.

Know the History of the Client

In addition to the questions asked as part of a traditional case history, there are questions particularly relevant to the assessment of CLD clients. Answers to certain questions offer insight into a client's current and past cultural linguistic environments.

Form 2-2, the "Multicultural Case History Form for Children," and Form 2-3, the "Multicultural Case History Form for Adults," are provided to help collect this information. They are intended to supplement the standard child and adult history forms provided in Chapter 3 of this manual. Be sensitive about how this information is obtained. In some cases, it may be best to gather it orally. For example, individuals with limited English proficiency may not understand the questions or be able to write the responses. Other respondents may be intimidated or offended by the personal nature of some of the questions. It may be most prudent to ask these questions after having met with the client and caregivers several times and to establish a positive rapport. It may be necessary to ask an interpreter to translate the forms.

Know the Normal Communicative Patterns of the Client's Dominant Language

It is important to be familiar with normal communication patterns associated with a cultural group; otherwise it will be difficult to determine whether a client is demonstrating a communicative disorder or a communicative difference. The appendices at the end of this chapter include several tables that provide information about normal speech-language patterns and development among African American English speakers, Spanish speakers, and Asian language speakers. Unfortunately, for many languages there are no published data that help identify what is normal versus what is delayed or disordered. In these situations, clinicians must do some investigating. This is usually accomplished by interviewing others who are very familiar with the cognitive and linguistic developmental patterns of the language. Sources of this information may include:

- Other professionals, especially speech-language pathologists
- Interpreters
- Teachers who have taught children who are of the same cultural background and age
- The client's family members
- Community members from the same culture

Within any language, there may be many dialects. Dialects are variations in grammatical and phonologic rules that are adhered to by identifiable groups of people. These subgroups may share a common ethnicity, socioeconomic history, or geography. In the United States, African American English (AAE) is a commonly spoken dialect among some members of the black community.

A dialect is not a disorder; therefore, it is important to know the characteristics of a client's dialect. Some individuals have been inappropriately placed in therapy or special education programs because dialectal differences were improperly diagnosed as language disorders.

Normal Patterns of Second-Language Acquisition

There are normal processes that occur during the acquisition of a second language. These are important to understand because they can help to differentiate between a language disorder and a language difference. Roseberry-McKibbin (2008) identified the following six normal processes of second-language acquisition:

1. *Interference or transfer.* This occurs when communicative behaviors from the first language are transferred to the second language.
2. *Fossilization.* This occurs when specific second-language errors become ingrained even after the speaker has achieved a high level of second-language proficiency.
3. *Interlanguage.* This occurs when a speaker develops a personal linguistic system while attempting to produce the target language. Interlanguage is constantly changing as the speaker becomes more proficient in the second language.
4. *Silent period.* This is a period of time when a second-language learner is actively listening and learning but speaking little.
5. *Code-switching.* This occurs when a speaker unknowingly alternates between two languages.
6. *Language loss.* This is a decline in a speaker's first-language proficiency while a second language is being learned.

Normal acquisition of a second language is dependent upon the continued development and proficiency of a speaker's first language. For this reason, it is advantageous for multilingual clients to develop and maintain proficiency in the primary language while learning the second language. These advantages also extend into other aspects of communication, including reading, writing, and cognition.

Proficient acquisition of a second language generally occurs in two stages, as described by Cummins (1992). The first is *basic interpersonal communication skills* (BICS). It is social communication, such as language used on a playground or lunchroom, at a party, or during a sporting event. Social language typically occurs in a meaningful context and is not cognitively demanding. The second stage is *cognitive academic language proficiency* (CALP). It is the more formal academic language required for success in school. CALP includes cognitively demanding forms of communication with little to no help from context or shared experience. According to Cummins, in ideal situations it takes approximately 2 years to develop BICS and 5 to 7 years to develop CALP. When evaluating multilingual clients, it is important to consider both social and academic language proficiency. A client may have strong BICS, yet struggle in school. In such a situation it is important to differentiate between normal academic language acquisition and possible learning disability.

PLANNING AND COMPLETING THE ASSESSMENT

After gaining the foundational knowledge of the client's cultural and linguistic background, an appropriate assessment can be planned and executed. In most cases, formal methods of assessment are not effective and in certain situations may even be detrimental to serving the best interest of the client. A thorough assessment will include elements of traditional assessment, although it may be necessary to evaluate these elements using creative and nontraditional methods.

Standardized tests are almost always inappropriate for use with culturally and linguistically diverse clients (although there is a slowly expanding repertoire of standardized tests that are written for specific cultural groups). Standardized tests are often culturally biased, usually favoring the mainstream, white culture. Some test writers have attempted to expand their stimulus materials and normative sample groups to include diverse populations. Unfortunately, these tests are still not appropriate for most CLD clients. It is imperative to critically review the standardization information included with a test to determine the appropriateness of using the test with diverse populations. It is also inappropriate to modify a standardized test by directly translating the assessment tasks. There may not be direct translations for certain words and concepts, salient words and concepts from the client's background that should be included may not be included, and images depicted in the test may be unfamiliar in the client's native culture.

Authentic assessment is a desirable alternative to standardized testing. Authentic assessment allows for the evaluation of a client's behaviors in real-life situations and contexts. Assessment materials can be tailored to reflect the client's culture. The approach is also dynamic. Assessments are completed over time and in different environments rather than in one or two sessions in a clinician's office. Data are maintained in an assessment portfolio to allow for ongoing evaluation. Authentic assessment allows clinicians to determine whether a client's functional communicative abilities are adequate to meet the demands of different communication situations.

When not fluent in the client's primary language, it may be advantageous to learn some basic vocabulary and social phrases even though an interpreter will assist with a majority of the communication. Speaking to the client and caregivers in their primary language, even a small amount, may help them feel more at ease and it will demonstrate effort in relating to them.

If the client is school-aged, it is often helpful to interview his or her teacher as part of the assessment process. Specific interview questions may include:

- How does the student interact with classmates?
- How well is the student able to follow directions?
- How well is the student able to communicate needs and ideas?
- How quickly is the student able to learn new skills as compared to other classmates?
- How well is the student able to stay on topic?
- How disorganized or confused does the student appear to be?
- How adept is the student at following classroom routines?
- How well does the student perform gross and fine motor tasks?
- What are some of the specific difficulties the student is experiencing in the classroom?
- To what extent does it seem the student's difficulties are related to limited English proficiency?
- Are there differences between this student and others from a similar educational and cultural linguistic background?

A good assessment incorporates all of the knowledge obtained thus far so that valid and reliable assessment data are obtained in a culturally sensitive manner. Take the following steps when planning and administering an evaluation:

1. *Use culturally appropriate assessment materials.* Use stimulus items that are familiar to the client, and do not use materials that might be offensive.

2. *Test in the client's dominant language and in English.* Test in one language at a time.

3. *Collect multiple speech-language samples.* Collect samples from a variety of contexts, such as home, school, playground, neighborhood, and work. Tape record or, preferably, video record the samples. Obtain samples of the client communicating with a variety of people, including siblings, parents, peers, and teachers. Also sample in a variety of academically and cognitively demanding situations.

4. *Use narrative assessment.* Evaluate the client's ability to construct and recall stories. Wordless storybooks may be particularly helpful.

5. *Focus on the client's ability to learn rather than focusing on what the client already knows.* This will help determine whether the client's current communicative patterns are due to limited experience with the language or due to an underlying language-learning disability.

6. *Be prepared to modify your assessment approach as you learn more about the client's abilities.* Allow the process to be dynamic and flexible.

7. *Consult with other professionals, such as physicians and teachers.* It is often helpful to review medical or academic records. Some teachers may have experience working with students of a similar age and background and can provide information about the client's behaviors in comparison to the client's peers.

8. *Consult with an interpreter.* An interpreter can provide insight into the client's speech, language, and cognitive behaviors in comparison to what may be considered normal in the culture. The interpreter can also help you synthesize information gathered from the client's caregivers and anticipate the amount of cooperation and support likely to be given if treatment is recommended.

9. *Be sensitive when meeting with clients or caregivers in an interview situation.* Make every effort to help them feel as comfortable as possible. Keep in mind that some clients or caregivers may not value the (re)habilitative process. If they are uncomfortable, they may not return for future appointments.

MAKING A DIAGNOSIS

It is important to differentiate between a communicative disorder and a communicative difference. Some CLD clients may demonstrate communicative difficulties that appear to be disorders. It will be necessary to determine whether the client is also experiencing difficulties in his or her predominant language(s). Legally and ethically, a *disorder* can be diagnosed only when the client demonstrates difficulties in all of his or her languages. If the difficulties are present only while speaking Standard American English (SAE), they are considered language *differences*. In most settings, clinicians cannot recommend therapy for clients who exhibit only communicative differences. It is acceptable, however, to provide therapy to clients who are *electively* receiving treatment for communicative differences. For example, a client may choose to receive therapy to modify a foreign accent. These situations are usually limited to private practices or university clinics.

To make a diagnosis, integrate all of the collected data as if putting the pieces of a puzzle together. When analyzing the assessment data:

- Examine the phonological, grammatical, semantic, and pragmatic aspects of the client's language both in English and in the predominant language.
- Determine the client's ability to effectively use language in various environments.
- Note the client's level of participation and appropriateness.
- Note whether the client is able to make requests and follow directions.
- Note whether the client's discourse is logical and organized.
- Determine the client's ability to describe events and objects.
- Determine the client's ability to make accurate predictions and judgments.
- Analyze how much the client is using contextual cues to comprehend discourse.
- Determine whether the client has difficulty learning new skills.

There are certain patterns of behavior that are more likely to be present in the case of a communicative disorder. When evaluating the speech-language samples, the presence of these behaviors may be indicators of a disorder:

- Nonverbal aspects of language are inappropriate.
- The client does not adequately express basic needs.
- The client rarely initiates verbal interaction with peers.
- When peers initiate interactions, the client responds sporadically.
- The client replaces speech with gestures and communicates nonverbally when talking would be more appropriate.
- Peers indicate that they have difficulty understanding the client.
- The client often gives inappropriate responses.
- The client has difficulty conveying thoughts in an organized, sequential manner that is understandable to listeners.
- The client shows poor topic maintenance.
- The client has word-finding difficulties that are caused by factors other than the client's limited experience using the language.
- The client fails to provide significant information to the listener.
- The client has difficulty taking turns appropriately during communicative interactions.
- The client perseverates on conversation topics.
- The client fails to ask and answer questions appropriately.
- The client needs to have information repeated, even when that information is easy to comprehend and expressed clearly.
- The client often echoes what is heard. (adapted from Roseberry-McKibbin, 2008)

It is important to remember that a client exhibits a disorder only when speech and language deficiencies occur in all languages the client speaks, even though the degree of severity may vary from one language to the next. If a disorder is diagnosed, speech-language therapy is warranted. In some cases, the client will not qualify for therapy, but may benefit from other programs such as English as a Second Language (ESL), bilingual assistance, tutoring, counseling, or parent and family education programs. These programs may be available through schools, churches, hospitals, and community organizations.

WORKING WITH INTERPRETERS

Interpreters are invaluable for providing knowledge and assistance. They also bring particular challenges. Consider the years speech-language pathologists have put into developing clinical expertise. When working with an interpreter clinicians effectively need to transfer aspects of their knowledge to the interpreter so that the information obtained is reliable and valid. Once accustomed to working with interpreters, clinicians will appreciate the tremendous benefits and insights they provide.

There are several guidelines that should be followed when selecting an interpreter. It may not be possible to find this "ideal" interpreter, but do follow these principles as much as possible:

1. Select an interpreter who is proficient in English and the language of the client, including the client's regional dialect.
2. Select an interpreter who is experienced and trained in cross-cultural communication. The interpreter should understand and respect the cultural customs and subtleties of both parties.
3. Select an interpreter who has training and knowledge of issues relevant to speech-language pathology.
4. Avoid using a child as an interpreter when communicating with adults, as this could violate culturally based child and adult societal roles.
5. Avoid using the client's family members or friends as interpreters, as it could violate family privacy, and it may preclude unbiased interpretation.

Some work environments have staff interpreters. In other settings, clinicians are responsible for finding an interpreter. Consider these potential sources:

- Local churches, synagogues, mosques, and embassies
- Community leaders from the client's cultural group
- Other professionals and staff members in the same work setting
- Other parents, if in a school setting (be sensitive to confidentiality issues)

Effective interpreters are hard to find. They should be treated with respect and appreciation, and they should be financially compensated for their professional services. Langdon and Cheng (2002) suggest that working with an interpreter involves a three-phase process summarized as Briefing, Interaction, and Debriefing. The *Briefing* is a meeting with the interpreter and the clinician only. It takes place prior to meeting with the client to accomplish the following goals:

- Review the agenda and purposes of the meeting, clarify expectations, and discuss potentially sensitive issues.
- Discuss technical information that will be addressed.

- Train the interpreter to administer any tests. Give the interpreter an opportunity to practice administering the test. This will allow both of you to clarify instructions and ensure that there is no undesirable prompting or cuing.

The *Interaction* takes place with all parties present and includes the following guidelines:

- At the beginning of the meeting, introduce yourself and the interpreter to the client. Explain in simple language what you will be doing and how the interpreter will be assisting.
- Talk to the client, not the interpreter. Maintain appropriate eye contact with the client even when the interpreter is speaking.
- Use brief sentences and a normal rate of speech. Pause regularly so that the interpreter can convey the information.

The *Debriefing* is another meeting with only the interpreter and the clinician. It takes place after the Interaction to accomplish the following goals:

- Discuss any difficulties that were encountered.
- Discuss the interpreter's impressions of the meeting and learn as much as you can about the client's communication and culture through the lens of the interpreter.
- Provide additional training, if necessary, to hone the interpreter's skills for future meetings.

Clinicians and the interpreters may benefit from special training to develop the skills necessary to work effectively together. The integrity of the assessment may depend upon it, so that false diagnoses are not made.

CONCLUDING COMMENTS

This chapter presented some specific considerations for the assessment of culturally and linguistically diverse clients. Before assessing CLD clients, clinicians need to become knowledgeable about the client's cultural values, beliefs, and communicative behaviors, and the client's social and linguistic history. Assessments need to be custom-designed to meet the unique needs and situations of the client. Collaboration with an interpreter is often necessary.

Although assessing culturally and linguistically diverse clients is more time consuming because it requires assessing performance in both languages, it is important to be thorough. Clinicians must differentiate between a communication disorder and a communication difference, because only the former warrants a treatment recommendation.

SOURCES OF ADDITIONAL INFORMATION

Print Sources

Battle, D. E. (2012). *Communication disorders in multicultural and international populations* (4th ed.). St. Louis: Mosby.

Langdon, H. W. (2007). *Assessment and intervention for communication disorders in culturally and linguistically diverse populations*. Clifton Park, NY: Cengage Learning.

Langdon, H. W., & Cheng, L. L. (2002). *Collaborating with interpreters and translators: A guide for communication disorders professionals.* Greenville, SC: Super Duper.

McCleod, S. (2007). *The international guide to speech acquisition.* Clifton Park, NY: Cengage Learning.

Roseberry-McKibbin, C. (2014). *Multicultural students with special language needs* (4th ed.). Oceanside, CA: Academic Communication Associates.

Electronic Sources

American Speech-Language-Hearing Association (search: Multicultural Affairs and Resources)
http://www.asha.org

National Center for Cultural Competence
http://nccc.georgetown.edu

Form 2-1.

Clinician's Cultural Competence Worksheet

Name: _____

Homeland: _____

Region: _____

Person(s) Providing Information: _____

_____

_____

Date: _____

Instructions: Research these questions to become more familiar with a client's cultural linguistic background. Always keep in mind that cultural stereotypes do not apply to all individuals from that culture.

Family Life

What is traditional home life like (e.g., extended family living in one home, grandmother is primary caregiver, children work to support the family)?

Do other relatives often live in the same neighborhood?

During familial interactions, who is the traditional family authority? Who will make decisions regarding a client's care?

What are the names and titles that are most appropriate to use when interacting with various members of a family?

(continues)

Form 2-1. continued

Customs and Beliefs

What is the predominant religion? What are the religious holidays and customs? How might a person's religion influence his or her attitudes toward speech-language pathology services?

What are the predominant beliefs concerning disabilities and interventions?

What are the traditional views of a woman's role? How is a female professional likely to be viewed? What might be the social expectations of a female clinician (e.g., is shaking a man's hand inappropriate)?

What are the traditional views of a child's role in learning? In interacting with adults?

Speech and Language

What are the normal nonverbal and pragmatic communicative patterns commonly associated with this group?

(continues)

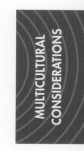

Form 2-1. continued

What are the normal phonologic patterns commonly associated with this group?

What are the normal morphologic and syntactic patterns commonly associated with this group?

What are the normal semantic patterns commonly associated with this group?

Is the prevalence of certain medical conditions associated with communicative disorders higher among members of this race or cultural group (e.g., middle ear problems, cleft palate, stroke)?

Testing Considerations

Will individuals from this cultural group possibly consider certain standard case history and interview questions to be too personal or offensive?

(continues)

Form 2-1. continued

What are some of the specific test administration challenges you might face? Will the testing environment be threatening or unfamiliar? Will the client be reluctant to respond to certain types of tests? Will it be necessary for the client to practice test-taking in advance?

What assessment materials and strategies will be most appropriate? Will an oral case history interview be preferable to a written case history?

What are some basic words and social phrases you can learn to facilitate a better rapport between you and your client or the client's caregivers?

Will you need to hire an interpreter to assist in the assessment process?

Form 2-2.

Multicultural Case History Form for Children

Name: _____ Age: _____ Date: _____

Informant's Name: _____

Relationship to the Child: _____

Instructions: Use this form as a supplement to a standard Child Case History Form, such as Form 3-1. Answer each question as thoroughly as possible.

In what countries, cities, and states has the child lived? For how long?

What is the predominant language spoken at home? In other settings (e.g., school, athletic programs, neighborhood, church)?

Are you concerned about your child's speech and language? Why or why not?

Was your child delayed in learning to speak?

(continues)

Form 2-2. continued

How does your child's speech and language differ from that of his or her siblings?

How well does your child follow directions?

How easily does your child learn new skills?

Form 2-3.

Multicultural Case History Form for Adults

Name: _____

Date: _____

Instructions: Use this form as a supplement to a standard Adult Case History Form, such as Form 3-2. Answer each question as thoroughly as possible.

In what countries, cities, and states have you lived? For how long?

Who lives in your home with you (parents, siblings, friends)?

What is the predominant language you speak at home? Other settings (e.g., work, social settings, gym, church)?

Why are you concerned about your speech and language?

How difficult is it for you to learn new skills?

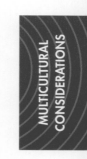

Appendix 2-A.

Speech and Language Characteristics of African American English

TABLE 2-1 **Characteristics of African American English Articulation and Phonology**

AAE FEATURE/CHARACTERISTIC	MAINSTREAM AMERICAN ENGLISH	AFRICAN AMERICAN ENGLISH
/l/ phoneme lessened or omitted	tool	too'
	always	a'ways
/r/ phoneme lessened or omitted	door	doah
	mother	mudah
	protect	p'otek
f/voiceless "th" substitution at end or middle of word	teeth	teef
	both	bof
	nothing	nufin'
t/voiceless "th" substitution in beginning of a word	think	tink
	thin	tin
d/voiced "th" substitution at the beginning, middle of words	this	dis
	brother	broder
v/voiced "th" substitution at the end of words'	breathe	breave
	smooth	smoov
Consonant cluster reduction	desk	des'
	rest	res'
	left	lef'
	wasp	was'
Differing syllable stress patterns	guitar	**gui** tar
	police	**po** lice
	July	**Ju** ly
Verbs ending in /k/ are changed	liked	li-tid
	walked	wah-tid
Metathesis occurs	ask	aks ("axe")
Devoicing of final voiced consonants	bed	bet
	rug	ruk
	cab	cap
Final consonants may be deleted	bad	ba'
	good	goo'
ɪ/ɛ substitution	pen	pin
	ten	tin

(continues)

Appendix 2-A. continued

TABLE 2-1 Characteristics of African American English Articulation and Phonology (continued)

AAE FEATURE/CHARACTERISTIC	MAINSTREAM AMERICAN ENGLISH	AFRICAN AMERICAN ENGLISH
b/v substitution	valentine	balentine
	vest	bes'
Diphthong reduction	find	fahnd
	oil	ol
	pound	pond
n/ng substitution	walking	walkin'
	thing	thin'

Note: Characteristics may vary depending on variables such as geographic region.

Source: *Multicultural Students with Special Language Needs*, 2nd ed. (pp. 63–64), by C. Roseberry-McKibbin, 2002, Oceanside, CA: Academic Communication Associates. Reprinted with permission.

(continues)

Appendix 2-A. continued

TABLE 2-2   Phonological Acquisition in Speakers of African American English*

Acquisition by Age 4

1. Mastery (90% accurate) of vowels and many consonants
2. Moderate occurrences (i.e., exhibited >10% of the time). Patterns are listed in descending order of occurrence (Haynes & Moran, 1989):
   a. palatal fronting
   b. fricative simplification
   c. cluster simplification
   d. final consonant deletion
   e. gliding
   f. cluster reduction
   g. velar fronting
3. Low occurrences (i.e., exhibited <10% of the time). Patterns are listed in descending order of occurrence (Haynes & Moran, 1989):
   a. velar assimilation and stopping
   b. nasal assimilation
   c. context sensitive voicing

Acquisition by Age 5

1. Mastery of most consonants
2. Periodic errors on the following consonants: /θ, ð, v, s, z/
3. Moderate occurrences (i.e., exhibited >10% of the time). Patterns are listed in descending order of occurrence (Haynes & Moran, 1989):
   a. stopping
   b. cluster simplification
   c. fricative simplification
   d. gliding
   e. final consonant deletion and cluster reduction
   f. velar fronting
   g. velar assimilation
4. Low occurrences (i.e., exhibited <10% of the time). Patterns are listed in descending order of occurrence (Haynes & Moran, 1989):
   a. context of sensitive voicing

Acquisition by Age 8

1. Mastery of all consonants
2. Low occurrences (i.e., exhibited <10% of the time). Patterns are listed in descending order of occurrence (Haynes & Moran, 1989):
   a. fricative simplification
   b. velar fronting
   c. final consonant deletion
   d. cluster reduction and stopping
   e. gliding
   f. context sensitive voicing

*True errors, that is, not attributable to dialect.

Source: Seymour and Seymour, 1981, and Washington, 1996, unless otherwise noted. As cited in *Cultural and Linguistic Diversity Resource Guide for Speech-Language Pathologists* (p. 13), by B. Goldstein, 2000, Clifton Park, NY: Singular Thomson Learning.

(continues)

Appendix 2-A. continued

TABLE 2-3   Characteristics of African American English Morphology and Syntax

AAL FEATURE/CHARACTERISTIC	MAINSTREAM AMERICAN ENGLISH	SAMPLE AAE UTTERANCE
Omission of noun possessive	That's the woman's car.	That **the woman** car.
	It's John's pencil.	It **John** pencil.
Omission of noun plural	He has 2 boxes of apples.	He got 2 **box** of **apple**.
	She gives me 5 cents.	She give me 5 **cent**.
Omission of third-person singular present-tense marker	She walks to school.	She **walk** to school.
	The man works in his yard.	The man **work** in his yard.
Omission of "to be" forms such as "is, are"	She is a nice lady.	**She a** nice lady.
	They are going to a movie.	**They going** to a movie.
Present-tense "is" may be used regardless of person/number.	They are having fun.	**They is** having fun.
	You are a smart man.	**You is** a smart man.
Utterances with "to be" may not show person number agreement with past and present forms.	You are playing ball.	You **is** playing ball.
	They are having a picnic.	They **is** having a picnic.
Present-tense forms of auxiliary "have" are omitted.	I have been here for 2 hours.	I been here for 2 hours.
	He has done it again.	He done it again.
Past-tense endings may be omitted.	He lived in California.	He **live** in California.
	She cracked the nut.	She **crack** the nut.
Past "was" may be used regardless of number and person.	They were shopping.	They **was** shopping.
	You were helping me.	You **was** helping me.
Multiple negatives (each additional negative form adds emphasis to the negative meaning.)	We don't have any more.	We **don't** have **no** more.
	I don't want any cake.	I **don't never** want **no** cake.
	I don't like broccoli.	I **don't never** like broccoli.
"None" may be substituted for "any."	She doesn't want any.	She don't want **none**.
Perfective construction; "been" may be used to indicate that an action took place in the distant past.	I had the mumps last year.	**I been had** the mumps last year.
	I have known her for years.	**I been known** her.
"Done" may be combined with a past-tense form to indicate that an action was started and completed.	He fixed the stove.	He **done fixed** the stove.
	She tried to paint it.	She **done tried** to paint it.

(continues)

Appendix 2-A. continued

TABLE 2-3 **Characteristics of African American English Morphology and Syntax**

AAL FEATURE/CHARACTERISTIC	MAINSTREAM AMERICAN ENGLISH	SAMPLE AAE UTTERANCE
The form "be" may be used as the main verb.	Today she is working. We are singing.	Today **she be** working. **We be** singing.
Distributive "be" may be used to indicate actions and events over time.	He is often cheerful. She's kind sometimes.	**He be** cheerful. **She be** kind.
A pronoun may be used to restate the subject.	My brother surprised me. My dog has fleas.	My brother, **he** surprise me. My dog, **he** got fleas.
"Them" may be substituted for "those."	Those cars are antiques. Where'd you get those books?	**Them** cars, they be antique. Where you get **them** books?
Future tense "is, are" may be replaced by "gonna."	She is going to help us. They are going to be there.	She **gonna** help us. They **gonna** be there.
"At" is used at the end of "where" questions.	Where is the house? Where is the store?	Where is the house **at**? Where is the store **at**?
Additional auxiliaries are often used.	I might have done it.	**I might could have done it.**
"Does" is replaced by "do."	She does funny things. It does make sense.	**She do** funny things. **It do** make sense.

Source: *Multicultural Students with Special Language Needs*, 2nd ed. (pp. 61–62), by C. Roseberry-McKibbin, 2002, Oceanside, CA: Academic Communication Associates. Reprinted with permission.

MULTICULTURAL CONSIDERATIONS

(continues)

Appendix 2-A. continued

TABLE 2-4   Acquisition of Morphosyntactic Features of African American English

FEATURE	EXAMPLE
At age 3	
present-tense copula	The girl in the house.
regular past tense	He eat the cookie.
remote past (e.g., "been")	He been had it.
third-person singular	Mary have some crackers.
At age 4	
indefinite article regularization	A egg.
multiple negation	He don't want none.
mean length of C-units* in words = 3.14	
mean length of C-units in morphemes = 3.48	
At age 5	
demonstrative pronoun	She want them books.
reflexive and pronomial regularization	They see theyselves.
mean length of C-units in words = 3.36	
mean length of C-units in morphemes = 3.76	
After age 5	
at (in questions)	Where my hat at?
be	He be scratching.
embedded questions	She asked Can she eat with us?
first-person future	I ma have it tomorrow.
go copula	There go my mom.
hypercorrection	Feets
past copula	They was angry.
plural	Three dog
present copula	We is bored.
second-person pronoun	You all get over here.
mean length of C-units in words = 3.81 (age 6)	
mean length of C-units in morphemes = 4.24 (age 6)	

*Information on MLU from Craig, Washington, and Thompson-Porter, 1998.

Source: Anderson and Battle, 1993; Stockman, 1986; Terrell and Terrell, 1993; examples after Anderson and Battle, 1993. As cited in *Cultural and Linguistic Diversity Resource Guide for Speech-Language Pathologists* (p. 16), by B. Goldstein, 2000, Clifton Park, NY: Singular Thomson Learning.

(continues)

Appendix 2-A. continued

TABLE 2-5   Acquisition of Complex Syntax by 4- and 5-Year-Old Speakers of African American English

COMPLETE FORMS	% OF SUBJECTS (N = 45)	EXAMPLE
Infinitive—same subject	93	He don't need to **stand up**.
Noninfinitive wh- clause	64	This **where they live at**.
and	58	This one happy **and** that one happy.
Noun phrase complement	53	I told you **there's a whopper**.
Let(s)/Lemme	44	**Lemme** do it.
Relative clause	36	That's the noise **that I like.**
Infinitive-different subject	31	The bus driver told the kids **to stop**.
Unmarked infinitive	29	I help **braid** it sometimes.
If	27	Nothing can stop me **if** I got this.
Wh- infinitive clause	22	She know **how to do a flip**.
Because	20	It ain't gonna come out **because** it's stuck.
Gerunds and participles	18	They saw **splashing**.
But	18	I like Michael Jordan **but** he ain't playin' on the team no more.
When	13	**When** you done with this you get to play with this one.
So	9	That go right there **so** it can shoot him.
Tag questions	7	These the french fries, **ain't it**.
While	7	They could be here **while** we's fixin' it, can't they?
Since	2	I'll open the stuff for them **since** they don't know how to do it.
before	2	Put him in there **before** he comes back out.
Until	2	I didn't know it **until** my brother said it.
Like	2	Act **like** we already cook ours.

Source: *Cultural and Linguistic Diversity Resource Guide for Speech-Language Pathologists* (p. 17), by B. Goldstein, 2000, Clifton Park, NY: Singular Thomson Learning. Adapted from "The Complex Syntax Skills of Poor, Urban, African-American Preschoolers at School Entry," by J. Washington and H. Craig, 1994, *Language, Speech, and Hearing Services in the Schools, 25,* 184–185.

MULTICULTURAL CONSIDERATIONS

Appendix 2-B.

Speech and Language Characteristics of Spanish

TABLE 2-6   The Consonants of General Formal Spanish

	LABIAL	LABIODENTAL	INTERDENTAL	DENTAL	ALVEOLAR	PALATAL	VELAR	GLOTTAL
Stops								
Voiceless	p			t			k	
Voiced	b			d			g	
Fricatives		f	θ^a		s	y	x^c	h^c
Affricates						tʃ		
Nasals	m				n	ɲ		
Liquids					l	$ʎ^b$		
Vibrants								
Simple					ɾ			
Multiple					r			

[a]The /θ/ is only used in dialects in Spain, not in American Spanish; in American Spanish /s/ or a variant of /s/ is employed.

[b]The palatal liquid /ʎ/ contrasts with the alveolar liquid /l/ in some dialects; however, this contrast is gradually being lost and the palatal liquid is usually not heard.

[c]Either the /x/ or the /h/ occur as a phoneme in any given dialect but not both.

Source: *Language Acquisition Across North America: Cross-Cultural and Cross-Linguistic Perspectives* (p. 163), by O. L. Taylor and L. B. Leonard, 1999, Clifton Park, NY: Singular Thomson Learning.

(continues)

Appendix 2-B. continued

TABLE 2-7 The Age of Acquisition of Spanish Consonants

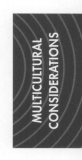

STUDY: ORIGIN OF PARTICIPANTS: CRITERION:	ACEVEDO (1993) TEXAS 90%	FANTINI (1985) TEXAS PRODUCED	JIMENEZ (1987B) CALIFORNIA 50%	LINARES (1981) CHIHUAHUA, MEXICO 90%	MELGAR (1976) MEXICO CITY 90%	ANDERSON & SMITH (1987) PUERTO RICO 75%	DE LA FUENTE (1985) DOMINICAN REPUBLIC 50%
p	3:6	1:6	<3:0	3:0	3:0–3:6	2:0	2:0
b	3:6	1:6	<3:0	6:0	4:0–4:6		2:0
t	3:6	1:6	<3:0	3:0	3:0–3:6	2:0	2:0
d	4:0		3:3	4:0			
k	4:0	2:0	<3:0	3:0	3:0–3:6	2:0	2:0
g	5:11+	1:6	3:3	3:0	4:0–4:6		2:6
β		2:0		6:0			
f	3:6	2:6	<3:0	4:0	3:0–3:6		2:0
ð		1:6		4:0			
ɣ							2:0
s	4:0	1:6	3:3	6:0	6:0–6:6		3:0
x	4:0	2:6	3:3				3:0
tʃ	4:6	2:0	<3:0	4:0	3:0–3:6		2:0
m	3:6	1:6	<3:0	3:0	3:0–3:6	2:0	2:0
n	3:6	1:6	<3:0	3:0	3:0–3:6	2:0	2:0
ñ	3:6	2:6	3:7	3:0	3:0–3:6	2:0	2:0
l	3:6	2:0	3:3	3:0	3:0–3:6		2:6
ɾ	4:6	4:5	3:7	4:0	4:0–4:6		3:0
r	5:11+	5:0	4:7	6:0	6:0–6:6		3:6
w	3:6	1:6	<3:0	5:0		2:0	
j	3:6	1:6	<3:0		3:0–3:6	2:0	2:6
h-x				3:0			

Source: *Language Acquisition Across North America: Cross-Cultural and Cross-Linguistic Perspectives* (p. 182), by O. L. Taylor and L. B. Leonard, 1999, Clifton Park, NY: Singular Thomson Learning.

(continues)

Appendix 2-B. continued

TABLE 2-8 Phonological Acquisition in Spanish Speakers

Acquisition by Age 4

1. Mastery (90% accurate) of vowels and many consonants
2. Consonants not typically mastered:
    a. g, f, s, ɲ, flap ɾ, (maɾtillo), trill r (rojo); consonant clusters (tɾen)

Acquisition by Age 5

1. Mastery of most consonants
2. Periodic errors on the following consonants:
    a. ð, x (reloj), s, ɲ, tʃ, ɾ, r, l; consonant clusters
3. Moderate occurrences of:

a. cluster reduction	/tɾen/ (train) → [ten]
b. unstressed syllable deletion	/elefante/ (elephant) → [fante]
c. stridency deletion	/sopa/ (soup) → [opa]
d. tap/trill /r/ deviation	/roo/ (red) → [doo]

4. Low occurrences of:

a. fronting	/boka/ (mouth) → [bota]
b. prevocalic singleton omission	/dos/ (two) → [os]
c. stopping	/sopa/ (soup) → [topa]
d. assimilation	/sopa/ (soup) → [popa]

Acquisition by Age 7

1. Mastery of all consonants
2. Infrequent errors on:
    a. x, s tʃ, ɾ, r, l; consonant clusters

Source: Acevedo, 1987, 1991; Eblen, 1982; Bleile and Goldstein, 1996; Goldstein and Eglesias, 1996a. As cited in *Cultural and Linguistic Diversity Resource Guide for Speech-Language Pathologists* (p. 26) by B. Goldstein, 2000, Clifton Park, NY: Singular Thomson Learning.

(continues)

Appendix 2-B. continued

TABLE 2-9 Articulation Differences Commonly Observed Among Spanish Speakers

ARTICULATION CHARACTERISTICS	SAMPLE ENGLISH PATTERNS
1. /t, d, n/ may be dentalized (tip of tongue is placed against the back of the upper central incisors).	
2. Final consonants are often devoiced.	dose/doze
3. b/v substitution	berry/very
4. Deaspirated stops (sounds like speaker is omitting the sound because it is said with little air release).	
5. ch/sh substitution	chew/shoe
6. d/voiced th, or z/voiced th (voiced "th" does not exist in Spanish).	dis/this, zat/that
7. t/voiceless th (voiceless "th" does not exist in Spanish).	tink/think
8. Schwa sound is inserted before word initial consonant clusters.	eskate/skate espend/spend
9. Words can end in 10 different sounds: a, e, i o, u, l, r, n, s, d	may omit sounds at the ends of words
10. When words start with /h/, the /h/ is silent.	'old/hold, 'it/hit
11. /r/ is tapped or trilled (tap /r/ might sound like the tap in the English word "butter").	
12. There is no /dʒ/ (e.g., judge) sound in Spanish; speakers may substitute "y."	Yulie/Julie yoke/joke
13. Spanish /s/ is produced more frontally than English /s/.	Some speakers may sound like they have frontal lisps.
14 The ñ is pronounced like a "y" (e.g., "baño" is pronounced "bahnyo").	
Spanish has 5 vowels: a, e, i, o, u (ah, E, ee, o, u) and few diphthongs. Thus, Spanish speakers may produce the following vowel substitutions:	
15. ee/ɪ substitution	peeg/pig, leetle/little
16. ɛ/ae, ah/ae substitutions	pet/pat, Stahn/Stan

Source: *Multicultural Students with Special Language Needs*, 2nd ed. (p. 85), by C. Roseberry-McKibbin, 2002, Oceanside, CA: Academic Communication Associates. Reprinted with permission.

(continues)

MULTICULTURAL CONSIDERATIONS

Appendix 2-B. continued

TABLE 2-10   Language Differences Commonly Observed Among Spanish Speakers

LANGUAGE CHARACTERISTICS	SAMPLE ENGLISH UTTERANCES
1. Adjective comes after noun.	The house green.
2. 's is often omitted in plurals and possessives.	The girl book is . . . Juan hat is red.
3. Past tense -ed is often omitted.	We walk yesterday.
4. Double negatives are required.	I don't have no more.
5. Superiority is demonstrated by using *mas*.	This cake is more big.
6. The adverb often follows the verb.	He drives very fast his motorcycle.

Source: *Multicultural Students with Special Language Needs*, 2nd ed. (p. 84), by C. Roseberry-McKibbin, 2002, Oceanside, CA: Academic Communication Associates. Reprinted with permission.

(continues)

Appendix 2-B. continued

TABLE 2-11   Lexical Acquisition in Spanish Speakers

Comprehension

Monolingual Speakers (Jackson-Moldonado, Marchman, Thal, Bates, & Gutierrez-Clellen, 1993; 328 monolingual Spanish speakers)

Age (months)	Comprehension (median number of words)
7–8	17
11–12	63
15–16	161
24	not available
28–31	not available

Expression

Monolingual Speakers (Jackson-Moldonado et al., 1993; 328 monolingual Spanish speakers)

Age (months)	Production (median number of words)
7–8	0
11–12	4
15–16	13.5
24	189
28–31	399

Bilingual Speakers

Pearson et al., 1993 (25 Spanish-English bilingual children and 35 monolingual Spanish children)

Age (months)	Mean Number of Words Produced	
	Bilingual	Monolingual
16–17	40 (SD=31)	44 (35)
20–21	168 (118)	109 (71)
24–25	190 (136)	286 (170)

Patterson, 1998 (102 Spanish-English bilingual children)

Age (months)	Production (mean number of words)	Range	Minimum for 90% of children
21–22	101	7–525	20
23–25	128	18–297	37
26–27	208	59–431	82

Source: *Cultural and Linguistic Diversity Resource Guide for Speech-Language Pathologists* (p. 32), by B. Goldstein, 2000, Clifton Park, NY: Singular Thomson Learning.

(continues)

MULTICULTURAL CONSIDERATIONS

Appendix 2-B. continued

TABLE 2-12   Acquisition of Morphology and Syntax in Spanish

	BY:	AGE 3	AGE 4	AGE 5	AGE 7
Comprehension					
Active word order			X		
Plural				X	
Number in verb phrases					X
Regular preterite					X
Passive word order					X
Expressive Language					
Personal Pronouns					
Yo		X			
Tú		X			
El/Ella		X			
Me		X			
Te		X			
Lo/La		X			
Se		X			
Morphology/Syntax					
Present indicative		X			
Regular preterite		X			
Imperative		X			
Copulas		X			
Present progressive		X			
Periphrastic (ir a + infinitive)		X			
Past progressive and Imperfect (Van a caminar)		X			
Indirect and direct object		X			
Transformations		X			
Verb–subject–direct object		X			
Verb–direct object–subject		X			
Subject–verb–direct object		X			
Demonstratives		X			
Articles		X			
Imperfect indicative (caminaba)			X		
Past progressive			X		

(continues)

Appendix 2-B. continued

TABLE 2-12   Acquisition of Morphology and Syntax in Spanish (continued)

	BY:	AGE 3	AGE 4	AGE 5	AGE 7
Present subjunctive (cuando caminemos)			X		
Conditional clauses			X		
Comparisons			X		
Tag questions			X		
Plural			X		
Possessive			X		
Prepositions			X		
Past subjunctive (Te dije que no lo hicieras asi.)				X	
Irregular preterite				X	
Number				X	
Conjunctives				X	
Relative clauses				X	
Noun clauses				X	
Adverbial clauses				X	
Gender				X	

Acquisition = use in 75% of obligatory contexts.

Source: Anderson, 1995; Bedore, 1999; Gonzalez, 1983, as cited in Kayser, 1993; Kvaal, Shipstead-Cox, Nevitt, Hodson, and Launer, 1988; Merino, 1992; Pérez-Pereira, 1989, 1991; and Schnell de Acedo, 1994, as cited in *Cultural and Linguistic Diversity Resource Guide for Speech-Language Pathologists* (p. 28), by B. Goldstein, 2000, Clifton Park, NY: Singular Thomson Learning.

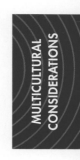

MULTICULTURAL CONSIDERATIONS

(continues)

Appendix 2-B. continued

TABLE 2-13 Norms for Morphosyntactic Development in Spanish

AGE RANGE	VERB MORPHOLOGY	NOUN PHRASE ELABORATION	PREPOSITIONAL PHRASES	SYNTACTIC STRUCTURE

2–3	Present indicative
	Simple preterite
	Imperative
	Periphrastic future
	Copulas ser/estar
		Indefinite and
		  definite
		  articles
		Article gender
		Plural /s/
		Plural /es/
			en
			con
			para
			a
			de
				Sentences with copula
				  verbs
				Use of clitic direct object
				Reflexives
				(S)VO sentences
				Yes/No questions
				Negative with *no* before
				  verb
				Imperative sentences
				Wh- questions
				  qué
				  quién
				  dónde
				  para qué
				  cuándo
				  por qué
				  cómo
				  de quién
				  con quién
				Embedded sentences
				Embedded direct object

3–4	Imperfect preterite
	Past progressive
	Ir progressive—
	  past/present
	Compound
	  preterite
		Grammatical
		  gender in nouns/
		  adjectives
		Use of quantifiers
			hasta
			
			entre
			desde
			sobre
				Wh- questions established
				
				Use of full set of negatives
				Embedding

4–5	Present subjunctive
	Past subjunctive
	Present perfect
	  indicative
		Gender in clitic third-
		  person pronouns		

Source: "Spanish Morphological and Syntactic Development" (pp. 41–47), by R. Anderson. In *Bilingual Speech-Language Pathology: An Hispanic Focus*, H. Kayser (Ed.), 1995, Clifton Park, NY: Singular Thomson Learning.

Appendix 2-C.

Speech and Language Characteristics of Asian Languages

TABLE 2-14   Articulation Differences Commonly Observed Among Asian Speakers

ARTICULATION CHARACTERISTICS	SAMPLE ENGLISH UTTERANCES	
In many Asian languages, words end in vowels only or in just a few consonants; speakers may delete many final consonants in English.	ste/step ro/robe	li/lid do/dog
Some languages are monosyllabic; speakers may truncate polysyllabic words or emphasize the wrong syllable.	efunt/elephant **di**versity/diversity (emphasis on first syllable)	
Possible devoicing of voiced cognates	beece/bees luff/love	pick/pig crip/crib
r/l confusion	lize/rise	clown/crown
/r/ may be omitted entirely.	gull/girl	tone/torn
Reduction of vowel length in words	Words sound choppy to Americans.	
No voiced or voiceless "th"	dose/those zose/those	tin/thin sin/thin
Epenthesis (addition of "uh" sound in blends, ends of words).	bulack/black	woodah/wood
Confusion of "ch" and "sh"	sheep/cheap	beesh/beach
/ae/ does not exist in many Asian languages	block/black	shock/shack
b/v substitutions	base/vase	Beberly/Beverly
v/w substitutions	vork/work	vall/wall

Source: *Multicultural Students with Special Language Needs*, 2nd ed. (p. 109), by C. Roseberry-McKibbin, 2002, Oceanside, CA: Academic Communication Associates. Reprinted with permission.

(continues)

Appendix 2-C. continued

TABLE 2-15 **Syntactic and Morphologic Differences Commonly Observed Among Asian Speakers**

LANGUAGE CHARACTERISTICS	SAMPLE ENGLISH UTTERANCES
Omission of plurals	Here are 2 piece of toast.
	I got 5 finger on each hand.
Omission of copula	He going home now.
	They eating.
Omission of possessive	I have Phuong pencil.
	Mom food is cold.
Omission of past tense morpheme	We cook dinner yesterday.
	Last night she walk home.
Past tense double marking	He didn't went by himself.
Double negative	They don't have no books.
Subject–verb–object relationship differences/omissions	I messed up it.
	He like.
Misordering of interrogatives	You are going now?
Misuse or omission of prepositions	She is in home.
	He goes to school 8:00.
Misuse of pronouns	She husband is coming.
	She said her wife is here.
Omission and/or overgeneralization of articles	Boy is sick.
	He went the home.
Incorrect use of comparatives	This book is gooder than that book.
Omission of conjunctions	You ____ I going to the beach.
Omission, lack of inflection on auxiliary "do"	She ____ not take it.
	He do not have enough.
Omission, lack of inflection on forms of "have"	She have no money.
	We ____ been the store.

Source: *Multicultural Students with Special Language Needs,* 2nd ed. (p. 108), by C. Roseberry-McKibbin, 2002, Oceanside, CA: Academic Communication Associates. Reprinted with permission.

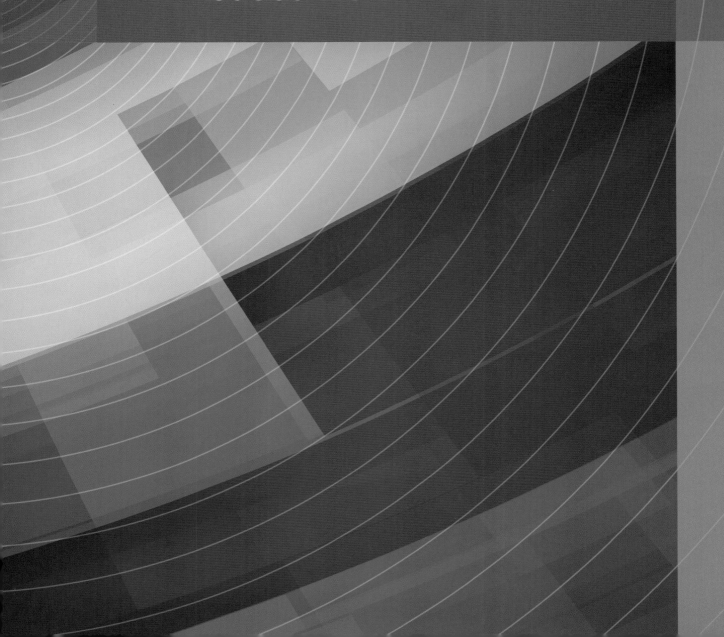

Part II

Obtaining, Interpreting, and Reporting Assessment Information

Chapter 3

OBTAINING PREASSESSMENT INFORMATION

Thorough assessments involve obtaining comprehensive information about clients and their communicative disorders. Collect as much information as possible before the actual assessment session is conducted. Primary sources of preassessment information include:

- A written case history
- An interview with the client, parents, spouse, or other caregivers
- Information from other professionals

The preliminary information gathered, combined with actual assessment results, will enable the clinician to make an accurate diagnosis and develop the most appropriate treatment recommendations.

WRITTEN CASE HISTORIES

The written case history is a starting point for understanding clients and their communicative problems. A case history form is typically completed by the client or a caregiver and reviewed by the clinician prior to the initial meeting. This enables the clinician to anticipate those areas that will require assessment, identify topics requiring further clarification, and preselect appropriate evaluation materials and procedures for use during the evaluation session. Be aware, though, that sometimes the value of a case history form as a preassessment tool is limited, due to potential problems such as:

1. *The respondent may not understand all the terminology on the form.* As a result, inaccurate or incomplete information may be provided.

2. *Insufficient time may be provided to complete the entire form.* Realize that it can take considerable time to collect certain requested information, such as dates of illnesses or developmental history.

3. *The respondent may not know, or may have only vague recall of, certain information.* Naturally, the amount and accuracy of information provided is related to the length and depth of the relationship between the client and the person completing the form. The client's parent, grandparent, spouse, sibling, social worker, teacher, or others will not all have equal knowledge of the client's history and communicative behavior.

4. *Significant time may have elapsed between the onset of the problem and the speech–language assessment.* Respondents will usually have a greater recollection of recent events than events that occurred months or even years ago.

5. *Other life events or circumstances may hinder the respondent's ability to recall certain information.* For example, the parent of an only child will probably remember developmental milestones more clearly than the parent who has several children. Or the parent of a child with multiple medical, communicative, and academic problems will likely be less focused on speech and language development than the parent of a child who has only a communication disorder.

6. *Cultural differences may interfere with accurate provision of information.* The respondent may not understand cultural innuendos reflected in the case history queries, or by their own responses.

Clearly, there are potential dangers to overrelying on the information obtained in a case history. However, when viewed cautiously, case histories provide an excellent starting point for understanding clients, the problems they have experienced, and the difficulties they are facing. No one knows a client's situation better than the client him- or herself, or in the case of a child, the child's parent or primary caregiver. The input provided is certainly an important piece of assessment data.

In the field of communicative disorders, a standard case history form used by all professionals does not exist. Practitioners in different settings typically develop or adapt forms that reflect the information they feel is needed. Form 3-1, "Child Case History Form," is a case history form for use with children, and Form 3-2, "Adult Case History Form," is designed for use with adults. These are basic forms that can be adapted for different practices or settings.

ALLERGY AWARENESS

Some clients may have mild to life-threatening allergies. For example, some clinicians use food products such as peanut butter to assess lingual range of motion. Obviously, this technique would not be appropriate for clients who are allergic to nuts. Form 3-3, "Allergy Alert Form," is reproducible for use in the clinic. Copy the form onto a brightly colored paper so that it is a prominent document in the client's file.

INFORMATION-GATHERING INTERVIEWS

Professionals in communicative disorders generally conduct three types of interviews. These are information-gathering, information-giving, and counseling interviews (Shipley & Roseberry-McKibbin, 2006). The information-gathering interview, sometimes called an intake interview, consists of three phases—the opening, the body, and the closing. The basic content of each phase is as follows:

Opening Phase

- Introductions
- Describe the purpose of the meeting.
- Indicate approximately how much time the session will take.

For example: "I am Mrs. Smith, the speech pathologist who will be evaluating Sarah's speech today. I'd like to begin by asking you some questions about her speech. Then I'll spend some time with Sarah by herself and get together with you again when we are finished. This should take about 90 minutes."

Body of the Interview

- Discuss the client's history and current status in depth. Focus on communicative development, abilities, and problems, along with other pertinent information such as the client's medical, developmental, familial, social, or educational history.
- If a written case history form has already been completed, clarify and confirm relevant information during this portion of the interview.

Closing Phase

• Summarize the major points from the body of the interview.
• Express your appreciation for the interviewee's help.
• Indicate the steps that will be taken next.

For example: "Thank you for all of the helpful information. Now I'd like to spend some time with Sarah and evaluate her speech. In about an hour we will get together again, and I'll share my findings with you."

The opening and closing phases are generally brief and succinct. A majority of the interview occurs in the second phase—the body of the interview—during which the major content areas are discussed. The content and length of this phase are directly influenced by the amount and type of information provided on the written case history, the concerns of the client or the caregiver, and the needs of the clinician to best understand the client and the problems he or she is experiencing.

Questions Common to Most Communicative Disorders

During an interview, both open-ended questions (e.g., *How would you describe your speech?*) and closed-ended questions (e.g., *Which sounds are difficult?*) are asked. Closed-ended questions typically elicit short, direct responses. Open-ended questions are less confining, allowing the respondent to provide more general and elaborate answers. It is usually best to begin an interview with open-ended questions. This will help identify primary concerns that often require further clarification and follow-up through closed-ended questions.

The following questions are often asked about most communicative disorders during the body of the interview. Some or all of these questions may be used with clients, their caregivers, or both. Select those that are appropriate and integrate them into the interview. Answers to these questions, when combined with information from the case history, provide insight into the client's communicative handicap and become a springboard for asking questions that are more specific to the presenting disorder.

• Please describe the problem.
• When did the problem begin?
• How did it begin? Gradually? Suddenly?
• Has the problem changed since it was first noticed? Gotten better? Gotten worse?
• Is the problem consistent or does it vary? Are there certain circumstances that create fluctuations or variations?
• How do you react or respond to the problem? Does it bother you? What do you do?
• Where else have you been seen for the problem? What did they suggest? Did it help?
• How have you tried to help the problem? How have others tried to help?
• What other specialists (physician, teachers, hearing aid dispensers, etc.) have you seen?
• Why did you decide to come in for an evaluation? What do you hope will result? (Shipley & Roseberry-McKibbin, 2006)

Questions Common to Specific Communicative Disorders

Once the general questions have been asked, more specific questions related to the presenting disorder can be introduced. Questions that are common to the disorders of articulation, language, fluency, or voice are listed here. Be aware that asking every question is not usually necessary. Ask the appropriate questions and adapt as needed to gain a more complete understanding of the client's problems. When questioning a parent or caregiver about a child, substitute the words *your child* or the child's name for *you* or *your*.

Articulation

- Describe your concerns about your speech.
- What is your native language? What language do you speak most often?
- What language is spoken most often at home? At school? At work?
- How long have you been concerned about your speech? Who first noticed the problem?
- Describe your speech when the problem was first noticed. Has it improved over time?
- Has your hearing ever been tested? When? Where? What were the results?
- As a child, did you have ear infections? How often? How were they treated?
- What do you think is the cause of your speech problem?
- What sounds are most difficult for you?
- Is it difficult for you to repeat what other people have said?
- Are there times when your speech is better than others?
- How well does your family understand you? Do they ask you to repeat yourself?
- How well do your friends and acquaintances understand you? Do they ask you to repeat yourself?
- Does your speech affect your interactions with other people? How does it affect your work? Your social activities? Your school activities?
- What have you done to try to improve your speech?
- Have you had speech therapy before? When? Where? With whom? What were the results?
- During the time you have been with me, has your speech been typical? Is it better or worse than usual?

Language (Child)

Use the child's name rather than "your child" whenever possible.

- Describe your concerns about your child's language.
- What is your child's native language? What language does your child speak most often?
- What language is spoken most often at home? At school? At work?
- Whom does your child interact with most often? What kinds of activities do they do together?
- Does your child seem to understand you? Others?
- How well do you understand your child?

- Does your child have a history of recurrent ear infections? At what age(s)? How were they treated?
- Has your child's hearing ever been tested? When? Where? What were the results?
- Does your child maintain eye contact?
- How does your child get your attention (through gestures, verbalizations, etc.)?
- How does your child express needs and wants?
- Approximately how many words does your child understand?
- Approximately how many words does your child use?
- Provide an estimate of your child's average sentence length. Approximately how many words does your child use in his or her longest sentences?
- Does your child follow:
     Simple commands (e.g., *put that away*)?
     Two-part commands (e.g., *get your shoes and brush your hair*)?
     Three-part commands (e.g., *pick up your toys, brush your teeth, and get in bed*)?
- Does your child ask questions?
- Does your child use:
     Nouns (e.g., *boy, car*)?
     Verbs (e.g., *jump, eat*)?
     Adjectives (e.g., *big, funny*)?
     Adverbs (e.g., *quickly, slowly*)?
     Pronouns (e.g., *he, they*)?
     Conjunctions (e.g., *and, but*)?
     -ing endings (e.g., *going, jumping*)?
     Past-tense word forms (e.g., *went, jumped*)?
     Plurals (e.g., *dogs, toys*)?
     Possessives (e.g., *my mom's, the dog's*)?
     Comparatives (e.g., *slower, bigger*)?
- Does your child appear to understand cause-and-effect relationships? The function of objects?
- Is your child able to imitate immediately? Following a short lapse of time? How accurate is the imitation?
- Can your child narrate or talk about experiences?
- Does your child know how to take turns in conversation?
- Is your child's speech usually appropriate to the situation?
- Does your child participate in symbolic play (e.g., use a stick to represent a microphone)?

Language (Adult)

- What is your native language? What language do you speak most often?
- Do you have a problem in your native language *and* in English?
- How long have you been concerned about your language? Who first noticed the problem?

- Describe your language abilities when the problem was first noticed. Have they improved over time?
- Do you read? How often? What kinds of books do you read?
- Describe your education. Did you have any problems learning?
- What do you think is the cause of your language problem?
- What does your family think about the problem?
- Does your language affect your interaction with other people? How does it affect your work? Your social activities?
- Have you had any accidents or illnesses that have affected your language?
- Have you ever had your hearing tested? When? Where? What were the results?
- What have you done to try to improve your language skills?
- Have you had language therapy before? When? Where? With whom? What were the results?

Stuttering

- Describe your concerns about your speech.
- When did you first begin to stutter? Who noticed it? In what type of speaking situations did you first notice it?
- Describe your stuttering when it was first noticed. How has it changed over time?
- Did anyone else in the family stutter (parents, brothers, sisters, grandparents, uncles, aunts, cousins, etc.)? Do they still stutter? Did they have therapy? If so, did it help?
- Why do you think you stutter?
- Does the stuttering bother you? How?
- How does your family react to the problem?
- How do your friends and acquaintances react to the problem?
- What do you do when you stutter?
- When you stutter, what do you do to try to stop it? Does your strategy work? If yes, why do you think it works? If no, why not?
- In what situations do you stutter the most (over the telephone; speaking to a large group; speaking to your spouse, boss, or someone in a position of authority; etc.)?
- In what situations do you stutter the least (speaking to a child, speaking to your spouse, etc.)?
- Do you avoid certain speaking situations? Describe these.
- Do you avoid certain sounds or words? Which ones?
- Does your stuttering problem vary from day to day? How does it vary? Why do you think it varies?
- What have you done to try to eliminate the stuttering (previous therapy, self-help books, etc.)? What were the results?
- Have you had speech therapy before? When? Where? With whom? What were the results?

OBTAINING PREASSESSMENT INFORMATION

- Does your stuttering give you difficulties at work, at school, or at home? Are there other places that it gives you trouble?
- Have you had any illnesses or accidents that seemed to affect your speech? Describe these.
- During the time you have been with me, has your speech been typical? Are you stuttering more or less than usual?

Voice

- Describe your concerns about your voice.
- How long have you had the voice problem? Who first noticed it?
- Describe your voice when the problem was first noticed. How has it changed over time?
- What do you think is the cause of your voice problem?
- Do you speak a lot at work? At home? On the telephone? At social events or in large groups?
- What types of activities are you involved in?
- Do you ever run out of breath when you talk? Describe those situations.
- In what speaking situations is your voice the worst?
- In what situations is your voice the best?
- Is your voice better or worse at different times of the day?
- How does your family react to your voice problem?
- How do your friends and acquaintances react to your voice?
- How does your voice affect your interactions with other people? How does it affect your work? Your social activities? School?
- What have you done to try to resolve the problem?
- Have you seen an ear, nose, and throat specialist? What were the results?
- Have you had speech therapy before? When? Where? With whom? What were the results?
- Have you had any illnesses or accidents that seemed to affect your voice? Describe these.
- During the time you have been with me, has your voice been typical? Is it better or worse than usual?

INFORMATION FROM OTHER PROFESSIONALS

Information is sometimes available from other professionals who have seen the client. Occasionally, such information is necessary before commencing treatment (as in the case of an otolaryngologic evaluation before the initiation of voice therapy), and this information is often helpful for understanding the disorder more thoroughly before making a diagnosis. There are many sources for such preassessment information, including other speech-language pathologists, audiologists, physicians (general or family practitioners, pediatricians, otolaryngologists, neurologists, psychiatrists, etc.), dentists or orthodontists, regular and special educators (classroom teachers, reading specialists, etc.), school nurses, clinical or educational psychologists, occupational or physical therapists, and rehabilitation or vocational counselors. Of course, this list is not all-inclusive. Professionals from other fields may also be involved with a client. Information from other professionals may help identify:

- The history or etiology of a disorder
- Associated or concomitant medical, social, educational, and familial problems
- Treatment histories, including the effects of treatment
- Prognostic implications
- Treatment options and alternatives

Be aware that information from other professionals can potentially lead to a biased view of a client's condition. It is important to maintain an objective position throughout the assessment, relying primarily on direct observation and evaluation results.

Federal law mandates that any information obtained from, or provided to, another person or agency must fall under the guidelines of the Health Insurance Portability and Accountability Act (HIPAA) Privacy Rule.[1] The Privacy Rule states that it is not legal to request information about a client that is not reasonably necessary for the client's care (nor is it appropriate to provide protected information to another provider that is not reasonably necessary). Although not mandated by the Privacy Rule, we also strongly recommend that you obtain client or caregiver authorization before contacting other professionals. A written permission is sometimes required and is always advisable. Licensure requirements in many states, ethical practice principles, and common sense dictate that students should never contact an outside professional or agency without the full knowledge and permission of their clinic supervisor. Virtually all speech and hearing clinics have specific procedures and protocols for contacting outside agencies. These are available by contacting the clinic supervisor, the office staff, or the clinic director.

A "Sample Release of Information," "Sample Request for Information," and "Sample Referral for Medical Evaluation" are provided in Appendices 3-A, 3-B, and 3-C at the end of this chapter. These can be adapted for different clinical situations.

CONCLUDING COMMENTS

Three primary sources of obtaining information about a client were discussed in this chapter. These were written case histories, information-gathering interviews, and information from other professionals. It is best to obtain as much information as possible to aid in diagnosing the communicative disorder, designing a treatment program, assessing prognosis, and preparing recommendations. Important information may include various histories of the disorder, current levels of functioning, and previous and current reports of evaluations or treatment. The amount, quality, and clinical applicability of the information collected will vary. Some information will be immensely helpful, whereas other information will be of less use. The degree of applicability is, of course, related to the information itself and to the clinician's ability to use it. Information can sometimes be like a computer—a dust collector to one person and an indispensable tool to another. Information and its use is, indeed, in the hands of the holder.

---

1. Contact the United States Department of Health and Human Services for complete information about HIPAA. Information can also be viewed online at http://www.hhs.gov

SOURCES OF ADDITIONAL INFORMATION

Print Sources

Haynes, W. O., & Pindzola, R. H. (2012). *Diagnosis and evaluation in speech pathology* (8th ed.). Needham Heights, MA: Allyn & Bacon.

Luterman, D. M. (2008). *Counseling persons with communicative disorders and their families* (5th ed.). Austin, TX: Pro-ed.

Shipley, K. G., & Roseberry-McKibbin, C. (2006). *Interviewing and counseling in communicative disorders: Principles and procedures* (3rd ed.). Austin, Tx: Pro-ed.

Stewart, C. J., & Cash, W. B. (2010). *Interviewing: Principles and practices* (13th ed.). Columbus, OH: McGraw-Hill.

Electronic Sources

ASHA:
http://www.asha.org

Form 3-1.

Child Case History Form

General Information

Child's Name: _____   Date of Birth: _____

Address: _____   Phone: _____

City: _____   Zip Code: _____

Does the Child Live with Both Parents? _____

If no, describe living arrangement _____

Mother's Name: _____   Email: _____

Mother's Occupation: _____   Cell Phone: _____

Father's Name: _____   Email: _____

Father's Occupation: _____   Cell Phone: _____

Referred by: _____   Phone: _____

Address: _____

Pediatrician: _____   Phone: _____

Address: _____

Family Doctor: _____   Phone: _____

Address: _____

Brothers and Sisters (include names and ages):

_____

_____

_____

_____

What languages does the child speak? What is the child's dominant language?

What languages are spoken in the home? What is the dominant language spoken?

(continues)

Form 3-1. continued

With whom does the child spend most of his or her time?

Describe the child's speech-language problem.

How does the child usually communicate (gestures, single words, short phrases, sentences)?

When was the problem first noticed? By whom?

What do you think may have caused the problem?

Has the problem changed since it was first noticed?

(continues)

Form 3-1. continued

Is the child aware of the problem? If yes, how does he or she feel about it?

Have any other speech-language specialists seen the child? Who and when? What were their conclusions or suggestions?

Have any other specialists (physicians, audiologists, psychologists, special education teachers, etc.) seen the child? If yes, indicate the type of specialist, when the child was seen, and the specialist's conclusions or suggestions.

Are there any other speech, language, or hearing problems in your family? If yes, please describe.

(continues)

OBTAINING
PREASSESSMENT
INFORMATION

Form 3-1. continued

Prenatal and Birth History

Mother's general health during pregnancy (illnesses, accidents, medications, etc.).

Length of pregnancy: _____   Length of labor: _____

General condition: _____   Birth weight: _____

Circle type of delivery: head first   feet first   breech   cesarean

Were there any unusual conditions that may have affected the pregnancy or birth?

Medical History

Provide the approximate ages at which the child suffered the following illnesses and conditions:

Asthma _____   Chicken pox _____   Colds _____

Croup _____   Dizziness _____   Draining ear _____

Ear infections _____   Encephalitis _____   German measles _____

Headaches _____   High fever _____   Influenza _____

Mastoiditis _____   Measles _____   Meningitis _____

Mumps _____   Pneumonia _____   Seizures _____

Sinusitis _____   Tinnitus _____   Tonsillitis _____

Other _____

Has the child had any surgeries? If yes, what type and when (e.g., tonsillectomy, tube placement)?

Describe any major accidents or hospitalizations.

(continues)

Form 3-1. continued

Is the child taking any medications? If yes, identify.

Have there been any negative reactions to medications? If yes, identify.

Developmental History

Provide the approximate age at which the child began to do the following activities:

Crawl _____ Sit _____ Stand _____

Walk _____ Feed self _____ Dress self _____

Use toilet _____

Use single words (e.g., *no, mom, doggie*) _____

Combine words (e.g., *me go, daddy shoe*) _____

Name simple objects (e.g., *dog, car, tree*) _____

Use simple questions (e.g., *Where's doggie?*) _____

Engage in a conversation _____

Does the child have difficulty walking, running, or participating in other activities that require small or large muscle coordination?

Are there or have there ever been any feeding problems (e.g., problems with sucking, swallowing, drooling, chewing)? If yes, describe.

(continues)

Describe the child's response to sound (e.g., responds to all sounds, responds to loud sounds only, inconsistently responds to sounds).

Educational History

School: _____ Grade: _____

Teacher(s): _____

How is the child doing academically (or preacademically)?

Does the child receive special services? If yes, describe.

How does the child interact with others (e.g., shy, aggressive, uncooperative)?

(continues)

Form 3-1. continued

Has an Individualized Education Plan (IEP) been developed?
If yes, list goals.

Provide any additional information that might be helpful in the evaluation or remediation of the child's problem.

Person completing form: _____

Relationship to client: _____

Signed: _____ Date: _____

Form 3-2.

Adult Case History Form

General Information

Name: _____   Date of Birth: _____

Address: _____   Zip Code: _____

City: _____   Home Phone: _____

Email: _____   Cell Phone: _____

Occupation: _____   Employer: _____

Referred by: _____   Phone: _____

Address: _____   Email: _____

Family Physician: _____   Phone: _____

Address: _____   Email: _____

Single _____ Widowed _____ Divorced _____   Spouse's Name: _____

Children (include names, gender, and ages):

_____

_____

_____

_____

Who lives in the home?

What languages do you speak? If more than one, which one is your dominant language?

What was the highest grade, diploma, or degree you earned?

(continues)

OBTAINING PREASSESSMENT INFORMATION

Form 3-2. continued

Describe your speech-language problem.

What do you think may have caused the problem?

Has the problem changed since it was first noticed?

Have you seen any other speech-language specialists? Who and when? What were their conclusions or suggestions?

Have you seen any other specialists (physicians, audiologists, psychologists, neurologists, etc.)? If yes, indicate the type of specialist, when you were seen, and the specialist's conclusions or suggestions.

Are there any other speech, language, or hearing problems in your family? If yes, please describe.

(continues)

Form 3-2. continued

Medical History

Provide the approximate ages at which you suffered the following illnesses and conditions:

Adenoidectomy _____	Asthma _____	Chicken pox _____
Colds _____	Croup _____	Dizziness _____
Draining ear _____	Ear infections _____	Encephalitis _____
German measles _____	Headaches _____	Hearing loss _____
High fever _____	Influenza _____	Mastoiditis _____
Measles _____	Meningitis _____	Mumps _____
Noise exposure _____	Otosclerosis _____	Pneumonia _____
Seizures _____	Sinusitis _____	Tinnitus _____
Tonsillectomy _____	Tonsillitis _____	Other _____

Do you have any eating or swallowing difficulties? If yes, describe.

List all medications you are taking.

Are you having any negative reactions to these medications? If yes, describe.

Describe any major surgeries, operations, or hospitalizations (include dates).

(continues)

OBTAINING PREASSESSMENT INFORMATION

Form 3-2. continued

Describe any major accidents.

Provide any additional information that might be helpful in the evaluation or remediation process.

Person completing form: _____

Relationship to client: _____

Signed: _____ Date: _____

Form 3-3.

Allergy Alert Form

Date: _____

Name: _____

Person to Contact in Case of Emergency: _____

Phone Number: _____

Does the client have any known allergies (e.g., to foods, medicines, environmental agents)? If yes, please list each allergen and describe the client's response to contact with the allergen(s).

Please describe immediate action to be taken in case of contact with allergen(s).

Person completing form: _____

Relationship to client: _____

Signed: _____ Date: _____

Appendix 3-A.

Sample Release of Information

ABC Clinic
123 Main Street
Anytown, CA 99999
(XXX)555-1529 • clinic@email.com

April 1, 20XX

Becky Posada, M.A.
321 Main Street
Anytown, CA 99999

Re: Kaylyn Jackson

Dear Ms. Posada:

You have my permission to provide the ABC Clinic with copies of all medical and clinical records for Kaylyn Jackson. The information will be used at the ABC Clinic for evaluating Kaylyn's speech-language and determining the most appropriate treatment for her.

Thank you,

Elizabeth Jackson
(Kaylyn's Mother)

Appendix 3-B.

Sample Request for Information

ABC Clinic
123 Main Street
Anytown, CA 99999
(XXX)555-1529 • clinic@email.com

September 12, 20XX

Timothy Aspinwall, M.A.
321 Main Street
Anytown, CA 99999

Re: Audiological records for Laura Tolle

Dear Mr. Aspinwall:

Please send a copy of your most recent audiological findings and other appropriate information about Laura's hearing to the ABC Clinic. The information will be used in the evaluation of Laura's speech.

Permission is hereby granted to release and forward this information by:

_____   _____
Name   Signature

_____   _____
Relationship to Client   Date

_____   _____
Address   Phone

_____   _____
Witness   Date

Thank you.

_____

Name of Professional Requesting Information

Title

Appendix 3-C.

Sample Referral for Medical Evaluation

Date: _____

Name: _____

Address: _____

Re: _____ Date of Birth: _____

Dear Dr. _____ :

_____ was seen for a speech-language evaluation on _____ .

My findings were:

A medical evaluation appears to be necessary for:

Please contact me with the results of your evaluation.

Thank you.

_____

Speech-Language Pathologist

_____

Address

_____

Telephone

Chapter 4

REPORTING ASSESSMENT FINDINGS

There are two primary methods for conveying clinical findings, conclusions, and recommendations: information-giving conferences and written reports. This chapter describes each method and provides examples that can be used and adapted for different practices. In many cases both information-giving conferences and written reports are used to convey assessment results and recommendations.

INFORMATION-GIVING CONFERENCES

Information-giving conferences are conducted with the client and the client's caregivers. They are typically completed in person, but can be conducted online or over the telephone in some cases. Information-giving conferences usually consist of an introduction, a discussion of findings, and a conclusion. The basic information in each phase includes:

Introduction

- Introduce the purpose of the meeting.
- Indicate approximately how much time the session will take.
- Report whether adequate information was obtained during the assessment.
- If reporting to caregivers, describe the client's behavior during the assessment.

For example: "Sarah was very cooperative and I enjoyed working with her. I was able to get all of the information I needed. I'd like to spend the next 10–15 minutes sharing my results and recommendations with you. Here's what I found. . . ."

Discussion

- Discuss the major findings and conclusions from the assessment.
- Keep your language easy to understand and jargon-free.
- Emphasize the major points so that the listener will be able to understand and retain the information you present.
- Provide a written reports that summarizes findings.
- Use illustrations, charts, and/or diagrams as needed to help explain and clarify certain materials.

Conclusion

- Summarize the major findings, conclusions, and recommendations.
- Ask if the listener has any further comments or questions.
- Thank the person for his or her help and interest.
- Describe the next steps that will need to be taken (e.g., seeing the client again, making an appointment with a physician, beginning treatment).

For example: "Thank you for bringing Sarah in today. Do you have any more questions before we finish? Once again, (restate major points). . . . That's why I think the next thing we should do is. . . ."

When working with children, it is important to listen carefully to the parent's or primary caregiver's responses and concerns throughout the conference. Although they are not proficient in professional issues of speech-language pathology, they certainly know their child better than the clinician does. Caregiver input is vital to the entire assessment and treatment process.

WRITING ASSESSMENT REPORTS

The precise format, style, scope, length, and degree of detail needed for a diagnostic report varies across settings, university programs, and even different supervisors in the same setting. In some situations (e.g., individualized family service plans [IFSPs] and individualized education plans [IEPs]), the structure of a report is dictated by a particular clinic or agency. In other situations, clinicians write reports according to their own style and preferences, regardless of the style of the report. Most assessment or diagnostic reports have a similar format and generally present the same basic information, which includes the following components:

Identifying Information

- Name
- Date of birth/age
- School/teacher/grade (if appropriate)
- Address
- Phone numbers
- Email addresses
- Physician(s)
- Billing party (if appropriate)
- Diagnostic code (if appropriate)
- Date of evaluation

Overview/Background/Presenting Complaint/Initial Status

- Referral source
- Dates and locations of previous evaluations and treatment
- Presenting complaint (unintelligible speech, disfluency, voice problem, etc.)

Histories

- Speech, language, and hearing
- Medical
- Educational
- Psychological/emotional
- Developmental/motor
- Familial
- Social
- Occupational (adult)

Assessment Information

Articulation and Phonological Processes

- Phoneme productions in isolation, syllables, words, phrases, and conversational speech
- Overall intelligibility
- Identification and analysis of sound errors
- Consistency of sound errors
- Influence of coarticulation
- Patterns of sound errors (error types, severity of errors, phonological processes)
- Stimulability for correct phoneme production

Language

- Receptive language, including information from formal and informal evaluations, primarily of semantics and syntax
- Expressive language, including information from formal and informal language samples of semantics, syntax, and morphologic features
- Pragmatics
- Literacy
- Cognition, including nonverbal cognitive abilities, use of metacognitive strategies, memory, and attention

Fluency

- Types and frequencies of disfluencies
- Associated motor behaviors (hand movements, eye blinking, etc.)
- Avoidance of sounds, words, or situations, anticipation of disfluency
- Speech rates with and without disfluencies
- Stimulability for fluent speech

Voice

- Pitch, quality, and loudness
- Resonance
- Breath support
- Muscular tension
- Stimulability for improved voice

Dysphagia

- Feeding
- Chewing
- Deglutition
- Food textures tolerated and/or not tolerated
- Position
- Graphic assessment
- Compensations

Orofacial Examination

- Structures and functions that affect speech and swallowing production
- Peripheral areas (if appropriate)—for example, hand and arm movements that indicate alternative communication potential

Hearing

- Hearing screening or summary of audiological assessment
- Middle ear status, including otoscopic findings

Summary

- Statement of diagnosis
- Concise statement of most significant findings
- Prognosis

Recommendations

- Treatment (including frequency, duration, and goals), no treatment, recheck at a later time
- Referral to other professionals
- Suggestions to the client and caregivers

Speech-Language Pathologist's Name and Signature

Three sample reports are included in Appendix 4-A. These sample reports vary in length and amount of detail provided. There are many other possible styles. Consult with a supervisor to determine specific expectations for report writing in each setting.

Although report styles do vary across clinical settings, there are some generally accepted standards for all reports. When preparing a written report, consider the following questions to check content and quality:

1. Does it contain all of the major information needed?

2. Is the information appropriately categorized? For example, is the historical information presented under a history heading or subheading? Is the information from language testing under language?

3. Is there redundancy of words, phrases, or topics?

4. Is it too wordy? Are any sentences too long?

5. Is all terminology used correctly? Are professional words used appropriately? Should professional terminology be used instead of lay terms?

6. Is the report written objectively?

7. Are the "facts" truly based on fact? Or are there facts that are actually interpretations or presumptions?

8. Is the focus on the major points? Are there any major points that have been omitted or underemphasized? Are secondary points overemphasized?

9. Does the report contain ambiguities that could be misinterpreted? Is it specific?

10. Is it written in a logical progression? Do introductory sections lead to assessment findings, which then lead to conclusions and recommendations?

11. Are the mechanics appropriate (spelling, punctuation, grammar, etc.)?

It may be tempting, especially for students learning to write reports, to ask peers or family members to read their reports for basic readability, organization, spelling, and grammar. Keep in mind that this is inappropriate for most clinical reports, as it would violate the client's confidentiality—whether or not the outside reader knows the client—and could subject the student to penalties imposed by Health Insurance Portability and Accountability Act (HIPAA) regulations.

WRITING IFSPs AND IEPs

The *Individualized Family Service Plan (IFSP)* and *Individualized Education Plan (IEP)* are written documents specific to children from birth through high school. They outline the disabilities and needs of an individual child, describe services to be provided, and emphasize the importance of family participation in the child's well-being. An IFSP is typically for infants and toddlers and should transfer somewhat seamlessly to an IEP at age three. Table 4-1 summarizes the major differences and similarities of IFSPs and IEPs. More detailed information can be found on the website of the National Dissemination Center for Children with Disabilities at www.nichcy.org.

TABLE 4-1 Differences and Similarities of the IFSP and IEP

Similarities:

- Services are authorized by law as part of the Individual with Disabilities Education Act (IDEA).
- Plans are individualized to meet the specific and unique needs of each child.
- The child's weaknesses are identified and goals are established to address the areas of weakness.
- A collaborating team of individuals writes goals, with the child's parents participating as integral members of the team.
- Written consent for services is required from the parent(s) or legal guardian.
- Plans describe how services will be delivered and how progress will be measured.

Differences:

IFSP	IEP
For early intervention with infants and toddlers from birth through age 2	For special education of preschool and school-age children ages 3–21
Identifies child's current levels of development	Identifies child's current levels of academic performance
States the natural environment where services will be provided	States the amount of time the student will receive services in and apart from the regular educational program.
Includes provisions for the family as recipients of services	Does not include provisions for the family
Identifies the early intervention services necessary to achieve expected outcomes	Identifies the special education services necessary to achieve goals
Supports the transition to a preschool program upon reaching 3 years of age	Supports the transition to adulthood upon or before reaching age 21
Plan is reviewed at least every 6 months	Plan is reviewed at least every 12 months
Services are coordinated through a county regional center	Services are coordinated through a local educational agency

IFSPs

Early intervention is provided to infants and toddlers with a disability or developmental delay, and their families. Services are coordinated through regional centers, where a service coordinator implements the IFSP. The IFSP is developed by a team, which includes, at minimum, the child's parent or parents, the service coordinator, one or more professionals who evaluates the child and family, and one or more professionals who provide early intervention services if needed. Professionals involved may be medical specialists, speech-language pathologists, occupational therapists, physical therapists, audiologists, nutritionists, psychologists, social workers, and others.

Although early intervention services are federally mandated, guidelines for determining qualifications and developing an IFSP are regulated by individual state agencies. Clinicians will need to research specific requirements in the states in which they practice. In general, the following information must be included in every IFSP:

- The child's present levels of functioning and needs in the areas of physical, cognitive, social/emotional, communicative, and adaptive development
- The parent's or legal guardian's concerns, priorities, and resources
- Description of intervention services the child will receive
- Results and outcomes expected
- Start date, frequency, duration, and location of services to be provided
- Who will pay for services
- The name of the service coordinator
- At the end of the IFSP period (usually age 3), transitional steps out of the early intervention and into another program if needed
- Written consent for services from the parents or legal guardian

The IFSP is reviewed every 6 months and is updated at least once per year. Revisions are made depending on growth and progress toward stated goals. A sample IFSP is provided in Appendix 4-B.

IEPs

Special education services for school-age children with a disability are coordinated through local educational agencies, typically school districts. The IEP is the written document that describes the services and educational goals that will best meet the child's individual needs. It is written by a team that includes the child's parents, the child's regular and special education teachers, a local educational agency (LEA) representative who disseminates services, an interpreter and integrator of assessment findings, other professionals with particular knowledge or expertise related to the child (such as a speech-language pathologist), and, when appropriate, the student for whom the IEP is provided. Each child's IEP contains the following information:

- The child's present levels of functioning and academic achievement, particularly relating to his or her success in school
- Measurable annual goals. Benchmarks or short-term objectives are required for those who take alternate assessments aligned to alternate achievement standards.
- Description of how progress toward meeting goals will be measured and when periodic progress report will be provided
- Description of special education or other services the child will receive
- Amount of time per school day the child will receive special education or special services separate from nondisabled peers
- If and how the child will participate in state- and district-wide standardized assessments, and what modifications will be allowed; if an alternate assessment is recommended, an explanation of why the specific alternate assessment is selected and why the child cannot participate in the regular assessment
- Start date, duration, frequency, and location of services to be provided
- Written consent for services from the parents or legal guardian

The IEP is reviewed annually; goals and services are updated to address changing needs. During the transition to adulthood, which starts when the child reaches age 16, the child becomes a mandatory member of the IEP team. A sample IEP is provided in Appendix 4-B. Additional samples can be found at http://specialchildren.about.com. From this home page, search "sample IEPs." This site provides sample IEPs for specific disabilities. Another helpful resource is the IEP Goal Bank, which is a shared collection of goals written by speech-language pathologists. It can be found at http://www.speakingofspeech.com/IEP_Goal_Bank.html.

CLINICAL CORRESPONDENCE

Sending letters or reports to other professionals is a common clinical practice. Recipients of clinical information may include physicians, social workers, mental health professionals, teachers, other school personnel, and family members. The Health Insurance Portability and Accountability Act (HIPAA) Privacy Rule mandates that clinical information can only be forwarded when it is essential and for the benefit of the client.[1] It is necessary to have a client's written approval before forwarding confidential information to another party. A "Sample Release of Information Form" is included in Appendix 4-C. It can be adapted for different clinical environments.

Written correspondences vary in length and scope depending on the client, the findings, and the recipient. Many professionals, particularly physicians, prefer a short report that simply gets to the point without excessive background or verbiage. Others prefer a lengthier report that provides a thorough description of the clinical findings. Three sample correspondences are presented in Appendix 4-D. The first is brief, the second is moderately detailed, and the third is very detailed.

WRITING SOAP NOTES

SOAP notes are often used in medical settings for reporting client information. They are used to facilitate communication among professionals, such as physicians, nurses, dietitian, and other therapists, who are involved with the same client. SOAP notes are used on an ongoing basis during the evaluative and treatment phases of a client's care and are written immediately after working with a client. These notes are part of the client's legal medical records.

SOAP is an acronym for *subjective, objective, assessment, plan.* The basic elements of a SOAP note are described next, followed by an example of a SOAP note.

- **Subjective:** This section contains nonmeasurable and historical information. Summarize the problem from the client's or caregiver's point of view. Include the current complaint and relevant past history and recent history. Include information about the client's level of concern, degree of cooperation, and overall affect.

- **Objective:** This section contains measurable findings. For an initial diagnostic session, document the examination results. For a treatment session, document objective performance measures on treatment tasks.

---

1. Contact the United States Department of Health and Human Services Office for Civil Rights for complete information about HIPAA. Information can also be viewed online at http://www.hhs.gov/ocr/hipaa.

- **A**ssessment: This section is a synthesis of the information in the subjective and objective sections. For a diagnostic session, write conclusions and recommendations. For a treatment session, record the client's current status in relation to his or her goals. Write the note in such a way that other professionals will understand the outcome of the session.

- **P**lan: Record your plan of action.

Sample SOAP Note

S: 69 YO male suffered acute Ⓛ CVA 27 days ago. Received ⓈⓉ *[speech therapy]* at hosp. Referred for cont of tx upon dc from hosp. Pt's wife reported good progress c̄ tx, although pt still unintelligible at x^s. Pt reported frustration c̄ word retrieval. Pt was very coop during eval.

O: Oral-facial exam revealed mild R facial droop. Lingual & labial strength & ROM mod ↓ on Ⓡ & slightly ↓ on Ⓛ. Tongue protruded to Ⓡ. Dentition WNL. Palatal weakness on Ⓡ noted during phonation of "ah" Hypernasality present. Speech intelligibility 98% during conv speech c̄ context known & 92% c̄ context unknown. Pt able to repeat 5-wd phrases c̄ 100% intelligibility. 50% acc for confrontational naming of common objects. Circumlocutions noted during conv speech. 100% acc for yes/no Qs & 3-part commands. Cognition, reading & writing WFL.

A: Dx: mod anomic aphasia & mild-mod flaccid dysarthria 2° CVA. Recommend speech tx 5x/week x 2 weeks to address the following goals: ① ↑ OM strength to WNL, ② ↑ conv speech intelligibility to 100% c̄ context unknown, ③ ↑ word finding during structured speech tasks to 100%, ④ ↑ word retrieval during conv speech to 98%. Excellent prognosis considering client's cognitive status, motivation, & stimulability during tx trials.

P: Initiate tx plan per Rx.

Learning to write (and read) SOAP notes can be challenging for beginning clinicians because of the medical abbreviations they contain. Refer to the common medical abbreviations provided in Table 4-2 to assist in this process. This is certainly not an exhaustive list, but it does define many of the most common abbreviations used by speech-language pathologists. Clinicians can also download apps that are free or very inexpensive. Two we recommend are:

- "MedAbbreviations: Medical Abbreviations Reference," by Evan Schoenberg

- "Medly—Medical Abbreviation, Terminology, and Prescription Reference," by AppBrew LLC

TABLE 4–2   Common Medical Abbreviations

ABBREVIATION	DEFINITION
Ⓐ	assisted
A&O	alert and oriented
ā	before
A/P	anterior-posterior

continued on the next page

Table 4-2, continued from the previous page

ABBREVIATION	DEFINITION
ac	before meals
ADL	activity of daily living
ama	against medical advice
b/s	bedside
Ba	barium
bib	drink
bid	twice per day
c̄	with
c/o	complaining of
c/w	continue with
ca	cancer
CC	chief complaint
CT	computerized tomography
CVA	cerebral vascular accident
CXR	chest x-ray
d	day
d/t	due to
dc	discontinue or discharge
dls	date last seen
DNR	do not resuscitate
DNT	did not test
dw	discussed with
dx	diagnosis
exam	examination
f/h	family history
f/u	follow up
fld	fluid
fx	fracture
gen	general
gi	gastrointestinal
h	hour
H & P	history and physical
h.d.	at bedtime
h/o	history of
hx	history
Ⓘ	independent
incr	increased, increasing

ABBREVIATION	DEFINITION
iv	intravenous
Ⓛ	left
liq	liquid
lx	larynx
m/h	medical history
MBSS	modified barium swallow study
med	medical or medication
min	minute
ml	milliliter
mod	moderate
MRI	magnetic resonance imaging
N&W	normal and well
NAD	no abnormality detected
neg	negative
NG	nasogastric
NKA	no known allergies
no.	number
NOS	not otherwise specified
npo	nothing by mouth
nyd	not yet diagnosed
O	oral
o	non, without
o/e	on examination
obs	observation
od *or* oid	once a day
OH	occupational history
oob	out of bed
OT	occupational therapy or therapist
ot.	ear
p̄	after
p/c	after meals
Path	pathology
PEG	percutaneous endoscopic gastrostomy
per	by or through
PET	positron emission tomography
PH	past history
PI	present illness

continued on the next page

Table 4-2, continued from the previous page

ABBREVIATION	DEFINITION
PLF	prior level of function
PMH	past medical history
pneu.	Pneumonia
po	by mouth
pos	positive
prm	according to circumstances
prn	whenever necessary
prod	productive
prog	prognosis
PT	physical therapy or therapist
pt	patient
PTA	prior to admission
Px	prognosis
q	every
qh	every hour
qid	four times a day
qol	quality of life
®	right
r/o	rule out
reg	regular
rehab	rehabilitation
ROM	range of motion
RT	respiratory therapy or therapist
Rx	therapy; prescription
s̄	without
s/p	status post
s/s	signs and symptoms
sec	second
SGA	small for gestational age
SH	social history
SI	stroke index
sig	marked or significant
sl	slightly
SLP	speech-language pathologist
sm	small
SOAP	subjective, objective, assessment, plan
SOB	short of breath

ABBREVIATION	DEFINITION
sp&h	speech and hearing
spont	spontaneous
SS	social service
ST	speech therapy
STAT	immediately
sx	symptom
T&A	tonsils and adenoids, tonsillectomy and adenoidectomy
TBI	traumatic brain injury
TIA	transient ischemic attack
tid	three times a day
trach	tracheostomy
tx	treatment
u/o	under observation
via	by way of
w/c	wheelchair
WFL	within functional limits
WNL	within normal limits
Wt	weight
wk	week
x	times (e.g., 2x = twice)
YO	year old
Δ	change
2°	secondary to
~	approximately
↓	reduce
↑	increase

CONCLUDING COMMENTS

Once assessment information is gathered and the diagnostic evaluation completed, it is time to begin the process of sharing results with the client, caregivers, and other professionals. Results and suggestions are typically conveyed through an information-giving conference, a clinical assessment report, a SOAP note, and/or specific correspondence to other professionals. In all cases, the effectiveness of the information conveyed depends on adequate assessment data, knowledgeable interpretations of the data, and the use of good oral or written reporting skills. Acceptable presentation and dissemination of clinical findings is extremely important. Remember that the best assessment in the world may have little effect unless the information is presented effectively to others.

SOURCES OF ADDITIONAL INFORMATION

Print Sources

Goldfarb, R., & Serpanos, Y. C. (2013). *Professional writing in speech-language pathology and audiolody* (2nd ed.). San Diego, CA: Plural.

Hegde, M. N. (2010). *A coursebook on scientific and professional writing in speech-language -pathology* (4th ed.). Clifton Park, NY: Delmar, Cengage Learning.

Hegde, M. N., & Davis, D. (2010). *Clinical methods and practicum in speech-language pathology* (5th ed.). Clifton Park, NY: Delmar, Cengage Learning.

Kettenbach, G. (2003). *Writing SOAP notes: With patient/client management formats* (3rd ed.). Los Angeles: F.A. Davis.

Pannbacker, M., Middleton, G., Vekovius, G. T., & Sanders, K. L. (2001). *Report writing for speech-language pathologists and audiologists* (2nd ed.). Austin, TX: Pro-ed.

Shipley, K. G., & Roseberry-McKibbin, C. (2006). *Interviewing and counseling in communicative disorders: Principles and procedures* (3rd ed.). Austin, TX: Pro-ed.

Stein-Rubin, C., & Fabus, R. (2012). *Clinical assessment and professional report writing in speech-language pathology.* Clifton Park, NY: Delmar, Cengage learning.

Stewart, C. J., & Cash, W. B. (2007). *Interviewing: Principles and practices* (12th ed.). Columbus, OH: McGraw-Hill.

Electronic Sources

Center for Parent Information and Resources:
http://www.parentcenterhub.org

U.S. Department of Education:
http://www.idea.ed.gov

"IEP Goals and Objectives with Common Core State Standards" app by NASET

"IEP Pal" app by Perceptum Solutions LLC

"MedAbbreviations: Medical Abbreviations Reference" app by Even Schoenberg

"Medly—Medical Abbreviation, Terminology, and Prescription Reference" app by App-Brew LLC

Appendix 4-A.

Three Sample Clinical Reports

Sample Report I

University Clinic
123 Main Street
Anytown, CA 99999
(xxx)555-1529 · clinic@email.com

Diagnostic Evaluation

Name: Adam McCune   **Date:** 9-14-20xx
Birthdate: 4-2-20xx   **Clinic File No.:** 12345
Age: 7 years, 5 months   **Diagnosis:** Fluency Disorder, 315.35
Address: 4574 E. 1st St.   **Phone:** (xxx)555-8942
       Anytown, CA 99999
School Status: 2nd grade, Holt Elementary

History and Presenting Complaint

Adam, a 7-year 5-month-old male, was seen for a speech-language evaluation at the University Clinic on September 14, 20xx. He was accompanied by his mother.

Adam attended Holt Elementary School and received speech therapy two times per week for remediation of disfluent speech. Mrs. McCune reported that Adam began stuttering at approximately 3 years of age. She also stated that his stuttering fluctuated and increased during stressful situations. Mrs. McCune stated that her father also stuttered.

Adam's medical history was unremarkable.

Assessment Findings

Speech: The *Goldman-Fristoe Test of Articulation-2* was administered to assess Adam's production of consonants in fixed positions at the word level. Adam lateralized /s/ and /z/ in all positions. He substituted /nk/ for /n/ in the medial and final positions. Adam was stimulable for /s/ and /z/ at the word level.

A 384-word conversational speech sample revealed similar errors. He also omitted /d/ and /t/ in the final position during connected speech. Adam was 100% intelligible during this sample.

Orofacial Examination: An orofacial examination was administered to assess the structural and functional integrity of the oral mechanism. Facial features were symmetrical. Labial and lingual strength and range of motion were normal during speech and nonspeech tasks. Lingual size and shape were normal. Appropriate velar movement was observed during productions of /a/.

Diadochokinetic syllable tasks were administered to assess rapid movements of the speech musculature. Adam repeated /pʌtəkə/ at a rate of 4.04 repetitions per second. This was within normal limits for a child his age.

(continues)

Language: The *Peabody Picture Vocabulary Test-IV* was administered to assess receptive vocabulary. A raw score of 92 and a standard score of 108 were obtained. Age equivalency was 8:0 and percentile rank was 70. The results indicated average to above-average receptive vocabulary skills.

Analysis of the conversational speech-language sample revealed appropriate expressive language skills. Syntactic, morphologic, and semantic structures of the language were appropriate. Adam's average length of utterance was 10.9 words.

Voice: Adam exhibited a normal vocal quality. An s/z ratio of 1.0 was obtained.

Fluency: A 384-word spontaneous sample was elicited to assess Adam's fluency rate, and he was 82% fluent on a word-by-word basis. Disfluencies averaged 2 seconds in duration with a range of .8 seconds to 4 seconds. Disfluencies included:

	# Disfluencies	Percentage
Sound Interjections	28	17.3%
Word Interjections	11	10.3%
Sound Repetitions	19	15.0%
Word Repetitions	18	12.1%
Phrase Repetitions	18	12.1%
Revisions	13	10.8%
Prolongations	12	10.5%
Total	**69**	**18.1%**

Adam was stimulable for fluent speech at the 3-syllable phrase level when he was required to use an easy onset and syllable stretching.

Hearing: A hearing screen was administered at 20 dB HTL for the frequencies of 250, 500, 1000, 2000, 4000, and 6000 Hz. Adam responded to all sounds bilaterally.

Summary and Recommendations
Adam exhibited moderate disfluency characterized by sound interjections and sound, word, and phrase repetitions. He was stimulable for fluent speech, which suggests a good prognosis for improvement with therapy. Adam also exhibited mild articulatory errors of substitutions and additions. He was stimulable for all phonemes. Expressive and receptive language abilities were age appropriate.

It was recommended that Adam receive speech therapy to train fluent speech and correct his articulation errors.

Stephen D. Marshall, M.A., CCC/SLP
Speech-Language Pathologist

(continues)

Appendix 4-A. continued

Sample Report 2

University Clinic
123 Main Street
Anytown, CA 99999
(xxx)555-1529 · clinic@email.com

Diagnostic Evaluation

Name: Lisa Breckenridge
Birthdate: 12-12-19xx
Age: 35
Address: 4574 Cedar Ave.
            Anytown, CA 99999
Occupation: High School Mathematics Instructor

Date: 6-2-20xx
Clinic File No.: 98765
Diagnosis: Voice Disorder, 784.42
Phone: (xxx)555-0809
Email: lbreckenridge@email.com

History and Presenting Complaint

Mrs. Breckenridge, a 35-year-old female, was referred to the University Clinic by Stuart Goehring, M.D., subsequent to the development of bilateral vocal nodules. The patient complained of a hoarse voice. She reported that the problem started about 5 months ago and had become especially problematic during the last 2 months.

At the time of the evaluation, Mrs. Breckenridge reported that she taught four periods of high school mathematics per day at San Joaquin High School. There were approximately 35 students per class. She stated that she needed to project her voice during that time.

Mrs. Breckenridge stated that she liked to sing, but did so rarely because it aggravated her voice problem. She reported that she did not smoke and consumed a minimal amount of alcohol (i.e., a glass of wine once in a while). She also stated that she did not yell excessively, use inhalants, talk in noisy environments (other than the classroom), or cough excessively. She did not report a history of allergies, asthma, or frequent colds. Caffeine intake included, at most, one or two iced teas per day.

Assessment Findings

Mrs. Breckenridge exhibited the symptoms of vocal nodules. Her voice was characterized by hoarseness, intermittent breathiness, pitch breaks, and intermittent glottal fry. The symptoms were exacerbated when she was asked to increase her vocal intensity. Attempts to increase her loudness levels were accompanied by increased feelings of discomfort in the laryngeal region.

Mrs. Breckenridge's fundamental frequency was approximately 220 Hz when sustaining "ah" for 15+ seconds. An increase in breathiness and the occurrence of pitch breaks were noted during the last 5+ seconds of these vocalizations.

She exhibited a low vertical focus in the use of her voice. This created a lower pitch and poor vocal projection. In an attempt to increase her projection, she increased her vocal effort. This type of vocal abuse is typically associated with the development of vocal nodules.

(continues)

REPORTING
ASSESSMENT
FINDINGS

Appendix 4-A. continued

With instruction and modeling, Mrs. Breckenridge was able to raise her vertical focus and produce clearer, louder, nonhoarse, and nonbreathy vocal productions. During these stimulability tasks, Mrs. Breckenridge reported that she was not feeling the vocal tension and aggravation that typically accompanied her speech and voice use. This indicated a good prognosis for improved voice quality with therapy.

Diagnosis and Recommendations

Mrs. Breckenridge was diagnosed with moderate dysphonia secondary to vocal nodules. She was stimulable for improved voice quality during trial therapy tasks. She was also counseled on improved vocal hygiene. Voice therapy two times per week for 8 weeks was recommended. Additional therapy will be considered at the end of the initial treatment period.

Autumn Noel, M.A., CCC/SLP
Speech-Language Pathologist

(continues)

Appendix 4-A. continued

Sample Report 3

University Clinic
123 Main Street
Anytown, CA 99999
(xxx)555-1529 · clinic@email.com

Diagnostic Evaluation

Name: Christopher Elvi

Birthdate: 12-12-19xx

Age: 38

Address: 4574 Finch Ave

Home Phone: (xxx)555-0809

Email: celvi@email.com

Date: 5-16-20xx

Employment: not employed

Diagnosis: mixed dysarthria and apraxia, 784.59

City: Anytown, CA 99999

Cell Phone: (xxx) 555-1741

Clinic File No: 98765

History and Presenting Complaint

Christopher Elvi, a 38-year-old male, was evaluated at the University Clinic on May 7, 9, 14, and 16, 20xx. His attendant accompanied him. Mr. Elvi suffered a closed head injury as a result of a motor vehicle accident on July 4, 20xx. At the time of the evaluation, he was enrolled in his fifth semester of speech therapy at the University Clinic for remediation of mixed dysarthria and apraxia.

General Observations

Mr. Elvi was confined to a wheelchair. He had right hemiparesis and reported that before the accident, he was right-handed. He frequently used fingerspelling as a means of communication when speech was especially difficult. Fingerspelling was also used as a self-cuing strategy to elicit sound productions. He often corrected his own errors of articulation and language.

Mr. Elvi exhibited a significant amount of inappropriate laughter during the initial diagnostic session. He was able to control his outbursts and laugh more appropriately during the last two diagnostic sessions.

Orofacial Integrity

An orofacial evaluation revealed a mild drooping of the left lip corner at rest and while smiling. Mild groping movements were noted during lip puckering and mandibular depression. Lingual and labial strength were within normal limits bilaterally with slight nasal emission noted during evaluation of labial strength. The tongue deviated to the left upon protrusion. Degree of mandibular range, elevation, and depression were normal, with apparent jerky movements and temporomandibular joint noises noted during depression. It was also noted that Mr. Elvi maintained an open mouth rest posture.

Asymmetrical velopharyngeal movement was observed during the production of /ɑ/ with deviation of the velum to the left. Nasality was also noted. Nasal emission was present during blowing, cheek puffing, and the production of /ɑ/. A gag reflex was not elicited.

Diadochokinetic syllable rates were slow and labored with irregular timing. Mr. Elvi produced 25 productions of /pʌ/ in 8.44 seconds and 19 productions of /bʌ/ in 9.91 seconds. He was able to produce three repetitions of both /tʌ/ and /kʌ/ in 3 seconds; 1.5 repetitions of /dɪpədɪdɪpədɪdu/, 1.5 repetitions of /lɪpədɪlɪpədɪdu/, and

(continues)

Appendix 4-A. continued

1.25 repetitions of /ɡɪpədɪɡɪpədɪɡu/ were completed in 3-second intervals. Severe groping behavior was noted during complex diadochokinetic syllable tasks.

Hearing
A hearing screening revealed hearing to be within normal limits.

Voice
Mr. Elvi was required to sustain the vowel /i/ over four trials to assess velopharyngeal efficiency. He exhibited nasal emission and significant variation in his ability to maintain the original pitch on each trial. On the fourth trial, he was asked to lower his pitch and was able to control his pitch with more accuracy. However, there was still significant pitch variability. The average vowel duration was 8 seconds (range 5–9 seconds), which indicated velopharyngeal insufficiency as compared to the normal average of 15 seconds.

Mr. Elvi exhibited a high-pitched, strained-strangled voice quality with frequent nasal emission and hypernasality. Other features include poor control of pitch, pitchbreaks, and audible inhalation. Mr. Elvi exhibited monostress during conversational speech. With training, stimulability of appropriate stress during contrastive stress drills was good.

A fundamental frequency indicator was used to assess Mr. Elvi's habitual pitch and pitch range during conversational speech. Habitual pitch was determined to be 250 Hz, which is significantly higher than the adult-male average of 124 Hz. His pitch range was determined to be 150–300 Hz.

Control of loudness was poor. Mr. Elvi was required to produce selected vowels with continuous phonation for each vowel while changing from soft to loud. He exhibited poor control of loudness and pitch during this task. Vowels that appeared especially difficult were /i/ and /u/, while better control was exhibited during the productions of /ɑ/, /e/, and /æ/.

The s/z ratio of sustained productions also revealed deficits in respiration. Nasal emission was noted on all productions. Productions were inappropriately high in pitch and continued to rise following vocal onset. Audible inhalation was also noted. Mr. Elvi was able to maintain the production of /s/ for an average of 8.86 seconds, which is significantly below the average of 20–25 seconds. The s/z ratio was 1.0. Results indicated severe respiratory inefficiency and reduced vital capacity.

Repetitions of progressively more complex phrases revealed deficits in short-term memory, fluency, and respiration. Mr. Elvi was unable to repeat entire phrases of over seven syllables in length without cues provided by the clinician. He completed a maximum of three words per breath, and inhaled after almost every word in longer phrases (seven to nine syllables). It was also noted that he took frequent breaths in conversational speech, rarely completing more than three words following inhalation.

Fluency
Mr. Elvi exhibited frequent pauses, hesitations, and sound prolongations secondary to verbal apraxia and poor respiratory control.

Articulation
Mr. Elvi exhibited a severe articulation disorder characterized by sound omissions, substitutions, additions, and distortions. Intelligibility in conversational speech was approximately 92% with context known. Mr. Elvi exhibited severe groping behavior during all verbal speech tasks.

(continues)

Appendix 4-A. continued

The *Goldman–Fristoe Test of Articulation Sounds in Words Subtest* was administered to assess Mr. Elvi's consonant production in fixed positions. The following errors were noted:

Initial	Medial	Final
		-n
m/b	m/b	
	-k	
-p		b/p, -p
v/f	v/f	-f
	dist. g	-g
	-d	
	-t	n/t
ts/s, t/s, n/s, d/s		t/s, -s
dist. r	dist. r, -r	
-v		-v
dʒ/z	d/z	tʃ/z, s/z, -z
		tʃ/dʒ
	tʃ/ʃ	tʃ/ʃ
n/ð	d/ð	
b/bl		
k/kl		
l/sl		
tw/tr		

Additionally, these errors were noted in conversational speech:

Initial	Medial	Final
	m/p, b/p	
		+n
w/f, -f	v/f	
	k/g	
m/b	m/b	
	g/k	
dist. l		-l
n/d	n/d, -d	-d
n/t		-t
n/s, dʒ/s, -s	z/s, t/s	tʃ/s
w/r		dist. r
	dist. tʃ	
	t/z, -z	
f/θ		-θ
		dʒ
s/sl		
ɔ/aɪ	ɑ/aɪ	
	ɔ/ɑ	
	-ɔ	
		-ɪ

(continues)

Mr. Elvi was stimulable for all sound errors. He exhibited notable difficulty contrasting between productions of voiced and voiceless phonemes when sounds were modeled in isolation by the clinician. He also exhibited difficulty initiating phonation when preceded by sounds without phonation (/h/ to /hɑ/). He was stimulable for articulation tasks with practice.

The *Apraxia Battery for Adults* was administered to assess volitional control of the limbs and the speech musculature during verbal and nonverbal speech tasks. Results indicated a mild-moderate limb apraxia, a mild-moderate oral apraxia, and a severe-profound verbal apraxia.

Language

Selected items of the *Western Aphasia Battery* were administered to assess auditory comprehension, repetition, naming, reading, writing, and apraxia. Mr. Elvi performed well on tasks of yes/no responses, word recognition, object naming, sentence completion, reading, matching written word to object, spelled word recognition, oral spelling, and volitional oral and limb movements. He exhibited mild difficulty with responsive speech, word fluency, sequential commands, and repetition. On the subtest requiring oral reading and performing of commands, Mr. Elvi did not read all of the commands orally although he performed all tasks with ease. It was assumed he did not read aloud because of his difficulty programming speech sounds. He responded that the task was "too hard" when the clinician asked why he did not read the commands orally. The writing subtest was the most difficult for Mr. Elvi. He struggled to write his first and last name and could not complete writing his address. He wrote with his left hand, which was not his dominant hand before the accident.

The *Boston Naming Test* was administered to assess Mr. Elvi's confrontational naming skills. The following results were obtained:

	Raw Score	% Correct
No cues provided:	36/60	60%
Stimulus cues provided:	0/8	0%
Phonemic cues provided:	16/22	73%
Total score:	44/60	73%

Scores indicated the presence of moderate anomia. The number of items that required phonemic cues was significant.

Mr. Elvi experienced much difficulty during oral reading of sentences. A conversational speech sample was taken to assess Mr. Elvi's mean length of response in connected speech. His mean length of response was 1.8 words or 2.2 morphemes.

Memory

Mr. Elvi exhibited short-term and long-term memory deficits as judged by informal assessment. He frequently could not recall what he had done or what he had eaten for a meal during the day of evaluation. He also had difficulty recalling words during conversational speech and would often give up because he was unable to remember the appropriate word to complete his message.

(continues)

Appendix 4-A. continued

Summary

Christopher Elvi was diagnosed with severe mixed dysarthria and concurrent verbal apraxia, severely reduced respiratory control, and moderate anomia. His speech and language were characterized by imprecise consonant productions, hypernasality, audible inhalations, monostress, a harsh and strained-strangled voice quality, and an abnormally high-pitched voice with severely reduced laryngeal control of pitch. He took frequent breaths and exhibited a significant amount of groping movements during volitional speech tasks. He also exhibited word retrieval difficulty during conversational speech and confrontational naming tasks.

Prognosis

Prognosis for improvement of speech and language abilities with treatment is good. He was stimulable for increased articulatory accuracy and for improved pitch and vocal stress during trial treatment tasks. Considering the extent of Mr. Elvi's neurological impairments and the length of time that has passed since onset, prognosis for complete recovery with treatment is poor.

Recommended Plan of Treatment

It was recommended that Mr. Elvi continue obtaining speech and language therapy. The following treatment goals and objectives for a 6-month treatment period were recommended:

1. Christopher Elvi will imitatively produce four-syllable phrases without laryngeal tension and with precise articulation with 90% accuracy.

Treatment will begin at the one-syllable word level. The clinician will model whispered productions of one-syllable words and Mr. Elvi will imitate. When he is able to precisely articulate a word in a whisper with no laryngeal tension, voicing will be added. Productions will be mildly breathy and soft in order to maintain the relaxed quality. The breathiness will be gradually eliminated when the client exhibits the ability to control laryngeal tension in single words with 90% accuracy.

Syllabic length of modeled phrases will systematically increase by one syllable when Mr. Elvi exhibits the ability to imitatively articulate phrases without laryngeal tension at each preceding level with 90% accuracy.

2. Christopher Elvi will imitatively produce four-syllable phrases in a single breath with 90% accuracy.

This goal will be addressed in conjunction with goal #1. Mr. Elvi will produce each phrase modeled by the clinician in a single breath. Syllabic complexity of each phrase will increase by one syllable when the 90% criterion is met at each preceding level.

3. Christopher Elvi will imitatively produce four-syllable phrases at a pitch level determined to be appropriate by the clinician with 90% accuracy.

This goal will also be addressed in conjunction with goal #1. The clinician will require the client to lower his pitch to an appropriate level. Each phrase that the client imitates must be produced at this predetermined pitch level. A criterion of 90% must be met at each level before proceeding to the next syllabic phrase level.

(continues)

REPORTING ASSESSMENT FINDINGS

Appendix 4-A. continued

---

4. Christopher Elvi will recall five activities he participated in during each current day of treatment with 90% accuracy in the absence of auditory or visual cues.

At the onset of each treatment session, Mr. Elvi's attendant will provide a list of activities the client participated in during the day. The clinician will then ask the client questions about what he did during the day. Phonemic and visual cues will be provided as necessary to elicit the appropriate responses.

Madeleine Loud, M.A., CCC/SLP
Speech-Language Pathologist

Appendix 4-B.

Sample IFSP

Early Start Program Main Street Regional Center
Individualized Family Service Plan (IFSP)
for Children Birth to 3 Years

Child's Name: _Janelle Martin_   Birthdate: _5/11/20xx_   Age: _23_ months   Gender: _F_

Parent(s)/Guardian(s): _Doug & Wendy Martin_   Email: _dwmartin@email.com_

Address: _7544 Tiptoe Lane_   City: _Anytown_   Zip Code: _99999_

Home Phone: _xxx-555-1964_   Mobile/Work: _xxx-555-7548_

School District of Residence: _Anytown Union School District_

IFSP Type: ☒ Initial IFSP   ☐ 6-month review   ☐ Annual review   ☐ Other review

IFSP Date: _4/30/xx_

Service Coordinator

Service Coordinator: _Lindsay Black_   Agency: _Main Street Regional Center_

Address: _794 Main Street, Anytown, CA 99999_   Phone: _xxx-555-2930_

Assessment Team

Name	Title	Contact Phone
Lindsay Black	Service Coordinator	xxx-555-1298
Doug & Wendy Martin	Parents	xxx-555-7548
Brenda Khan	Speech-Language Pathologist	xxx-555-1785

Family's Priorities, Concerns, Resources:

Janelle was referred to the Early Start Program by her pediatrician due to concerns about her slow communicative development. She was accompanied to the clinic by both of her parents. The parents shared that she is not talking as much as other children her age and communicates mostly by gesturing. They reported that she seems to understand what is said to her.

The family lives in a remote region of the city. The mother is able to provide transportation to a clinic if in-home services are not available. Medical needs are provided through People's Healthcare.

Natural Environment

Janelle lives at home with both parents and her older brother, Timothy (age 5). The primary language spoken in the home is English. Both parents also speak fluent French. Her dad works full-time outside of the home. Her mom is home full-time. Janelle enjoys frequent visits to the library and the park with her mom and brother. Grandparents also live nearby and visit regularly.

(continues)

Appendix 4-B. continued

Present Levels of Functioning

Janelle was evaluated on 4/21/xx at the Early Start clinic. Assessment information was gathered via observation, parent interview, record review, and administration of the *Battelle Developmental Inventory, 2nd edition* (BDI-2).

General Health

Janelle's overall health is good. Her mother reports no significant illnesses or injuries. Vision and hearing are normal. Janelle weighs 26 pounds and is 33 inches tall.

Gross and Fine Motor

Gross and fine motor skills are within normal expectations for her age. She is able to run without falling, kick a ball forward, point with her index finger, scribble linear and circular patterns, and use the pads of her fingers to grasp a pencil. She is able to turn book pages independently, place rings on a post, and stack three cubes. She requires some assistance to walk up and down stairs or fasten her clothing. Her parents report that she sometimes has a hard time stabbing her food with a fork.

Cognitive

Cognitive abilities are within normal expectations for her age. Janelle is an inquisitive little girl and seemed to enjoy exploring and manipulating test items during the assessment. She shows interest in age-appropriate books, points to pictures in a book, searches for missing objects, and attends to learning tasks for 5 minutes or more. She is able to match some colors, and can nest objects with demonstration. She seems to understand that she is the cause of certain events. She completes age-appropriate puzzles with assistance.

Communicative

Janelle's receptive language skills are similar to those of an 18-month-old. She identifies family members when named, associates words with common objects or actions, and responds to her name when called. She can identify her own eyes, nose, ears, mouth, and feet when prompted. She sometimes follows one-step verbal and/ or gestural commands. She enjoys being read to, and will point to familiar items in a book when prompted.

Janelle's expressive language skills are similar to those of a 15-month-old. She primarily communicates using sounds and gestures. She says the names of family members (*mama, dad*) and calls her brother Timothy *Im*. She named (approximated) the following items from a picture book during the assessment: *dog, duck, ball, baby*. Her parents reported that she also says *no, bye-bye, some, beebee* (for blanket), and *hold-you* (spoken as a single word). She does not use two-word phrases with the exception of *bye-bye Mama*. During the assessment, Janelle babbled with long chains of unintelligible jargon-like speech. At times, she did not seem to be talking to anyone in the room.

Social/Emotional

Social and emotional abilities are within normal expectations for her age. She is somewhat shy around unfamiliar people, but warms up quickly. She looks to her mother regularly for reassurance in unfamiliar situations. She enjoys having stories read to her and allows others to participate in her activities. She responds positively to familiar adults, and is helpful with simple household tasks, such as putting dishes in the dishwasher or putting her diaper in the garbage. Other than her brother, she does not have a lot of interaction with other children. She sometimes plays cooperatively with him, but seems to prefer to play by herself. She does imitate his play behaviors.

(continues)

Appendix 4-B. continued

Adaptive/Self Help

Janelle's adaptive/self-help skills are within normal expectations for her age. She is able to feed herself bite-size pieces of food with her fingers and sometimes uses utensils. She can drink from a cup with minimal spilling. She removes her clothes by herself, but needs assistance to put them on. Janelle is not yet potty trained but is showing an emerging awareness of bowel movements, as she sometimes sneaks behind a chair to soil her diaper. She puts her toys away when asked and seems to demonstrate caution and avoid common dangers.

Summary

Janelle is a delightful little girl. At the beginning of the session, she was somewhat reserved, but quickly warmed up to the clinician and was cooperative with assessment tasks. Parents provided developmental information for behaviors not elicited in the clinic, and also reported that the behaviors observed were typical. Current findings are considered an accurate reflection of her skills at this time.

Outcomes Expected

Communication Outcome

Janelle will demonstrate age-appropriate receptive and expressive communication skills.

Criteria 1. Janelle will follow simple two-step commands in 4/5 opportunities.

Responsible agency: ☐ Parent(s)   ☐ Service Coordinator

☒ Other: SLP

Criteria 2. Janelle will imitate simple CV, VC, CVC, and CVCV words during play and structured language activities in 4/5 opportunities.

Responsible agency: ☐ Parent(s)   ☐ Service Coordinator

☒ Other: SLP

Criteria 3. Janelle will increase her functional vocabulary to 30 words and will use words for a variety of communicative purposes (e.g., request, label, protest, greet, call attention, comment).

Responsible agency: ☐ Parent(s)   ☐ Service Coordinator

☒ Other: SLP

Early Intervention Services

Service	Specialist	Frequency & Duration	Natural Environment*	Start	End
1. Speech-Language Services	SLP	1 hr/week	Clinic	5/12/xx	10/30/xx

*Justification if not providing services in natural environment: No itinerant SLPs available that provide services in the family's neighborhood.

(continues)

Appendix 4-B. continued

Funding

Parents were requested to pursue insurance within 40 days of this IFSP for the recommended services. Parents will provide the SC with a written copy of the insurance decision within 30 days of this IFSP. Early Start funding of services will be determined by the insurance coverage approved.

Follow-Up and/or Transition

Current IFSP to be reviewed in 6 months on ___10/30/xx___

On or before 02/11/xx (90 days before third birthday), a transition-planning meeting will take place to discuss transition of services to the local school agency.

Signatures and Parent Consent

IFSP Meeting Participants

Wendy Martin	4/30/xx
Parent/Guardian	Date
Doug Martin	4/30/xx
Parent/Guardian	Date
Lindsay Black	4/30/xx
Service Coordinator	Date
Brenda Khan	4/30/xx
Speech-Language Pathologist	Date

Consent

I/we have participated in the development of the IFSP for my/our child, Janelle Martin. I/we agree with the concerns and priorities presented in this document and, therefore, give permission to Early Start Program to implement and coordinate services.

Wendy Martin	4/30/xx
Signature of Parent/Guardian	Date
Doug Martin	4/30/xx
Signature of Parent/Guardian	Date

(continues)

Appendix 4-B. continued

Sample IEP

Anytown Union School District
Individualized Education Program (IEP)

Child's Name: <u>John Stuart</u>   Birthdate: <u>7/25/20xx</u>   Age:<u> 5 </u>   Gender: <u> M </u>

Parent(s)/Guardian(s): <u>Timothy & Mandy Stuart</u>   Email: <u>tmstuart@email.com</u>

Address: <u>4555 Cedar Ave</u>   City: <u>Anytown</u>   Zip Code: <u>99999</u>

Home Phone: <u>xxx-555-2746</u>   Mobile/Work: <u>xxx-555-9851</u>

Current School: <u> Lincoln School </u>   Grade: <u> Kindergarten </u>

Student Number: <u> 123-45-6789 </u>   Primary Language: <u> English </u>

Initial IEP Meeting Date: <u>   9/15/20xx </u>   Current IEP: <u> 9/15/20xx </u>

Classification: <u> Speech-Language Impaired (fluency disorder) </u>   Eligible for services: <u> yes </u>

Family Environment and Background Information

John lives at home with both parents and with his 2-year old sister, Anna. His father works outside the home as a building contractor. His mother is a part-time accountant and works out of their home office so she can take care of her children. John has had a healthy childhood to date. Developmental milestones have been met within normal expectations. There is no known history of stuttering in John's family.

IEP Development Team

Name	Title
Doug Stuart	Parent
Wendy Stuart	Parent
Derek Ramirez	Principal, District Representative
Barbara Stahl	General Education Teacher
Brenda Khan	Speech-Language Pathologist
Jonathon Manning	Psychologist

Strengths and Concerns

Strengths

John works hard in school and is well liked by his classmates. He is cooperative with classroom activities. So far, he is adjusting well to his kindergarten schedule.

(continues)

REPORTING ASSESSMENT FINDINGS

Appendix 4-B. continued

Concerns

John's parents report that he started stuttering at the age of 3. They were hopeful the behavior would resolve on its own, but it has not. They are concerned that he is shutting down at school over embarrassment and fear of talking in front of other people. His teacher reports that he is a quiet boy and rarely volunteers to speak in the classroom or on the playground. She concurred that he may be avoiding speech situations because of the stuttering.

Present Levels of Performance

John is currently performing within age expectation in all academic areas. A fluency evaluation was completed by the speech-language pathologist. Multiple speech samples were taken, including in the school's speech therapy room, in the classroom, and on the playground. His mother provided video-recorded speech samples from home. A total disfluency index of 14% was calculated. Prevalent disfluency types were part-word repetitions and prolongations. Both environments were similar in terms of fluency; however, it is significant that John spoke at home much more freely than he did at school. He did not demonstrate associated motor behaviors.

John's oral mechanism was evaluated and all oral structures appeared normal. Other aspects of speech and language, including voice quality, receptive and expressive language, and articulation, were informally assessed and appeared within normal limits for his age.

Annual Goals and Measurement

Goal 1. John will demonstrate increased control of fluency in academic and social environments at school.

Benchmark 1. John will learn and apply stuttering modification and fluency-enhancing strategies with 80% accuracy during moments of stuttering in structured activities. *Measurement:* Data collection by SLP

Benchmark 2. John will interact with his teacher and peers without perceived avoidance 5 times per day. *Measurement:* Observation by SLP and/or classroom teacher

Benchmark 3. John will demonstrate knowledge about stuttering by passing a quiz on stuttering facts. *Measurement:* Test administered by SLP

Services and Accommodations

	Services	**Duration**	**Frequency**	**Location**
Speech-Language Therapy	30-min	3x/week	ST room*	

*The speech-language pathologist will work with John in a non-therapy room (e.g., classroom, library, cafeteria, playground) at least 2x/month to promote carryover into other environments.

Accommodations

No specific accommodations are recommended at this time.

Follow-Up and/or Transition

Current IEP to be reviewed within 12 months, on or before ___9/15/xx___

(continues)

Appendix 4-B. continued

Signatures and Parent Consent

IEP Meeting Participants

Timothy Stuart	9/15/xx
Parent/Guardian	Date
Mandy Stuart	9/15/xx
Parent/Guardian	Date
Derek Ramirez	9/15/xx
District Representative	Date
Barbara Stahl	9/15/xx
Teacher	Date
Brenda Khan	9/15/xx
Speech-Language Pathologist	Date
Jonathon Manning	9/15/xx
Psychologist	Date

Consent for Services

I/we have participated in the development of the IEP for my/our child, <u>John Stuart</u>. I/we agree with the concerns and priorities presented in this document and, therefore, give permission to Lincoln School to implement and coordinate services.

Timothy Stuart	9/15/xx
Parent/Guardian	Date
Mandy Stuart	9/15/xx
Parent/Guardian	Date

Appendix 4-C.

Sample Release of Information Form

University Clinic
123 Main Street
Anytown, CA 99999
(xxx)555-1529 · clinic@email.com

Client name: _____

Address: _____

Date of birth: _____

I authorize University Clinic to release any or all clinical records, reports, therapy notes, test results, or other information pertaining to the clinical care of the above-named client to the persons or entities listed below for the sole purpose of benefiting the client. If there is clinical information I do not want disclosed, I have identified it on this form. I acknowledge this authorization is voluntary and refusal to sign will not affect the commencement, continuation, or quality of the above-named client's care at University Clinic. I understand I have the right to revoke consent except to the extent that action has already been taken based on this authorization. I also understand that University Clinic cannot guarantee that confidential information will not be re-disclosed by a recipient. This *Release of Information* will remain in effect unless revised or terminated by me in writing.

_____   _____
Print Name   Date

_____   _____
Signature   Relationship to Client (if under 18)

Clinical information, if any, for which disclosure is not permitted: _____

Client information may be released to the following recipients:

School Professional _____

Address_____

_____

Medical Professional _____

Address_____

_____

Other_____

Address_____

_____

Appendix 4-D.

Sample Clinical Correspondences

A Brief Example

ABC Clinic
123 Main Street
Anytown, CA 99999
(xxx)555-1529 · clinic@email.com

January 13, 20xx

Curtis Clay, M.D.
4242 W. Oak Street
Anytown, CA 99999

Re: Peggy Kiskaddon (DOB: 4-2-20xx)

Dear Dr. Clay:

Peggy was seen for an evaluation on January 12, 20xx. She has difficulty producing several speech sounds—specifically *r*, *l*, *th*, and most consonant blends (such as *br*, *pl*, and *thr*).

I was able to stimulate several sounds during the session, and she could produce these new sounds in several words and short phrases. Peggy will be enrolled for therapy to improve her misarticulations beginning in two weeks. Her prognosis for improvement with therapy is good.

I will forward a complete report of my findings if it would be helpful to you. Please let me know if you would like a copy. Thank you very much.

Sincerely,

Linda J. Rees, M.A., CCC/SLP
Speech-Language Pathologist

cc: Mr. and Mrs. Kiskaddon

REPORTING ASSESSMENT FINDINGS

(continues)

A Moderately Detailed Example

ABC Clinic
123 Main Street
Anytown, CA 99999
(xxx)555-1529 · clinic@email.com

January 19, 20xx

Mark Lapsley, M.D.
7772 1st Street, Suite 12
Anytown, CA 99999

Re: Eric Armstrong (DOB: 10-13-20xx)

Dear Dr. Lapsley:

Thank you for referring Eric to our clinic. His speech was evaluated on January 17, 20xx. He was cooperative throughout the 75-minute evaluative session and a good sample of his speech was obtained.

Eric exhibited a severe stuttering disorder. His speech was approximately 40% disfluent and included five different types of disfluencies. Eric and his mother confirmed that his stuttering was bothersome to both of them, that he avoids certain speaking situations, and that the stuttering patterns have become more prominent during the last 6 months.

Several techniques (particularly an easier onset of speech and a slower rate) resulted in fluent speech in the clinic. Eric's and his mother's levels of concern, their motivation, and the child's ability to produce fluent speech were considered good signs for teaching him a more fluent speech pattern with therapy. He will be enrolled for 40-minute sessions three times per week beginning this June.

Other areas of communication (articulation, hearing, language, and voice) were normal or above normal. Thus, I will focus only on his ability to produce fluent speech.

A more detailed report of my findings has been written. Please contact me if this is of interest to you. I will send you periodic reports of Eric's progress in treatment.

Again, thank you for referring Eric to us.

Sincerely,

Darlene Blackwood, M.A., CCC/SLP
Speech-Language Pathologist

cc: Mr. and Mrs. Armstrong

(continues)

Appendix 4-D. continued

A Detailed Example

ABC Clinic
123 Main Street
Anytown, CA 99999
(xxx)555-1529 · clinic@email.com

May 11, 20xx

Elizabeth Rees, M.D.
1998 Purdue Drive
Anytown, CA 99999

Re: Timothy Mathias
DOB: 7-25-19xx

Dear Dr. Rees,

Thank you for referring Timothy Mathias, a 73-year-old male, to our clinic. A complete dysphagia evaluation was completed at the Our Lady of Mercy Skilled Nursing Facility, where Mr. Mathias has been a resident for the past 7 months. Prior to his residence at the SNF, he was residing at home with his wife (who died 10 months ago).

Nurses at the facility reported that Mr. Mathias lost 7 pounds in the last 3 weeks and has been complaining of difficulty chewing his food. His medical history includes chronic obstructive pulmonary disease (COPD), emphysema, and a mild stroke that occurred 3 years ago. At the time of his stroke, he experienced oral dysphagia, characterized by reduced oral motor strength and range of motion, primarily on the right side. At that time, he received speech therapy services by another speech-language pathologist affiliated with the ABC Clinic and made a full recovery. Until recently, he has not experienced any additional chewing or swallowing difficulties.

Assessment:

The current evaluation took place during Mr. Mathias's afternoon meal. Mr. Mathias was seated in his wheelchair. He was served a hamburger, tomato soup, watermelon, pudding, and iced tea. He was in good spirits and was very cooperative. His cognitive status was excellent. Mr. Mathias reported that he preferred to eat in his room and occasionally ate while sitting up in his bed. He said that he has not been able to complete his meals in the past 4 to 5 weeks because of difficulty chewing his food. He said that hard foods, such as meats and raw vegetables, were usually most difficult for him to eat. He also reported that he often feels pressed for time during meals because the kitchen staff comes by to pick up the lunch trays about 30 minutes after delivering them, and sometimes he has not finished eating yet. When I asked him if he experiences coughing episodes during or immediately after meals, he said no.

A complete orofacial examination revealed adequate lingual and labial range of motion. Lingual strength was reduced bilaterally. Labial strength was adequate. Dentition was within normal limits for his age, with an upper partial plate in place. He was able to produce a dry swallow. Laryngeal elevation and timing appeared within normal limits. Dry cough was also within normal limits.

(continues)

REPORTING ASSESSMENT FINDINGS

Appendix 4-D. continued

Mr. Mathias managed puree and liquid textures without difficulty. No coughing or choking was noted. Laryngeal elevation and timing was good. When he attempted to eat his hamburger, I noticed that he paused frequently while chewing and his breathing was slightly more labored. I suggested that he take the meat out of the hamburger and chop it into smaller bites. Mr. Mathias reported that the smaller bites were easier for him to manage. I noted that he still took frequent pauses while chewing, but he was improved compared to the prior trial. Laryngeal elevation and timing of the swallows were within normal limits. Pocketed food was noted under the tongue. He was unable to clear the pocketed food on subsequent swallows. He also had difficulty moving a moderately sized hamburger bolus from side to side.

He said he normally eats about one-third of his meals. During the examination, he was able to eat about three-quarters of the meal. I did ask the kitchen staff to come back later for his tray when they arrived at the door to check on his progress because Mr. Mathias was not finished yet. I recommended that he do the same in the future. He said he feels a bit shy to do so, but he will start letting them know he would like more time to eat. I also recommended that he chop his food into smaller pieces, as he had done today, when he has difficulty chewing it.

Diagnosis:

Mr. Mathias presented with mild-moderate oral dysphagia characterized by reduced lingual strength and difficulty chewing solid food textures.

Recommendations:

- Change diet to a chopped-solids diet.
- Allow extra time for Mr. Mathias to eat his meals.
- Serve all meals while Mr. Mathias is seated upright in his wheelchair or with his bed fully raised so that his back and hips are at a 90° angle.
- Dysphagia therapy five times per week for 2 weeks to address the following goals.

Treatment goals:

- Increase lingual strength to within normal limits.
- Educate caregivers and Mr. Mathias about his dysphagia and train them to follow the recommendations listed above.
- Upgrade chopped-solids diet to regular diet upon completion of therapy.

Prognosis:

Prognosis for completion of goals is excellent considering Mr. Mathias's motivation and cognitive status stimulability for improvement, and the mild-moderate severity of the dysphagia.

A copy of this report was placed in Mr. Mathias's medical chart and I personally reviewed my recommendations with the head nurse and the dietitian. At the end of the treatment period, I will send you an updated report on his progress and condition.

Thank you again for the referral. Please contact me if you would like any further information.

Sincerely,

Janelle Davis, M.A., CCC/SLP
Speech-Language Pathologist

Chapter 5

ASSESSMENT PROCEDURES COMMON TO MOST COMMUNICATIVE DISORDERS

This chapter describes methods for assessing most speech and language disorders. Not every procedure is necessary for each client, although a majority of assessments will include several, if not most, of the procedures described here.

OROFACIAL EXAMINATION

The "Orofacial Evaluation Form" (Form 5-1) is an important component of a complete assessment. Its purpose is to identify or rule out structural or functional factors that relate to a communicative disorder or dysphagia. The materials in this section pertain primarily to communicative function. Because the orofacial component of a dysphagia examination is more specific to chewing and swallowing, it is presented in greater detail in Chapter 15.

At minimum, the clinician will need disposable gloves, a stopwatch, a small flashlight, and a tongue depressor to complete an orofacial examination. A bite block (to disassociate tongue and jaw movements), cotton gauze (to hold the tongue in place), an applicator stick (to assess velopharyngeal movement), a toothette, or a mirror may also be needed. When evaluating young children, especially those who are reluctant to participate, a sucker may be used in place of a tongue depressor or toothette. Foods such as peanut butter or applesauce can also be strategically placed in the oral cavity to help assess lip and tongue movements. Keep in mind that some children have allergies to certain foods. Be sure to obtain parental permission before giving a food product.

Precautions should always be followed to protect all parties from possible contact with body fluids and infectious materials. The Centers for Disease Control and Prevention (CDC) has mandated Universal Precautions (UP) to be followed to reduce a person's exposure to diseases that are spread by blood and certain body fluids. Specific precautions that are relevant to settings in which speech-language pathologists work are listed here. Always assume clients, and possibly other staff, are an infectious risk and use appropriate barrier practices, such as:

- Sterilize all equipment that is used in the mouth.
- Wash hands before and after contact.
- Wear gloves if there will be any contact with body fluids, mucous membranes, or broken skin.
- Remove gloves promptly without touching the outside of them (turn them inside out when removing), and then safely dispose of them.
- Wash hands after removing gloves.
- Wear eye and mouth protection if any body fluids are likely to splash or spray.
- Wear a gown and shoe coverings if clothing is likely to come in contact with body fluids.
- Change your clothing if another person's blood or body fluid gets onto your clothes.
- Never use single-use equipment (e.g., gloves, tongue depressor, toothette, etc.) more than once.
- Follow facility or campus infection control policies regarding procedures for disinfecting and cleaning various surfaces and instruments.

Interpreting the Orofacial Examination

The primary oral structures are presented in Figure 5-1. Valid interpretation of findings from an orofacial examination requires an understanding of the anatomic, physiologic, and neurologic bases of the orofacial structures and their functions. It also requires knowledge of the relationship between orofacial integrity and communicative function. Sophistication in administering these examinations takes time and a good deal of experience to develop.

Several common observations from an orofacial examination and possible clinical implications are described on the next page. Recognize that this is not an all-inclusive list, nor does it exhaust the potential implications of each finding.

- *Abnormal color of the tongue, palate, or pharynx:* A grayish color is normally associated with muscular paresis or paralysis. A bluish tint may result from excessive vascularity or bleeding. A whitish color present along the border of the hard and soft palate is a symptom of a submucosal cleft. An abnormally dark or a translucent color on the hard palate may be an indication of a palatal fistula or a cleft. Dark spots may indicate oral cancer.

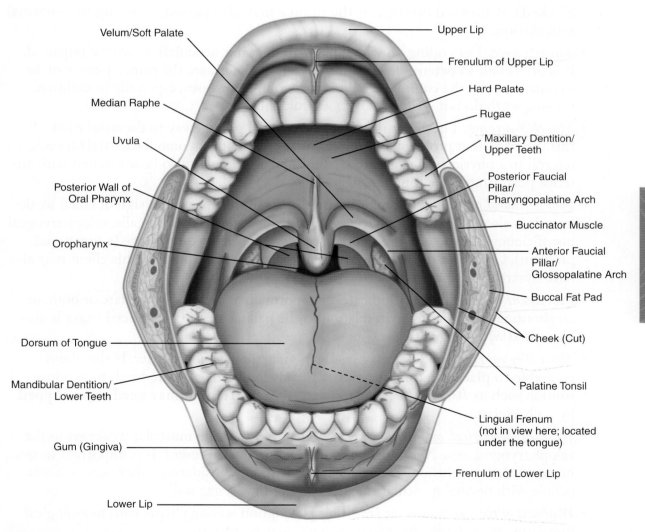

FIGURE 5-1. Oral Structures

- *Abnormal height or width of the palatal arch:* The shape of the palatal arch may vary considerably from client to client. If the arch is especially wide or high, the client may experience difficulties with palatal-lingual sounds. An abnormally low or narrow arch in the presence of a large tongue may result in consonant distortions.

- *Asymmetry of the face or palate:* This is often associated with neurological impairment or muscle weakness.

- *Deviation of the tongue or uvula to the left or right:* This may indicate neurological involvement. If so, the tongue may deviate to the weaker side because the weaker half of the tongue is unable to match the extension of the stronger half. On phonation, the uvula may deviate to the stronger side as the palatal muscles on that strong side pull the uvula farther toward the velopharyngeal opening. Facial asymmetry is also likely to be present. The client may exhibit concomitant aphasia, dysarthria, or both.

- *Enlarged tonsils:* Many children have large tonsils with no adverse affect on speech production. In some cases, however, enlarged tonsils interfere with general health, normal resonance, and hearing acuity (if the eustachian tubes are blocked). A forward carriage of the tongue may also persist, resulting in abnormal articulation.

- *Missing teeth:* Depending on which teeth are missing, articulation may be impaired. It is important to determine whether the missing teeth are the primary cause of, or a contributor to, the communicative disorder. In most cases, especially in children, missing teeth do not seriously affect articulation.

- *Mouth breathing:* The client may have a restricted passageway to the nasal cavity. If this is a persistent problem and the client also exhibits hyponasal (denasal) speech, a referral to a physician is warranted. Mouth breathing may also be associated with anterior posturing of the tongue at rest.

- *Poor intraoral pressure:* Poor maintenance of air in the cheeks is a sign of labial weakness. It is also a sign of velopharyngeal inadequacy—more specifically, velopharyngeal insufficiency (a structural problem) or velopharyngeal incompetence (a functional problem). Check for nasal emission or air escaping from the lips. This client may also have dysarthria, hypernasality, or both.

- *Prominent rugae:* This may indicate an abnormally narrow or low palate or both, or an abnormally large tongue in relation to the palatal areas. Pronounced rugae is also associated with tongue thrust.

- *Short lingual frenum:* This may result in an articulation disorder. If the client is unable to place the tongue against the alveolar ridge or the teeth to produce sounds such as /t/, /d/, /n/, /l/, /tʃ/, and /dʒ/, the frenum may need to be clipped by a physician.

- *Weak, asymmetrical, or absent gag reflex:* This may indicate muscular weakness in the velopharyngeal area. Neurological impairment may be present. It is important to note, however, that conclusions cannot be made without considering other factors. Some people with normal muscular integrity do not have a gag reflex.

- *Weakness of the lips, tongue, or jaw:* This is common among clients with neurological impairments. Aphasia, dysarthria, or both, may be present.

Assessing Diadochokinetic Syllable Rate

Diadochokinetic (DDK) syllable rate is the measure of a client's ability to make rapidly alternating speech movements. It may also be called alternating or sequential motion rate. DDK rate provides information about a client's motor and speech-planning ability. It is important to note the client's ability to sequence same and different syllables, accuracy of productions, fluency, rhythm, voicing, rate, and coordination of respiration, phonation, and articulation. DDK rate is measured in one of two ways: (1) counting the syllables produced within a predetermined number of seconds, or (2) measuring the seconds it takes to produce a predetermined number of syllables. The latter is the more traditional method used.

The "Diadochokinetic Syllable Rates Worksheet," Form 5-2, provided in this text is based on the research of Fletcher (1972) and provides norms for children ages 6 through 13. Administration follows the second method just described. More specifically:

1. Instruct the client to repeat the target syllable (e.g., /pʌ/, /tʌ/, /kʌ/) as quickly as possible until told to stop.

2. Model the sequence and allow the client to practice to be sure the instruction is understood.

3. Say *go* and start the stopwatch.

4. Say *stop* and stop the stopwatch after 20 repetitions.

5. Redo the sequence if the client stops or slows down intentionally before the task is completed.

6. After assessing each syllable individually, evaluate the client for 10 repetitions of /pʌtʌkʌ/.

7. Record findings on the worksheet.

Young children may have difficulty sequencing /pʌtʌkʌ/. In this case, have the child repeat a familiar word such as *pattycake* or *buttercup* instead. It may also be helpful to record the test for review at a later time to increase confidence that the findings are accurate.

SPEECH AND LANGUAGE SAMPLING

Speech-language samples are invaluable in the assessment of a client's communicative abilities and disorders. They can be the basis for determining whether a problem exists and, if so, identifying the client's specific deficiencies and needs. A speech-language sample should be long enough to obtain a truly, representative sample of the client's speech and language. A minimum of 50–100 distinct utterances is needed for a language sample, and we emphasize the word *minimum*. Collecting 50–100 utterances does not guarantee an adequate sample; rather, 200 or more different utterances will provide a better data set.

To obtain a reliable and valid speech-language sample, utilize the following recommendations:

- Strive for a long sample.
- Establish a positive relationship before collecting a sample.
- Be as unobtrusive as possible; minimize interruptions and distractions.
- Be willing to wait for the client to talk. Do not talk to fill the silence.

COMMON COMMUNICATION

- Preselect materials and topics that will be interesting to the client, and follow the client's lead in elaborating or changing topics.
- Vary the subject matter of the sample.
- Seek out multiple environments (e.g., clinic, playground, home, workplace).
- Alter the contexts (e.g., conversation, narratives, responses to pictures).
- Use a good-quality digital recorder. Videorecord if possible.
- In situations where it is not practical to record samples (e.g., home, classroom, workplace), ask another person, such as a spouse, parent, or teacher, to provide recorded samples.
- Ask questions that elicit lengthier responses, such as "tell me about . . .," "what happened?," or "why?"
- Avoid yes/no questions or other questions that can be answered with only a few words.
- Make natural contributions to the conversation.
- Consider the client's age and cultural background; avoid questions that could be considered demeaning or offensive.

Specific analysis of the speech sample is dependent upon the focus of the assessment. For information on analyzing aspects of the speech samples, consult these materials in other chapters within this manual:

- Identifying sound errors from a speech sample
- Evaluating rate of speech
- Determining intelligibility
- Comparison of sound errors from an articulation test and connected speech
- Language sampling and analysis
- Determining the mean length of utterance
- Assessment of semantic skills
- Determining the type-token ratio
- Assessment of syntactic skills
- Assessment of morphologic skills
- Examining the voice
- Identifying dysarthria
- Identifying apraxia

Conversation Starters for Eliciting a Speech-Language Sample

Obtaining an adequate speech-language sample from an adult client is usually an uncomplicated task. If the client is verbal and the clinician uses open-ended stimuli to elicit responses, (e.g., "tell me about . . ."), an adequate sample may be collected during the information-getting interview. If this does not occur, however, ask specific questions about the client's interests (e.g., hobbies, occupation, sports, family, current events) to encourage lengthier conversation.

Obtaining a representative speech-language sample is usually a bigger challenge with children, particularly if they are quiet by nature or are reticent about the situation. We have provided sample stimulus questions and statements to help elicit a speech-language sample. Adapt them as needed to obtain the best speech-language sample possible.

- Tell me what you would do if you won a million dollars.
- Have you ever been to a hospital? Tell me about it.
- Have you ever been in an airport? Tell me about it.
- Have you even gotten lost at the store? Tell me about it.
- Does your brother/sister ever make you really mad? What does he/she do to make you mad?
- Pretend I've never had pizza before. Describe it to me.
- Pretend I've never been to a library. Describe one to me.
- What is your favorite food? How do you make it?
- Tell me the story of the *Three Little Pigs* (or other children's story).
- Do you have a pet? Tell me about it.
- What would you get at the grocery store if you were going to make dinner for your family?
- Tell me how to make popcorn.
- Tell me what you and your friends play (or talk about) together.
- Tell me about your favorite movie (or TV show).
- Tell me about your favorite video game.

With younger children, introduce different activities, objects, or toys into the environment to elicit speech or vocalizations. For example, play *pat-a-cake* or *peek-a-boo*; use animals, cars, planes, dolls, or other toys; play matching games; or use a puppet to name common objects or body parts.

Pictures

Pictures are often useful for eliciting a speech-language sample. They provide a known context, which may be helpful when assessing clients with significantly impaired intelligibility. It is important to use pictures that illustrate a variety of activities. Pictures that show little action, depict few things to talk about, or elicit naming-only responses are of little use. When possible, use pictures to transition to more natural dialogue. For example, ask "Has that ever happened to you?" after the client describes a scenario. Figures 5-2 through 5-5 in Appendix 5-B are provided to help elicit a speech-language sample.

Narratives

An important form of a speech-language sample is a narrative, or story. Narrative production differs from conversational production in that the client must use certain rules of cognitive organization and language sequencing to relay events that have a beginning, middle, and end. One method of assessing narrative production is by telling a story and having the client tell it back. Figures 5-6 and 5-7 in Appendix 5-B are narratives with pictures that are helpful

COMMON COMMUNICATION

for narrative sampling. After reading each story, encourage the client to retell it with as much detail as possible. Other sources of narratives include:

- *Stories for Oral Language Development* (Mattes & Schuchardt, 2000)
- *Narrative Story Cards* (Helm-Estabrooks & Nicholas, 2003)
- *Narrative Toolbox* (Hutson-Nechkash, 2001)
- Sequencing picture cards
- Wordless storybooks
- Wordless videos

READING PASSAGES

Information obtained during oral reading is valuable for making many assessment decisions because it allows the clinician to observe the client's articulation, voice, fluency, and reading abilities. Compare oral reading results with those evoked from single-word or short-phrase utterances and conversational speech samples. Eight reading passages that vary in difficulty and age appropriateness are provided in Appendix 5-A. The first five passages are intended for children. All of the consonant phonemes of the English language are included in each passage. The following reading grade levels are guidelines only; they are not intended to assess the reading skills of clients.

- *Swimming* — Kindergarten to first grade
- *Grandma is Coming* — First grade to second grade
- *Nicknames* — Third grade to fourth grade
- *The Amazing Spider* — Third grade to fifth grade
- *The Toothbrush* — Fourth grade to sixth grade

There are also three adult reading passages. The *Grandfather* and the *Rainbow Passage* have been used for clinical and research purposes in our field for many years. The third adult passage is a portion of the *Declaration of Independence*. Two of the children's passages, *The Amazing Spider* and *The Toothbrush*, are also appropriate for some adults. Other sources of reading materials for children and adults include children's books, grade-level readers, general textbooks, popular magazines, newspapers, and reading apps.

EVALUATING RATE OF SPEECH

A client's speech rate can directly affect articulation, intelligibility, voice production, and fluency. With some clients, obtaining periodic rates will be necessary as a measure of improvement (e.g., such as with fluency) or deterioration (e.g., such as intelligibility associated with myasthenia gravis) over time.

It is important to note that speech rates vary tremendously among normal speakers. This statement is reinforced by the data in Table 5-1, which presents findings from several speech-rate studies. Some people who use seemingly slow speech rates have excellent speech, whereas others with the same rate struggle with a communicative disorder. Some people who speak exceedingly fast may have excellent intelligibility and control of their speech, whereas others exhibit communicative impairments due to the rapid speech rate.

TABLE 5-1   Normal Rates of Speech

	AVERAGE	RANGE	STUDY
Reading—Adult		160–180 wpm	Calvert & Silverman (1983)
		220–302 spm	Venkatagiri (1999)
Spontaneous Speech—Adult	270 wpm		Calvert & Silverman (1983)
		220–410 wpm	Weiner (1984)
		114–247 spm	Venkatagiri (1999)
Spontaneous Speech—First grader*	125 wpm		Purcell & Runyan (1980)
Spontaneous Speech—Fifth grader*	142 wpm		Purcell & Runyan (1980)

wpm: words per minute; spm: syllables per minute
*Purcell and Runyan (1980) studied children in first through fifth grade and reported an incremental increase in average speech rate at each grade level.

The importance of measuring the speech rate is not to compare it with preestablished norms, which only indicate whether the speech rate is normal, faster than normal, or slower than normal. The value of assessing rate of speech is that it allows the clinician to evaluate its effect on the client's communicative abilities. Consider the rate of speech and its effects on the articulation of sounds, intelligibility, voice production, and fluency. Will the use of a faster or slower rate result in better communication? Can a better speech rate be elicited? Can it be maintained? These are important questions to consider when assessing the implications of speech rate on communication.

Determining Speech Rate

To determine a client's speech rate, record a sample of connected speech (devoid of significant pausing) in oral reading, in conversational speech, or both. In a 60-second interval, count the number of words produced and divide by 60 (or 120 for a 2-minute sample, 180 for a 3-minute sample, etc.). For example, 200 words produced in 60 seconds is 200 words per minute (wpm). If there are no 60-second intervals of connected speech, use the following procedures to calculate the speech rate. Use a stopwatch to time the speech intervals.

1. Time the sample (e.g., 20 seconds).
2. Count the number of words produced (e.g., 62 words).
3. Divide the number of seconds in a minute (60) by the number of seconds in the sample (20 seconds in the example): $60 \div 20 = 3$.
4. Multiply the number of words in the sample (62 in the example) by the number in Step 3 (3 in the example): $62 \times 3 = 186$. The wpm is 186.

Greater reliability in wpm calculations is possible by collecting several samples. The following is based on three samples:

1. The three samples are 20, 25, and 30 seconds, which equals a total of 75 seconds.
2. The number of words in the respective samples are 15, 20, and 25, which equals a total of 60 words.

COMMON
COMMUNICATION

3. The number of seconds in 3 minutes (60 seconds per minute times three samples) is 180 seconds. Divide the number of seconds (180) by the number of seconds in the three samples (75): 180 ÷ 75 = 2.4.

4. Multiply the number of words in the sample (60) by the number in Step 3 (2.4): 60 × 2.4 = 144. The wpm is 144.

The same procedure can be followed to determine syllables per minute (spm) by counting syllables instead of words.

DETERMINING INTELLIGIBILITY

Calculating intelligibility is necessary when considering the need for treatment, identifying factors that contribute to poor intelligibility, selecting treatment goals, recording baseline information, and monitoring the effects of treatment over time. An "Assessing Intelligibility Worksheet," Form 5-3, is provided to help calculate intelligibility.

The speech sample used to determine intelligibility must be an adequate, representative sample of the client's speech in order to obtain a valid intelligibility rating. Refer to "Speech and Language Sampling" and "Conversation Starters for Eliciting a Speech-Language Sample" earlier in this chapter for specific suggestions for collecting a sample. Audio or video recording the sample is helpful for analysis and future comparison. The speech-language sample used can be from a clinical session, from the client's home, or from another environment (e.g., classroom, workplace, etc.). It is best to obtain representative samples from different environments.

When analyzing the speech sample, realize that there are many factors that can negatively influence intelligibility. These include:

- The number of sound errors. Generally, the greater the number of sound errors, the poorer the intelligibility.
- The type of sound errors. For example, omissions and additions sometimes result in poorer intelligibility than substitutions or distortions.
- Inconsistency of errors.
- Vowel errors.
- The rate of speech, especially if it is excessively slow or fast.
- Atypical prosodic characteristic of speech, such as abnormal intonation or stress.
- The length and linguistic complexity of the words and utterances used.
- Insufficient vocal intensity, dysphonia, hypernasality, or hyponasality.
- Disfluencies, particularly severe disfluencies that disrupt the context.
- The lack of gestures or other paralinguistic cues that assist understanding.
- The testing environment (such as at home versus in the clinic).
- The client's anxiety about the testing situation.
- The client's lack of familiarity with the stimulus materials.
- The client's level of fatigue. Fatigue particularly affects very young children, elderly clients, and clients with certain neurological disorders.
- The clinician's ability to understand "less intelligible" speech.

- The clinician's familiarity with the client and the client's speaking context.

In most cases, there are multiple factors—some client-related, some clinician-related, and some environmentally related—that influence overall intelligibility. This means that clinicians need to:

- Identify factors that affect intelligibility.
- View the intelligibility rating as being approximate, rather than absolute or definitive.
- Take more than one speech-language sample, and seek varied environments when possible.
- Secure a representative sample of speech. The client or the client's caregiver can usually help you determine whether a particular sample was a typical representation of the client's speech.

We also recommend that clinicians:

- Use a high-quality recording device.
- Avoid stimulus items that tend to elicit play rather than talk (e.g., blocks, doll houses, puzzles).
- Use open-ended stimuli (e.g., "Tell me about the car.") rather than closed-ended stimuli (e.g., "What is that?" "What color is it?" "What is it used for?").
- Consider reporting intelligibility in ranges (e.g., 65–75%), particularly when intelligibility varies. For example, a child may be 90–100% intelligible when speaking in utterances of one to three syllables. However, the same child may be only 50% intelligible in utterances of four or more syllables.
- Compare intelligibility on word-by-word and utterance-by-utterance bases. For some clients, the results will be very similar. For others, they may be considerably different. For example, a client whose loudness and articulation deteriorate in longer utterances may have many intelligible words, particularly at the beginning of individual utterances. But the end of the child's utterances may be unintelligible. A child with a pragmatic or organizational language disorder may produce many intelligible words, but the connected discourse may be unintelligible. Jargon aphasic speech may also contain many intelligible words, but be contextually illogical.

SYLLABLE-BY-SYLLABLE STIMULUS PHRASES

Clinicians use verbal phrases as stimuli for a variety of sampling tasks. They are especially valuable for evaluating stimulability, assessing the maintenance of newly learned target behaviors in the clinical setting, and determining the client's maximum phrase length for optimal speech production. Syllable-by-syllable phrases are useful for assessing many disorders. The following are just a few examples of clinical questions that can be answered by using syllable-by-syllable phrases:

- Can the hyponasal (denasal) client maintain appropriate nasal resonance across increasingly longer phrases containing nasal sounds?
- Can the hypernasal client produce the nonnasal phrases without nasality?
- What speech rate is optimal for the client to be able to articulate all sounds correctly in phrases of increasing length?

COMMON
COMMUNICATION

- Are there specific syllable lengths at which the client's speech begins to deteriorate?
- Are there specific syllable lengths at which the client's articulation becomes less intelligible?
- Can fluency be maintained in increasingly longer phrases?
- Can a desired voice quality (e.g., nonhoarse) be maintained in increasingly longer phrases?

Syllable-by-syllable phrases are versatile and can be used with different disorders. Articulation, rate, prosody, inflection, and intonation can all be sampled across a variety of disorders using these phrase lists. The phrases in Table 5-2 can be imitated from the clinician's model, read by the client, or both. Note the syllable lengths at which the desired behavior (e.g., fluent speech, appropriate voice, articulatory accuracy) can be maintained, as well as the lengths at which the desired behavior cannot be maintained. Also identify contexts that may be either easier or more difficult for the client. The phrase levels where breakdowns occur are often good starting points for treatment when therapy is initiated.

TABLE 5-2   Syllable-by-Syllable Stimulus Phrases

TWO-SYLLABLE PHRASES	
With Nasals	*Without Nasals*
at noon	Back up.
brown car	big boy
Come in.	blue sky
Down, please.	dog house
front door	hot dog
I'm fine.	Keep out.
in here	Pull hard.
my jam	Push it.
Show me.	red car
Thank you.	too slow

THREE-SYLLABLE PHRASES	
With Nasals	*Without Nasals*
Good morning.	apple pie
hot and cold	catch the bus
jumping rope	far to go
make it up	How are you?
moon and stars	Hurry up.
more and more	Laugh loudly.
Please call me.	Leave the house.
run and jump	red roses
shoes and socks	see the cat
yes or no	slept all day

FOUR-SYLLABLE PHRASES

With Nasals

bacon and eggs
Do it right now.
Do it for him.
It's a fine day.
Leave him alone.
My hands are cold.
Open it up.
salt and pepper
table and chairs
The meal was fine.

Without Nasals

after he left
Do it this way.
He has a coat.
Here is the key.
I like to read.
I told you so.
Keep to the left.
Show her the way.
Tell her okay.
The bus was full.

FIVE-SYLLABLE PHRASES

With Nasals

a piece of candy
a long vacation
He wants the money.
Look out the window.
My mother said no.
Please open the door.
She is very nice.
The dogs are barking.
The weather is fine.
We cut down the tree.

Without Nasals

a pair of scissors
Beware of the dog.
Did you hit the ball?
He would if he could.
How did you do it?
Let's go to the park.
She is very shy.
The car was dirty.
The weather is cold.
We sat by the trees.

SIX-SYLLABLE PHRASES

With Nasals

a nickel and a dime
Give them each a muffin.
How much more will it cost?
I haven't heard from them.
just beyond the corner
Leave the window open.
Put everything away.
Shut the door behind you.
The farmers needed rain.
We can go after lunch.

Without Nasals

Are you ready to go?
Do you have the address?
Go to the library.
He rushed to catch the bus.
He is very happy.
I have lost the car keys.
The potatoes were cold.
What size shoe do you wear?
Where did you put her coat?
Will you keep it secret?

continued on the next page

COMMON COMMUNICATION

Table 5-2, continued from the previous page

SEVEN-SYLLABLE PHRASES

With Nasals	*Without Nasals*
Come and see us when you can.	Did you read today's paper?
Come inside and close the door.	He has a good idea.
He wants more cake and ice cream.	I thought it would start at four.
I don't know what happened here.	I would like a cup of tea.
I wonder why she said that.	Put it back where you got it.
Is it time for the movie?	She is a very good cook.
Please knock before you enter.	They like to sit at the park.
She is not very happy.	Why did they go to the show?
What is it you want to know?	You did the best you could do.
When does the next show begin?	You should tell her about it.

EIGHT-SYLLABLE PHRASES

With Nasals	*Without Nasals*
Can you hear the television?	Did you see the keys to the car?
Come over as soon as you can.	Give it to that boy over there.
Do you want another one now?	He will pick you up after school.
Leave the window open tonight.	I have a lot of work to do.
The children are playing outside.	I would like to do it for you.
The melons are from our backyard.	She has to buy food for supper.
They are going to the movie.	The letter arrived yesterday.
We live just around the corner.	They all ate breakfast together.
We went to the animal farm.	We already heard about it.
When will you come to visit us?	We are so happy to see you.

CHARTING

Charting is useful for both diagnostic and treatment activities. It provides a method of scoring a client's responses and objectively identifying the client's communicative abilities and deficits. Desirable behaviors (e.g., correct sound productions, fluent speech) or undesirable behaviors (e.g., misarticulations, throat clearing) can be charted. This information provides an assessment baseline for diagnostic decisions, and demonstrates progress in treatment. Virtually any behavior can be charted during an evaluation. For example:

- Correct and incorrect productions of a particular sound at a specified syllable or word level
- Frequency of specific disfluency types

- Instances of motor behaviors associated with stuttering (e.g., facial grimaces)
- Groping or pre-posturing behaviors in clients with apraxia
- Specific language features (e.g., copula verbs, plural morphemes, verb phrases)
- Word-finding problems or circumlocutions in clients with aphasia
- Correct phonatory behaviors, such as nonhoarse vocal productions
- Inappropriate vocal behaviors, such as throat clearing or harsh phonatory onset

Charting is also appropriate for behaviors that are important in treatment but not necessarily caused by the communicative disorder. For example, record each time a child responds to a stimulus, stays in the chair for 30 seconds, and so forth. There are several ways to chart behaviors, including:

1. *Note each time a preselected behavior is exhibited.* For example, record each instance of throat clearing, each associated motor behavior, every interjection (e.g., "OK" or "uh"), and so forth. In this method, opposite behaviors (e.g., the absence of throat clearing) are not recorded. The result is a count of the number of times a specified behavior occurred within the time interval sampled.

2. *Note each instance of both correct and incorrect behaviors.* Use a check (✔) or plus (+) for each desirable production, and a zero (0) or a minus (−) for every undesirable production. For example, after 10 productions of a given sound, perhaps 7 were correct and 3 were incorrect. This yields a percentage (70% in this case) that can be compared with previous or future results.

3. *Note behaviors according to one of several preselected criteria.* For example, when charting articulation, a specified sound may be omitted (O), approximated (A), or produced correctly (C). Percentages can then be determined for each type of response.

Various forms are available that are simple to use and appropriate for different clients. Two such worksheets are provided in this manual. Form 5-4, "Charting Worksheet I," allows the clinician to chart up to 200 responses. A different target response can be entered on each row so progress on different stimulus items can be monitored. The worksheet is appropriate for charting children, adolescents, or adults.

Form 5-5, "Charting Worksheet II," is designed especially for children. A total of 100 responses can be charted on the sheet. Children enjoy receiving a star, stamp, happy face, or sticker in each box when they correctly produce the target behavior. It is also an enjoyable way to teach children to chart their own responses.

CONCLUDING COMMENTS

The procedures described in this chapter are used to assess many different communicative disorders. Most of these procedures, or some variation of them, are included in diagnostic sessions. This does not mean that each procedure has to be used during every assessment. For example, it may not be necessary to evaluate a client's speech rate or include a reading task during every evaluation.

The procedures described here, although common to most communicative disorders, do not focus on specific problems associated with each disorder. The information and procedures applicable for specific disorders are found in other chapters of this text. Information from this chapter is to be used along with the material from the chapters that follow.

SOURCES OF ADDITIONAL INFORMATION

Print Sources

Dworkin, J. P., & Culatta, R. A. (1996). *Dworkin-Culatta oral mechanism examination & treatment system*. Nicholasville, KY: Edgewood Press.

Hegde, M. N., & Maul, C. A. (2006). Language disorders in children: An evidence-based approach to assessment and treatment. Boston, MA: Pearson Education.

Owens, R. E. (2010). *Language disorders: A functional approach to assessment and intervention* (5th ed.). Needham Heights, MA: Allyn & Bacon.

Retherford, K. S. (2000). *Guide to analysis of language transcripts* (3rd ed.). Eu Claire, WI: Thinking Publications.

St. Louis, K., & Ruscello, D. (2000). *Oral speech mechanism screening examination* (3rd ed.). Austin, TX: PRO-ED.

Electronic Sources

American Speech-Language-Hearing Association: *http://www.asha.org*

Dworkin-Culatta Oral Mechanism Examination and Treatment System: *http://www20.csueastbay.edu/class/departments/commsci/files/docs/pdf/Dworkin-Culatta_Oral_Mech_Exam.pdf*

Speaking of Speech Data Forms: *http://www.speakingofspeech.com/Lesson_Plans___Data_Form.html*

"Chronological Age Calculator" app by Home-Speech-Home.com

"Diadochokinetics Assessment" app by Seth Koster

"Word Vault" app by Home-Speech-Home.com

Form 5-1.

Orofacial Examination Form

Name: _____ Age: _____ Date: _____

Examiner's Name: _____

Instructions: Check and circle each item noted. Include descriptive comments in the right-hand margin.

Evaluation of Face

_____ Symmetry: normal/droops on right/droops on left _____

_____ Abnormal movements: none/grimaces/spasms _____

_____ Mouth breathing: yes/no _____

_____ Other _____

Evaluation of Jaw and Teeth

Tell client to open and close mouth.

_____ Range of motion: normal/reduced _____

_____ Symmetry: normal/deviates to right/deviates to left _____

_____ Movement: normal/jerky/groping/slow/asymmetrical _____

_____ TMJ noises: absent/grinding/popping _____

_____ Other _____

Observe dentition.

_____ Teeth: all present/dentures/teeth missing (specify) _____

_____ Arrangement of teeth: normal/jumbled/spaces/misaligned _____

_____ Hygiene _____

_____ Other _____

Evaluation of Lips

Tell client to pucker.

_____ Range of motion: normal/reduced _____

_____ Symmetry: normal/droops bilaterally/droops right/droops left _____

_____ Strength (press tongue blade against lips): normal/weak _____

_____ Other _____

(continues)

COMMON COMMUNICATION

Form 5-1. continued

Tell client to smile.

_____ Range of motion: normal/reduced _____

_____ Symmetry: normal/droops bilaterally/droops right/droops left _____

_____ Other _____

Tell client to puff cheeks and hold air.

_____ Lip strength: normal/reduced _____

_____ Nasal emission: absent/present _____

_____ Other _____

Evaluation of Tongue

_____ Surface color: normal/abnormal (specify) _____

_____ Abnormal movements: absent/jerky/spasms/writhing/fasciculations _____

_____ Size: normal/small/large _____

_____ Frenum: normal/short _____

_____ Other _____

Tell client to protrude the tongue.

_____ Excursion: normal/deviates to right/deviates to left _____

_____ Range of motion: normal/reduced _____

_____ Speed of motion: normal/reduced _____

_____ Strength (apply opposing pressure with tongue blade): normal/reduced _____

_____ Other _____

Tell client to retract the tongue.

_____ Excursion: normal/deviates to right/deviates to left _____

_____ Range of motion: normal/reduced _____

_____ Speed of motion: normal/reduced _____

_____ Other _____

Tell client to move tongue tip to the right.

_____ Excursion: normal/incomplete/groping _____

_____ Range of motion: normal/reduced _____

_____ Strength (apply opposing pressure with tongue blade): normal/reduced _____

_____ Other _____

(continues)

Form 5-1. continued

Tell client to move the tongue tip to the left.

_____ Excursion: normal/incomplete/groping _____

_____ Range of motion: normal/reduced _____

_____ Strength (apply opposing pressure with tongue blade): normal/reduced _____

_____ Other _____

Tell client to move the tongue tip up.

_____ Movement: normal/groping _____

_____ Range of motion: normal/reduced _____

_____ Other _____

Tell client to move the tongue tip down.

_____ Movement: normal/groping _____

_____ Range of motion: normal/reduced _____

_____ Other _____

Observe rapid side-to-side movements.

_____ Rate: normal/reduced/slows down progressively _____

_____ Range of motion: normal/reduced on left/reduced on right _____

_____ Other _____

Evaluation of Pharynx

_____ Color: normal/abnormal _____

_____ Tonsils: absent/normal/enlarged _____

_____ Other _____

Evaluation of Hard and Soft Palates

_____ Color: normal/abnormal _____

_____ Rugae: normal/very prominent _____

_____ Arch height: normal/high/low _____

_____ Arch width: normal/narrow/wide _____

_____ Growths: absent/present (describe) _____

_____ Fistula: absent/present (describe) _____

(continues)

COMMON COMMUNICATION

Form 5-1. continued

Evaluation of Hard and Soft Palates (continued)

_____ Clefting: absent/present (describe) _____

_____ Symmetry at rest: normal/lower on right/lower on left _____

_____ Gag reflex: normal/absent/hyperactive/hypoactive _____

_____ Other _____

Tell client to phonate using /ɑ/.

_____ Symmetry of movement: normal/deviates right/deviates left _____

_____ Posterior movement: present/absent/reduced _____

_____ Lateral movement: present/absent/reduced _____

_____ Uvula: normal/bifid/deviates right/deviates left _____

_____ Nasality: absent/hypernasal _____

_____ Other _____

Summary of Findings

Form 5-2.

Diadochokinetic Syllable Rates Worksheet

Name: _____ Age: _____ Date: _____

Examiner's Name: _____

Instructions: Time the number of seconds it takes your client to complete each task the prescribed number of times. The average number of seconds for children from 6 to 13 years of age is reported on the right-hand side of the table.

The standard deviation (SD) from the mean is also represented. Subtract the SD from the norm to determine each SD interval. For example, using the /pʌ/ norm with a 6-year-old, 3.8 (4.8–1.0) is one SD, 2.8 (4.8–2.0) is two SDs, 2.3 (4.8–2.5) is two-and-a-half SDs, etc. Therefore, a 6-year-old child who needed 2.6 seconds to complete the /pʌ/ sequence would be two SDs below the mean.

			Norms in seconds for diadochokinetic syllable rates							
			Age							
Task	**Repetitions**	**Seconds**	6	7	8	9	10	11	12	13
pʌ	20	_____	4.8	4.8	4.2	4.0	3.7	3.6	3.4	3.3
tʌ	20	_____	4.9	4.9	4.4	4.1	3.8	3.6	3.5	3.3
kʌ	20	_____	5.5	5.3	4.8	4.6	4.3	4.0	3.9	3.7
		Standard Deviation:	1.0	1.0	0.7	0.7	0.6	0.6	0.6	0.6
pʌtəkə	10	_____	10.3	10.0	8.3	7.7	7.1	6.5	6.4	5.7
		Standard Deviation:	2.8	2.8	2.0	2.0	1.5	1.5	1.5	1.5

Comments:

COMMON COMMUNICATION

Norms are from "Time-by-Count Measurement of Diadochokinetic Syllable Rate," by S. G. Fletcher, 1972, *Journal of Speech and Hearing Disorders, 15*, pp. 763–770. Copyright by the American Speech-Language-Hearing Association. Reprinted with permission.

Form 5-3.

Assessing Intelligibility Worksheet

Name: _____ Age: _____ Date: _____

Examiner's Name: _____

Testing Situation

Stimuli (conversation, materials used, etc.): _____

Client's level of anxiety: _____

Talkative/Not talkative: _____

Prompts used: _____

Representativeness of sample: _____

Instructions

1. Write out each word in each utterance (use phonetics if possible).

2. Use a dash (—) to indicate each unintelligible word.

3. An utterance is considered intelligible only if the entire utterance can be understood.

4. Calculate intelligibility for words and utterances.

Example:

Utterances	# Intelligible Words	Total Words	# Intelligible Utterances	Total Utterances
1. hi wɛnt hom	3	3	1	1
2. ar ju— tu go	4	5	0	1
3. — — θɪn	1	3	0	1
4. pwiz pwe wɪf mi	4	4	1	1
5. aɪ want tu go hom	5	5	1	1
Totals	**17**	**20**	**3**	**5**

$$\frac{\text{intelligible words}}{\text{total words:}} \quad \frac{17}{20} = 85\%$$

$$\frac{\text{intelligible utterances:}}{\text{total utterances:}} \quad \frac{3}{5} = 60\%$$

(continues)

COMMON COMMUNICATION

Form 5-3. continued

Utterances	# Intelligible Words	Total Words	# Intelligible Utterances	Total Utterances
1. _____	_____	_____	_____	___
2. _____	_____	_____	_____	___
3. _____	_____	_____	_____	___
4. _____	_____	_____	_____	___
5. _____	_____	_____	_____	___
6. _____	_____	_____	_____	___
7. _____	_____	_____	_____	___
8. _____	_____	_____	_____	___
9. _____	_____	_____	_____	___
10. _____	_____	_____	_____	___
11. _____	_____	_____	_____	___
12. _____	_____	_____	_____	___
13. _____	_____	_____	_____	___
14. _____	_____	_____	_____	___
15. _____	_____	_____	_____	___
16. _____	_____	_____	_____	___
17. _____	_____	_____	_____	___
18. _____	_____	_____	_____	___
19. _____	_____	_____	_____	___
20. _____	_____	_____	_____	___
21. _____	_____	_____	_____	___
22. _____	_____	_____	_____	___
23. _____	_____	_____	_____	___
24. _____	_____	_____	_____	___
25. _____	_____	_____	_____	___
26. _____	_____	_____	_____	___
27. _____	_____	_____	_____	___
28. _____	_____	_____	_____	___
29. _____	_____	_____	_____	___

(continues)

Form 5-3. continued

Utterances	# Intelligible Words	Total Words	# Intelligible Utterances	Total Utterances
30. _____	_____	_____	_____	___
31. _____	_____	_____	_____	___
32. _____	_____	_____	_____	___
33. _____	_____	_____	_____	___
34. _____	_____	_____	_____	___
35. _____	_____	_____	_____	___
36. _____	_____	_____	_____	___
37. _____	_____	_____	_____	___
38. _____	_____	_____	_____	___
39. _____	_____	_____	_____	___
40. _____	_____	_____	_____	___
41. _____	_____	_____	_____	___
42. _____	_____	_____	_____	___
43. _____	_____	_____	_____	___
44. _____	_____	_____	_____	___
45. _____	_____	_____	_____	___
46. _____	_____	_____	_____	___
47. _____	_____	_____	_____	___
48. _____	_____	_____	_____	___
49. _____	_____	_____	_____	___
50. _____	_____	_____	_____	___
Totals	_____	_____	_____	___

Findings

Average # Words per Utterance: _____

% Intelligibility—Words: _____

% Intelligibility—Utterances: _____

Factors contributing to reduced intelligibility: _____

_____

_____

COMMON COMMUNICATION

Form 5-4.

Charting Worksheet I

Name: _____ Age: _____ Date: _____

Examiner's Name: _____

Charted Behavior: _____

Stimulus	**Trials**	**% Correct**
_____	____, ____, ____, ____, ____, ____, ____, ____, ____, ____	_____
_____	____, ____, ____, ____, ____, ____, ____, ____, ____, ____	_____
_____	____, ____, ____, ____, ____, ____, ____, ____, ____, ____	_____
_____	____, ____, ____, ____, ____, ____, ____, ____, ____, ____	_____
_____	____, ____, ____, ____, ____, ____, ____, ____, ____, ____	_____
_____	____, ____, ____, ____, ____, ____, ____, ____, ____, ____	_____
_____	____, ____, ____, ____, ____, ____, ____, ____, ____, ____	_____
_____	____, ____, ____, ____, ____, ____, ____, ____, ____, ____	_____
_____	____, ____, ____, ____, ____, ____, ____, ____, ____, ____	_____
_____	____, ____, ____, ____, ____, ____, ____, ____, ____, ____	_____
_____	____, ____, ____, ____, ____, ____, ____, ____, ____, ____	_____
_____	____, ____, ____, ____, ____, ____, ____, ____, ____, ____	_____
_____	____, ____, ____, ____, ____, ____, ____, ____, ____, ____	_____
_____	____, ____, ____, ____, ____, ____, ____, ____, ____, ____	_____
_____	____, ____, ____, ____, ____, ____, ____, ____, ____, ____	_____
_____	____, ____, ____, ____, ____, ____, ____, ____, ____, ____	_____
_____	____, ____, ____, ____, ____, ____, ____, ____, ____, ____	_____
_____	____, ____, ____, ____, ____, ____, ____, ____, ____, ____	_____
_____	____, ____, ____, ____, ____, ____, ____, ____, ____, ____	_____

Total Trials: _____   Total Correct: _____   % Correct: _____

FORM 5-1

Charting Worksheet 1

Name _____ Age/ _____ Date _____

Examiner Name _____

Charted Behavior _____

Stimulus	Trials		% Correct

Total Trials		Total Correct	% Correct

Form 5-5.

Charting Worksheet II

Name: _____   Age: _____

Examiner's Name: _____   Date: _____

Target									

COMMON COMMUNICATION

Charting Worksheet II

Appendix 5-A.

Reading Passage

Swimming

I like to swim when it is hot outside. It is very fun. I swim in a big pool. I can jump in the water. I get all wet. I can float on my back. I can float on my tummy too. I open my eyes under the water. I can see my brother. I can see my mom. They watch me. I think the water is cool. It feels good. I like to splash and blow bubbles and yell. After I swim, I dry off with my towel. My towel is yellow. It has a picture of a treasure chest on it.

COMMON COMMUNICATION

Appendix 5-A. continued

Reading Passage

Grandma Is Coming

Grandma is coming for a visit. She is coming in her big car. Timothy made a picture for her. Anna is going to show her a dance. They are hoping she will arrive soon. They want to go to the park. Grandma will push Timothy and Anna in the swing. When they go down the slide, Grandma will take their picture. On the way home, they will get an ice cream cone.

Grandma plays the piano. Timothy and Anna like to sing. They like it when she plays "Big Rock Candy Mountain." When Grandma comes, they will play and sing. Then Grandma will read each of them a story. Timothy has a new book he wants her to read. It is called *Mr. Shim's Measuring Machine.* Anna wants her to read her favorite book, *The Jolly Cat.*

Anna and Timothy are waiting for Grandma by the window. "Is she here yet?" they ask. They are looking for her big car. Finally, they see it. Grandma is here! They run out the front door and give her a big hug.

Appendix 5-A. continued

Reading Passage

Nicknames

The word nickname means "added name." Nicknames are used in place of a person's real name. Some nicknames are based on a person's first name. For example, Matt is a nickname for Matthew. Some nicknames are based on what a person has done. John Chapman traveled around the country handing out apple seeds. Now he is known as Johnny Appleseed.

Nicknames can also be based on how a person looks. A person with red hair might be called Red or Carrot-top. A lot of people in politics have nicknames. Some are nice nicknames. Some are not very kind. Many people who liked Abraham Lincoln called him Honest Abe. People who didn't like him called him Old Abe.

Some people are given nicknames based on where they were born. For example, a person from Texas might be called Tex. If you are an American, you might be called a Yankee. Sometimes people are given special, loving nicknames. Some moms and dads call their children Precious or Sweetie. Moms and dads often use nicknames, like Honey or Dear, when they talk to each other, too. It is not unusual to have a nickname. Do you have one?

COMMON COMMUNICATION

Appendix 5-A. continued

Reading Passage

The Amazing Spider

A spider is an amazing animal. It can build its own home and it doesn't even have to chop wood or buy a saw. Before the spider begins to build, it looks for the perfect spot. A spider usually likes to live in a grassy area where lots of insects can get caught in its web. Then the spider eats the insects for dinner. The spider also has to figure out which way the wind is blowing. The wind has to be on the spider's back before it is able to make its house.

After it finds a good place to live, it is ready to spin its webs. The spider has glands in its stomach that produce a silky liquid. It jumps from one side of the house and is carried by a rush of wind to the other side. As it travels through the air, the liquid comes out. As soon as the liquid hits the air it becomes solid, making a fine, tough thread. The spider uses the first thread as a bridge to travel from one side to the other. Then it continues to build its web strand by strand until its home is complete.

Appendix 5-A. continued

Reading Passage

The Toothbrush

Did you know that the toothbrush was invented in a prison? One morning in 1770, a man in an English jail woke up with a new idea. He thought it would be better if he could use a brush to clean his teeth, rather than wipe them with a rag. At dinner he took a bone from his meat and kept it. Then he told the prison guard about his unusual idea. The guard gave him some bristles to use for the brush. The prisoner made holes in the bone and stuffed the bristles into the holes. It was a success! The prisoner was so excited about his new invention that he went into the toothbrush making business when he got out of jail.

For more than 200 years we have used toothbrushes similar to the one the prisoner invented. Toothbrushes are not made out of bones anymore. They come in all kinds of colors, shapes, and sizes. The next time you brush your teeth, think about the prisoner in England who invented the toothbrush.

COMMON COMMUNICATION

Appendix 5-A. continued

Reading Passage

Grandfather

You wished to know all about my grandfather. Well, he is nearly ninety-three years old; he dresses himself in an ancient black frock coat, usually minus several buttons, yet he still thinks as swiftly as ever. A long, flowing beard clings to his chin, giving those who observe him a pronounced feeling of the utmost respect. When he speaks, his voice is just a bit cracked and quivers a trifle. Twice each day he plays skillfully and with zest upon our small organ. Except in winter when the ooze or snow or ice prevents, he slowly takes a short walk in the open air each day. We have often urged him to walk more and smoke less, but he always answers, "Banana oil!" Grandfather likes to be modern in his language.

Appendix 5-A. continued

Reading Passage

Rainbow Passage

When the sunlight strikes raindrops in the air they act like a prism and form a rainbow. The rainbow is a division of white light into many beautiful colors. These take the shape of a long round arch, with its path high above, and its two ends apparently beyond the horizon. There is, according to legend, a boiling pot of gold at one end. People look, but no one ever finds it. When a man looks for something beyond his reach, his friends say he is looking for the pot of gold at the end of the rainbow.

Throughout the centuries men have explained the rainbow in various ways. Some have accepted it as a miracle without physical explanation. To the Hebrews, it was a token that there would be no more universal floods. The Greeks used to imagine that it was a sign from the gods to foretell war or heavy rain. The Norsemen considered the rainbow as a bridge over which the gods passed from earth to their home in the sky. Other men have tried to explain the phenomenon physically. Aristotle thought that the rainbow was caused by reflection of the sun's rays by the rain. Since then, physicists have found that it is not reflection, but refraction by the raindrops which causes the rainbow. Many complicated

(continues)

Reading Passage, continued

ideas about the rainbow have been formed. The difference in the rainbow depends considerably upon the size of the water drops, and the width of the colored band increases as the size of the drops increases. The actual primary rainbow observed is said to be the effect of superposition of a number of bows. If the red of the second bow falls upon the green of the first, the result is to give a bow with an abnormally wide yellow band, since red and green lights when mixed form yellow. This is a very common type of bow, one showing mainly red and yellow, with little or no green or blue.

Appendix 5-A. continued

Reading Passage

Declaration of Independence

We hold these truths to be self-evident, that all men are created equal, that they are endowed by their Creator with certain unalienable rights, that among these are life, liberty and the pursuit of happiness. That to secure these rights, governments are instituted among men, deriving their just powers from the consent of the governed, that whenever any form of government becomes destructive of these ends, it is the right of the people to alter or abolish it, and to institute new government, laying its foundation on such principles and organizing its powers in such form, as to them shall seem most likely to effect their safety and happiness.

Prudence, indeed, will dictate that governments long established should not be changed for light and transient causes; and accordingly all experience has shown, that mankind are more disposed to suffer, while evils are sufferable, than to right themselves by abolishing the forms to which they are accustomed. But when a long train of abuses and usurpations, pursuing invariably the same object evinces a design to reduce them under absolute despotism, it is their right, it is their duty, to throw off such government, and to provide new guards for their future security.

COMMON COMMUNICATION

Appendix 5-B.

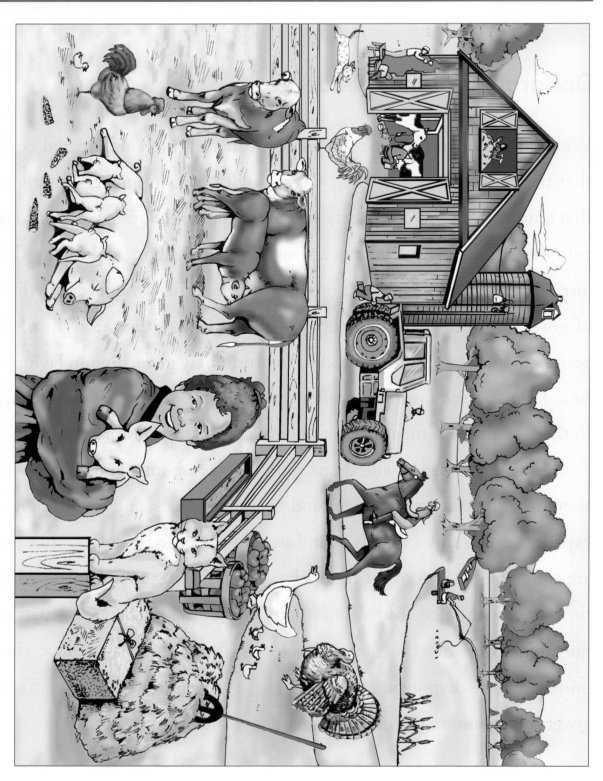

FIGURE 5-2. Speech-Language Sample Stimulus—Farm

Appendix 5-B. continued

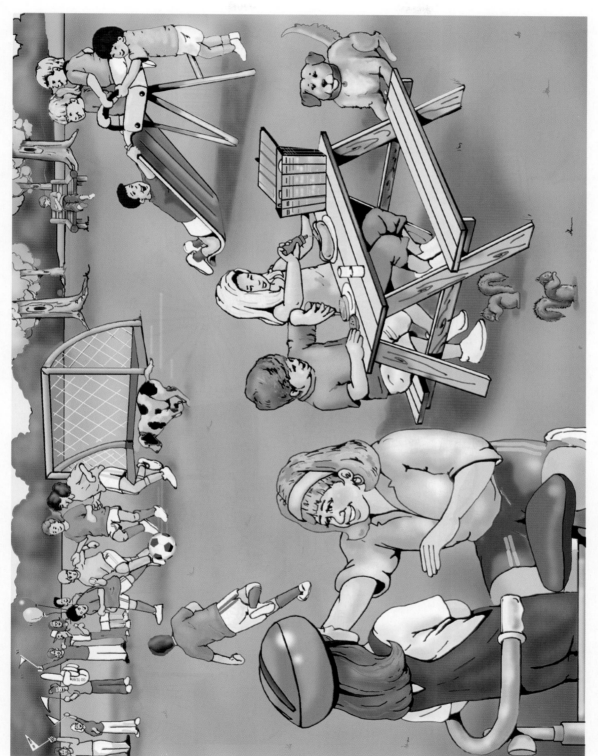

FIGURE 5-3. Speech-Language Sample Stimulus—Park

COMMON COMMUNICATION

Appendix 5-B. continued

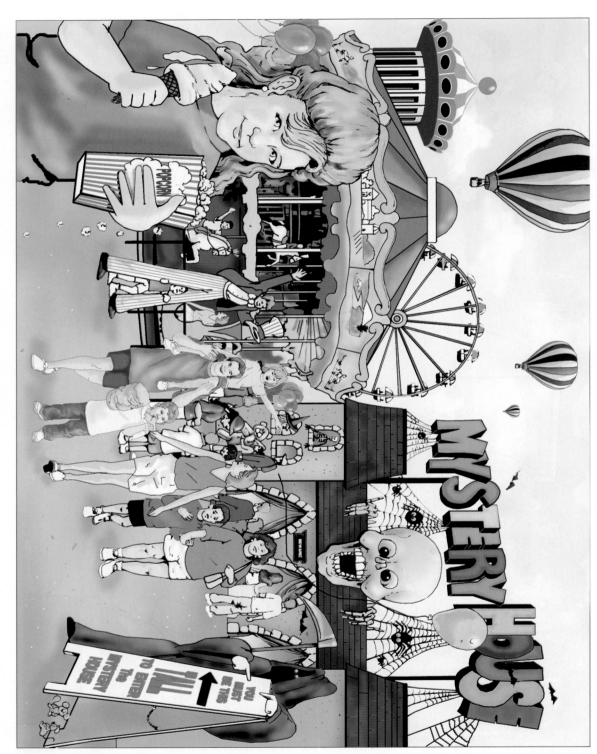

FIGURE 5-4. Speech-Language Sample Stimulus—Amusement Park

Appendix 5-B. continued

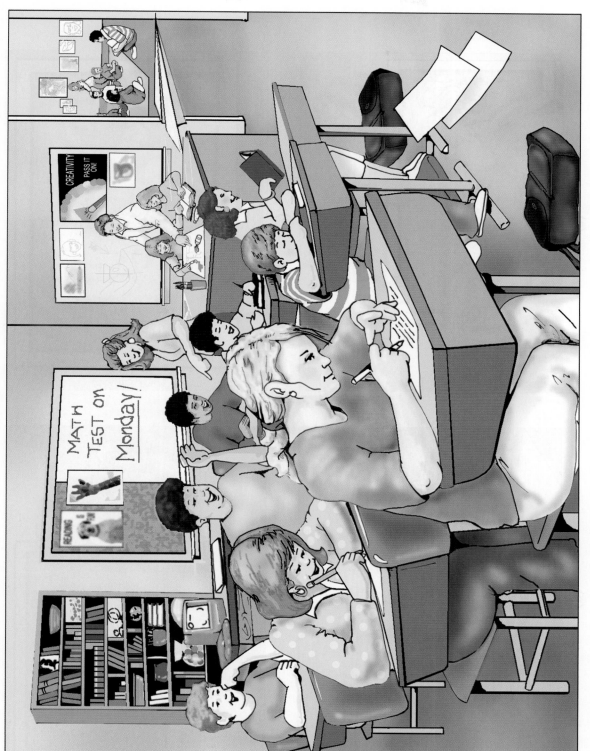

FIGURE 5-5.   Speech-Language Sample Stimulus—Classroom

COMMON
COMMUNICATION

Appendix 5-B. continued

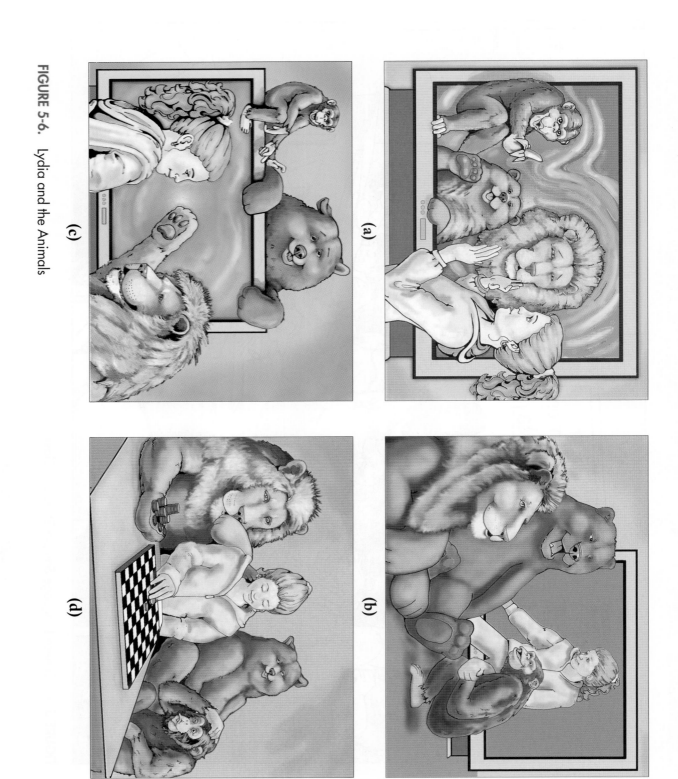

FIGURE 5-6. Lydia and the Animals

(continues)

FIGURE 5-6.   Lydia and the Animals

(a)   One day when Lydia was watching television, an amazing thing happened. The animals on the screen came to life in her living room! A bear, a monkey, and a lion were looking right at her. Lydia was very scared. She tried to yell for her mom, but nothing came out of her mouth.

(b)   Then the animals started talking all at once. Finally, in a quiet voice she said, "Where did you come from?"

(c)   The lion pointed to the TV and said, "We came from your television set. We want to play with you." She could tell from his voice that he was a friendly lion. She wasn't afraid anymore.

(d)   "Do you want to play checkers?" Lydia asked. All the animals looked at each other and nodded. Lydia got out the checker game and taught them to play.

Appendix 5-B. continued

FIGURE 5-6. Lydia and the Animals (Continued)

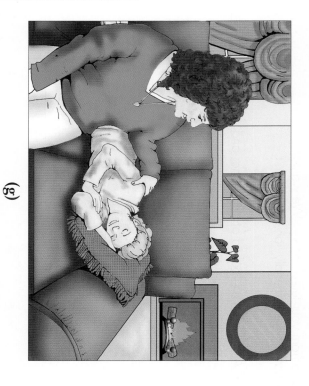

(g)

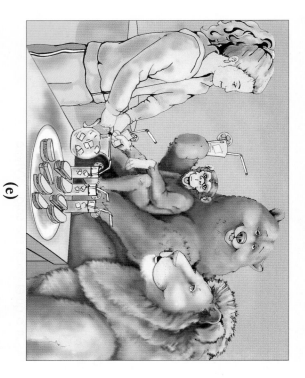

(e)

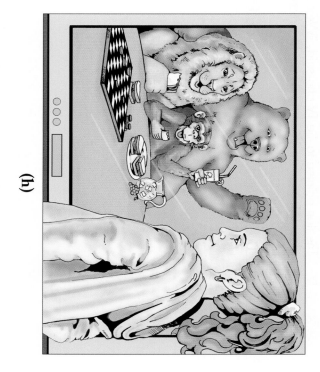

(h)

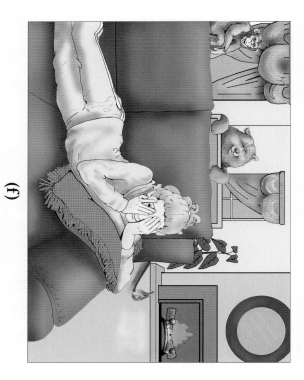

(f)

FIGURE 5-6.   Lydia and the Animals *(Continued)*

(e)   After a while, Lydia asked, "Are you hungry? I'll bring you some sandwiches." The animals nodded, so Lydia and the animals all sat down and ate sandwiches and drank lemonade.

(f)   Next, they decided to play hide-and-go-seek. Lydia was "it." "Stay in this room," she said, "I don't want my mom to see you!" While the animals were hiding, she fell asleep.

(g)   A little while later, Lydia's mom came in and woke her up. Lydia looked around the room. The TV was on, the checkerboard was put away, and there were no cups and plates on the table. Was it all a dream?

(h)   Then Lydia looked at the television. There she saw the animals giggling as they gazed up at her. The bear, the monkey, and the lion were drinking lemonade, eating sandwiches, and playing checkers on TV!

COMMON
COMMUNICATION

Appendix 5-B. continued

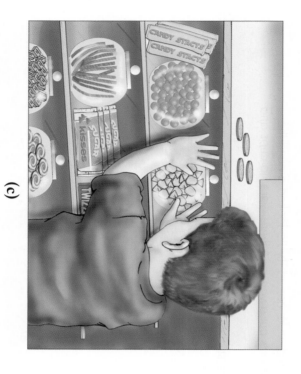

(c)

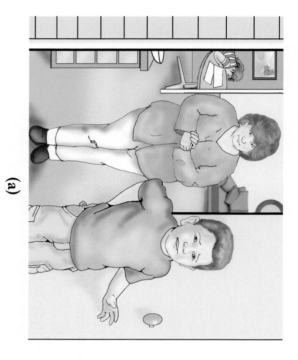

(a)

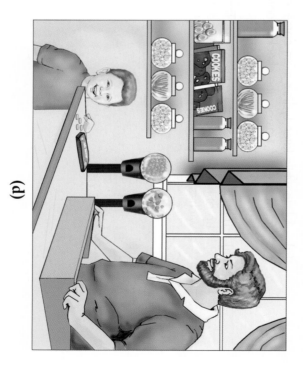

(d)

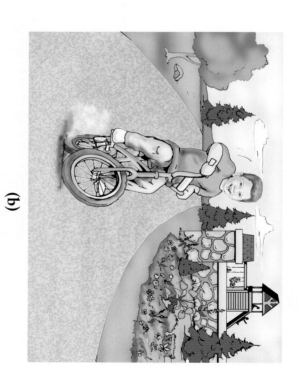

(b)

FIGURE 5-7.   Jacob's Day

(continues)

Appendix 5-B. continued

FIGURE 5-7. Jacob's Day (Continued)

(a) Jacob was a young boy who had two big brothers and one big sister. He didn't like being the smallest boy in the family because he never got to do things by himself. One day Jacob asked his mom if he could go to the store to buy a candy bar. Of course she said, "Not by yourself, Jacob." That made Jacob very mad. Jacob said sadly, "Okay, I guess I'll go play outside."

(b) Once Jacob got outside, he got an idea. He thought, "I'll just go by myself anyway. I can get there and back without Mom ever knowing I was gone." So Jacob counted the money in his pocket to make sure he had enough and then got on his bicycle and pedaled to the store as fast as he could.

(c) He went inside the store and looked for the candy bar aisle. "Oh, look at all the choices!" he thought to himself. He was so excited! Jacob finally picked his favorite candy bar and stepped toward the counter.

(d) As he was paying for the candy the cashier asked, "Aren't you a little young to be here alone?" "Oh no, I'm older than I look," he said with a smile. He felt so grown up.

Appendix 5-B. continued

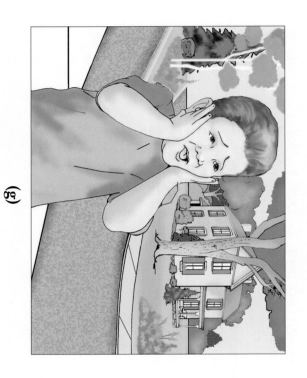

(g)

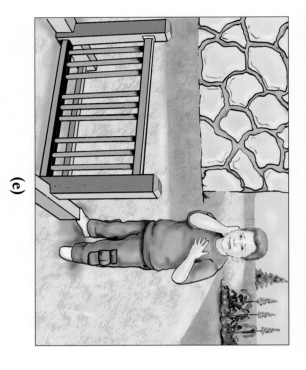

(e)

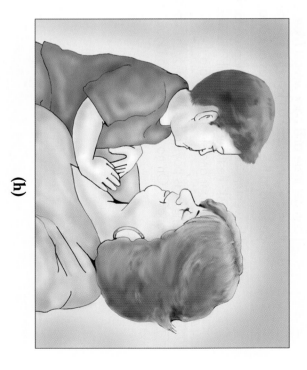

(h)

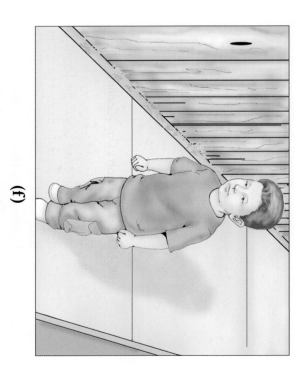

(f)

FIGURE 5-7. Jacob's Day (Continued)

FIGURE 5-7.   Jacob's Day (Continued)

(e)   Well, Jacob's excitement turned to fear when he went outside to go home. His bike was gone! How could he get home before his mom found out he had left? Jacob looked all around for his bike, but it was nowhere to be found. Somebody had stolen it.

(f)   It was a long walk home for Jacob. He knew he was in big trouble. Somehow he didn't feel very grown up anymore. And he no longer wanted to eat his candy bar.

(g)   When he turned onto the street where his house was, he could hear his mother calling out his name. He was afraid to tell his mom what happened. He felt scared.

(h)   Jacob realized that he really was too young to be out alone and started running toward home. His mother gave him a big hug and said, "Where did you go? I was so worried!" Jacob cried as he told his story. After that, he didn't mind it so much that he never got to do things by himself.

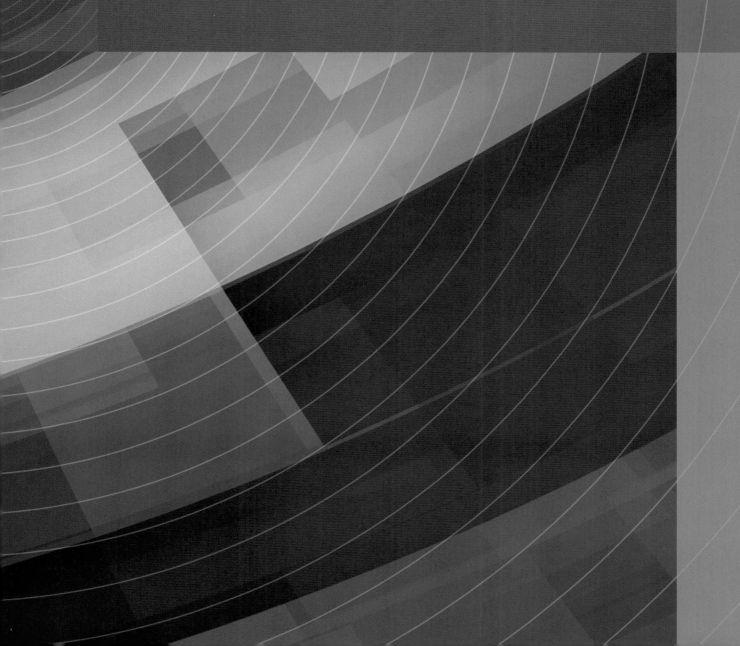

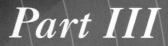

Part III

Resources for Assessing
Communicative Disorders

Chapter 6

ASSESSMENT OF SPEECH SOUND DISORDERS

OVERVIEW OF ASSESSMENT

Normal speech production requires a series of coordinated actions. It requires exact placement, sequencing, timing, direction, and force of the articulators. This occurs simultaneously with precise airstream alteration, initiation or halting of phonation, and velopharyngeal action. Articulation errors occur when this complex process is disrupted.

Articulatory problems result from organic (a known physical cause) or functional (no known physical cause issues such as) etiologies. Some organically based articulatory or phonological disorders are related to hearing loss, cleft lip or palate, cerebral palsy, ankyloglossia (tongue-tie), apraxia, or dysarthria. There are also many articulation disorders of a functional etiology. Clinicians attempt to identify physical causes, particularly during the oral-facial examination. However, in many cases, the precise cause of a speech sound disorder is unknown.

The primary purposes of an assessment of articulation and phonological processes include:

- Describing the articulatory or phonological development and status of the client
- Determining whether the individual's speech sufficiently deviates from normal expectations to warrant concern or intervention
- Identifying factors that relate to the presence or maintenance of the speech disorder
- Determining the direction of treatment
- Making prognostic judgments about change with and without intervention
- Monitoring changes in articulatory or phonological abilities and performance across time (Bernthal & Bankson, 2004, p. 202)

The outline below identifies several important components of a complete evaluation of articulation and phonological processes.

History of the Client

    Procedures

        Written Case History
        Information-Gathering Interview
        Information from Other Professionals

    Contributing Factors

        Hearing Impairment
        Medical or Neurological Factors
        Dental Problems
        Maturation and Motor Development
        Intelligence, Sex, Birth Order, Motivation and Concern, Dialect

Assessment of Speech Sound Disorders

    Procedures

        Screening
        Formal and Informal Tests

Speech Sampling
Stimulability of Errors
Analysis
Number of Errors
Error Types (substitutions, omissions, distortions, additions)
Form of Errors (distinctive features, phonological processes)
Consistency of Errors
Intelligibility
Rate of Speech
Prosody
Orofacial Examination
Hearing Assessment
Language Assessment
Determining the Diagnosis
Providing Information (written report, interview, etc.)

Assessment of articulation and phonological disorders requires knowledge of the phonetic symbols of the English language. These are presented in Table 6-1.

TABLE 6–1   Phonetic Symbols of the English Language

CONSONANTS				VOWELS			
VOICED		**UNVOICED**				**R-CONTROLLED**	**DIPHTHONGS**
/b/ as in big		/p/ as in pin		/i/ as in meet		/ɝ/ as in sure (stressed)	/aɪ/ as in bye
/d/ as in dog		/t/ as in tie		/ɪ/ as in it		/ɚ/ as in mother (unstressed)	/eɪ/ as in crayon
/g/ as in go		/k/ as in cat		/e/ as in eight			/ɑʊ/ as in out
/v/ as in vase		/f/ as in far		/ɛ/ as in met		/ɪɚ/ as in ear	/ɔɪ/ as in boy
/z/ as in zoo		/s/ as in sit		/æ/ as in ask		/ɛɚ/ as in hair	/oʊ/ as in mode
/ð/ as in this		/θ/ as in think		/ə/ as in control (unstressed)		/ɔɚ/ as in or	
/ʒ/ as in measure		/ʃ/ as in shake				/ɑɚ/ as in car	
/dʒ/ as in jump		/tʃ/ as in chip		/ʌ/ as in country (stressed)			
/m/ as in mop		/h/ as in hi					
/n/ as in no				/u/ as in too			
/ŋ/ as in sing				/ʊ/ as in book			
/l/ as in light				/o/ as in go			
/r/ as in rake				/ɔ/ as in dog			
/j/ as in yes				/ɑ/ as in saw			
/w/ as in wet							

SCREENING

The purpose of a screening is to quickly identify those people who communicate within normal limits and those who *may* have a communicative disorder. People in the second group are seen or referred for a complete evaluation. A screening is not an in-depth assessment and should not take more than a few minutes. Screenings most commonly occur in the schools, where large numbers of children in the early grades are screened for communicative disorders.

An articulation or phonological processes screening test does not have to be formal. Many clinicians listen to the person's speech and have him or her perform simple tasks, such as counting, reciting the days of the week, reading, naming objects or colors, and so on. Other clinicians prefer to use published tests. There are several available, including:

- *Diagnostic Evaluation of Articulation and Phonology (DEAP)* (Dodd, Hua, Crosbie, Holm, & Ozanne, 2006)
- *Fluharty Preschool Speech and Language Screening Test (Fluharty-2)* (Fluharty, 2000)
- *Hodson Assessment of Phonological Patterns (HAPP-3)* (Hodson, 2004)
- *Phonological Screening Assessment* (Stevens & Isles, 2011)

Clinicians can develop their own screening instruments by using some of the resources in this manual, such as the reading passages and the pictures in Chapter 5. If using picture stimuli, be sure to select pictures that will elicit the later-developing sounds. Refer to "Developmental Norms for Phonemes and Blends" and "The Frequency of Occurrence of Consonants" in selecting appropriate target sounds when screening articulation.

FORMAL TESTS

There are many standardized tests that clinicians use to identify articulation errors. The website of the American Speech-Language-Hearing Association (ASHA) includes an extensive directory of assessment instruments. Some of the more widely used traditional tests include:

- *Arizona Articulation Proficiency Scale (Arizona-3)* (Fudala, 2000)
- *Clinical Assessment of Articulation and Phonology (CAAP)* (Secord, Donohue, & Johnson, 2002)
- *Diagnostic Evaluation of Articulation and Phonology (DEAP)* (Dodd, Hua, Crosbie, Holm, & Ozanne, 2006)
- *Goldman-Fristoe Test of Articulation 2* (Goldman & Fristoe, 2000)

These tests, and others like them, assess sounds in the initial, medial, and final positions (e.g., the /l/ in *light*, *balloon*, and *ball*), allowing the clinician to identify the number and types of errors.

Articulation tests are used to identify a client's articulation errors in a relatively quick and systematic fashion. They are popular and useful assessment tools. However, they do have limitations. For example, consider these drawbacks:

- These tests usually elicit phonemes in only one phonetic context within a preselected word. Even if the client produces the sound correctly, there may be other contexts and words in which the client cannot produce the target sound correctly. Or, an error may be elicited that is not reflective of a general pattern in other contexts.

- Most articulation tests elicit phonemes at the word level for the assessment of initial, medial, and final position productions. However, conversational speech is made up of complex, coarticulated movements in which discrete initial, medial, and final sounds may not occur. Thus, sound productions in single words may differ from those in spontaneous speech.

- Some articulation tests examine only consonants, yet accurately produced vowels are also important for well-developed speech.

- These tests provide only an inventory of the sounds sampled. They do not yield certain diagnostic information, such as whether a particular sound error might be developmentally appropriate.

- The reliability of findings may be questionable with disorders that result in variable sound productions. For example, a key feature of childhood apraxia of speech (CAS) is inconsistently produced sounds. Many clients with CAS produce a sound or word correctly one time and incorrectly the next. With a variable disorder, the clinician who samples a given word once or only a few times may draw conclusions that are not accurate.

When evaluating clients with moderate to severe articulation disorders, tests of phonological processes may prove more diagnostically valuable than traditional articulation tests. Phonological processes are described later in this chapter. Some of the tests commonly used to examine these processes include:

- *Assessment Link Between Phonology and Articulation—Revised (ALPHA-R)* (Lowe, 2000*)
- *Clinical Assessment of Articulation and Phonology (CAAP)* (Secord & Donohue, 2002)
- *Comprehensive Test of Phonological Processing (CTOPP-2)* (Wagner, Torgesen, & Rashotte, 2009)
- *Diagnostic Evaluation of Articulation and Phonology (DEAP)* (Dodd, Hua, Crosbie, Holm, & Ozanne, 2006)
- *Hodson Assessment of Phonological Patterns (HAPP-3)* (Hodson, 2004)
- *Kahn-Lewis Phonological Analysis—2nd ed. (KLPA-2)* (Khan & Lewis, 2003)
- *Smit-Hand Articulation and Phonology Evaluation (SHAPE)* (Smit & Hand, 1997).

Electronic assessment tools are helpful for automatically generating a phonemic and phonologic profile. Some tools allow the clinician to select from different assessment levels, and results can be stored in a client's digital file for future retrieval. Keep in mind that not all electronic resources are standardized and/or norm-based, and results must be considered with this limitation in mind. Some electronic assessment tools are:

- *"Articulation Test Center"* (app by Little Bee Speech)
- *"Sunny Articulation and Phonology Test"* (app by Smarty Ears)
- *Computerized Articulation and Phonology Evaluation System (CAPES)* (Masterson & Bernhardt, 2001)
- *Computerized Profiling for Phonology (PROPHET)* (Long, Fey, & Channell, 2006)
- *Hodson Computerized Analysis of Phonological Patterns (HCAPP)* (Hodson, 2003)

*Robert Lowe, the author, has made this assessment available for download as a free gift to the profession. It can be retrieved at http://www.speech-language-therapy.com/alpha.html

IDENTIFYING SOUND ERRORS FROM A SPEECH SAMPLE

Procedures for collecting a speech-language sample were described in Chapter 5. The speech sample is especially important for accurately diagnosing disorders of speech sound production. After obtaining one or more representative samples of the client's speech, analyze the sample with a focus on the following behaviors:

- Number of errors
- Error types
- Consistency of errors between the speech sample and the articulation test, within the same speech sample, and between different speech samples
- Correctly produced sounds
- Intelligibility
- Speech rate
- Prosody

Most articulation tests allow for easy identification of sound errors. This is a more difficult task with speech samples because they may not elicit all of the phonetic sounds unless the sample is elicited in a systematic manner. To complete a thorough diagnostic evaluation, the clinician will need to compare errors made during the articulation test to those errors made during connected speech. For some sounds, there may be multiple error types. It is also necessary to inventory correctly produced sounds. Form 6-1, "Comparison of Sound Errors from an Articulation Test and Connected Speech," will help to identify the errors produced during the speech sample and then compare the results with errors identified on the articulation test. Typically, more sound errors will be found during the connected speech sample. Also note that initial, medial, and final sound positions are not as definitive in connected speech.

STIMULABILITY

Stimulability refers to a client's ability to produce a correct (or improved) production of an erred sound. The client attempts to imitate the clinician's correct production, often after receiving specific instructions regarding the articulatory placement or manner of sound production. For example, the clinician may hold the client's lips together to form a /p/, or touch the client's hard palate with a tongue depressor to show tongue placement for the production of /t/. In some cases, a mirror is helpful for eliciting the target sound.

The assessment of stimulability provides important prognostic information. If the clinician is able to stimulate a target behavior at the sound level or word level during the diagnostic session, it is more likely that the desired behavior will be trainable at more complex levels. Those behaviors that are most easily stimulated provide excellent starting points in therapy because they often lead to treatment success quicker than other, less stimulable behaviors.

The ability to stimulate erred sounds is based on a good working knowledge of phonetics. The clinician must know what needs to be changed in order to improve the production. It is also important to realize that, in some cases, there is more than one way to correctly articulate a sound. For example, a "textbook description" of /t/ will state that it is a lingua-alveolar sound produced by tapping the tongue on the hard palate. However, some people produce a good /t/ by tapping the tongue on the front teeth.

Another key to stimulability is visually observing the client's erred productions. Even though not *all* sounds are visible, many are. Beginning clinicians tend to *listen* to speech more than *watch* speech, but seeing an error can help identify what needs to change in order to produce a better sound.

There are resources that provide helpful instructions for stimulating each phoneme. These are some that we recommend:

- *Applied Phonetics: The Sounds of American English* (3rd ed.) (Edwards, 2003)
- *Manual of Articulation and Phonological Disorders* (2nd ed.) (Bleile, 2004)
- *Eliciting Sounds: Techniques and Strategies for Clinicians* (2nd ed.) (Secord, Boyce, Donohue, Fox, & Shine, 2007)

Once a sound is stimulated at the sound or syllable level, sample it at the word and phrase levels. The words and phrases in Appendix 6-A are provided for this purpose. The "Syllable-by-Syllable Stimulus Phrases" in Chapter 5 can also be used to assess stimulability in phrases of increasing length (Secord, Boyce, Donohue, Fox, & Shine, 2007).

Form 6-2, "Sounds That Are Stimulable," can be used to summarize stimulability assessment findings. In many cases, the form will help identify patterns of stimulable sounds at different levels, providing potential starting points for therapy. The clinician may also get a clearer picture of specific error types that may be more amenable to earlier treatment (e.g., bilabials may be more stimulable than velars).

DEVELOPMENTAL NORMS FOR PHONEMES AND BLENDS

Clinicians often use normative data to determine whether or not a child is developing within normal expectations. Although norms are helpful, consider these limitations of overreliance on developmental norms:

- A norm is only an average age at which a behavior occurs. It refers, therefore, to a hypothetical child who does not, and never did, exist.
- True norms are collected from and apply to a normal, randomly selected sample. These exact representative samples rarely exist in the real world.
- Different norms are rarely in agreement with each other. The differences are caused by many factors, including when the study was conducted, where the study was conducted, the size and characteristics of the sample, the research design followed, and the mastery criteria used.

Despite these limitations, norms are useful for estimating approximately how well a child's sounds are developing. In current practice, the more recent studies presented in Table 6-2 are referred to most frequently. Generally, the later studies indicate an earlier development of consonants than the earlier studies from the 1930s. The following notes are offered as a general explanation of the material in Table 6-2:

- Wellman, Case, Mengurt, and Bradbury's (1931) study represents the earliest age at which 75% of the 204 children tested (ages 2 to 6 years) correctly produced the consonant phoneme in the initial, medial, and final positions.

- Poole's (1934) study represents the earliest age at which 100% of the 140 children tested (ages 2;6 to 8;5) correctly produced the consonant phoneme in all three positions.
- Templin's (1957) study represents the earliest age at which 75% of the 480 children tested (ages 3 to 8) correctly produced the consonant phoneme in all three positions.
- Sander's (1972) data represent a reinterpretation of Templin's (1957) and Wellman et al.'s (1931) research based on a criterion of 51% accuracy in two out of three positions.
- Prather et al.'s (1975) study represents the earliest age at which 75% of the 147 children tested (ages 2 to 4) correctly produced the consonant in the initial and final positions.

TABLE 6-2   Five Commonly Cited Norms for Consonant Development

CONSONANT	WELLMAN ET AL. (1931)	POOLE (1934)	TEMPLIN (1957)	SANDER (1972)	PRATHER ET AL. (1975)
m	3;0	3;6	3;0	before 2;0	2;0
n	3;0	4;6	3;0	before 2;0	2;0
h	3;0	3;6	3;0	before 2;0	2;0
p	4;0	3;6	3;0	before 2;0	2;0
f	3;0	5;6	3;0	3;0	2;0–4;0
w	3;0	3;6	3;0	before 2;0	2;0–8;0
b	3;0	3;6	4;0	before 2;0	2;0–8;0
ŋ		4;6	3;0	2;0	2;0
j	4;0	4;6	3;6	3;0	2;0–4;0
k	4;0	4;6	4;0	2;0	2;0–4;0
g	4;0	4;6	4;0	2;0	2;0–4;0
l	4;0	6;6	6;0	3;0	3;0–4;0
d	5;0	4;6	4;0	2;0	2;0–4;0
t	5;0	4;6	6;0	2;0	2;0–8;0
s	5;0	7;6	4;6	3;0	3;0
r	5;0	7;6	4;0	3;0	3;0–4;0
tʃ	5;0		4;6	4;0	3;0–8;0
v	5;0	6;6	6;0	4;0	4;0
z	5;0	7;6	7;0	4;0	4;0
ʒ	6;0	6;6	7;0	6;0	4;0
θ		7;6	6;0	5;0	4;0
dʒ			7;0	4;0	4;0
ʃ		6;6	4;6	4;0	3;0–8;0
ð		6;6	7;0	5;0	4;0

The data from the normative studies in Table 6-2 resulted in a specific age of development, but these ages do not reflect normal and acceptable developmental variability. Sander (1972) reinterpreted the data collected by Templin (1957) and Wellman et al. (1931) and compiled the age ranges presented in Figure 6-1. It is important to view ranges, because they provide useful information about developmental variations. For example, compare Table 6-2 with Figure 6-1. In Table 6-2, Sander suggests that /p/ develops before age 2. However, in Figure 6-1, you can see he also found that /p/ in normal development may continue to develop until age 3.

Keep in mind that normative data only tell part of the story, as certain errors are developmentally appropriate whereas others are not. For example, consider two different errors involving /s/. A substitution of /t/ for /s/ is acceptable at age 2 but not at age 4, but a /θ/ for /s/ at age 4 may not be a concern. Remember to interpret normative data for individual sounds relative to their overall patterns.

Normative data for the development of consonant clusters is presented in Table 6-3. The information is based on research by Smit, Hand, Frelinger, Bernthal, and Byrd (1990). The data reflect the ages at which at least 50% (first column) or 75% (second column) of the children in the sample group accurately produced each consonant cluster in the initial position of words.

TABLE 6-3   Age of Acquisition of Consonant Clusters in Word Initial Positions

CLUSTER	50%	75%	CLUSTER	50%	75%
tw	3;0	3;6	pr	4;0	6;0
kw	3;0	3;6	br	3;6	6;0
sp	3;6	5;0	tr	5;0	5;6
st	3;6	5;0	dr	4;0	6;0
sk	3;6	5;0	kr	4;0	5;6
sm	3;6	5;0	gr	4;6	6;0
sn	3;6	5;6	fr	3;6	6;0
sw	3;6	5;6	θr	5;0	7;0
sl	4;6	7;0	skw	3;6	7;0
pl	3;6	5;6	spl	5;0	7;0
bl	3;6	5;0	spr	5;0	8;0
kl	4;0	5;6	str	5;0	8;0
gl	3;6	4;6	skr	5;0	8;0
fl	3;6	5;6			

Source: *Manual of Articulation and Phonological Disorders*, 2nd ed. (p. 104, Table 3-7), by K. M. Bleile, 2004, Clifton Park, NY: Delmar Cengage Learning. Adapted from "The Iowa Articulation Norms Project and Its Nebraska Replication" by A. Smit, L. Hand, J. Frelinger, J. Bernthal, & A. Byrd, 1990, *Journal of Speech and Hearing Disorders*, 55, 779–798.

SPEECH SOUND DISORDERS

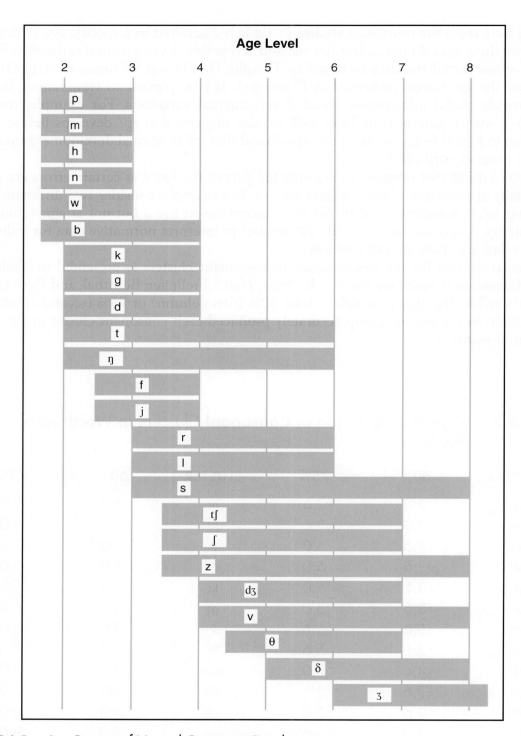

FIGURE 6-1.   Age Ranges of Normal Consonant Development

Average age estimates and upper age limits of customary consonant production. The bar corresponding to each sound starts at the median age of customary articulation; it stops at an age level at which 90% of all children are customarily producing the sound (data from Templin, 1957; Wellman et al., 1931). From "When Are Speech Sounds Learned?" by E. Sander, 1972, *Journal of Speech and Hearing Disorders, 37,* 55–63. Copyright 1972 by the American Speech-Language-Hearing Association. Reprinted with permission.

FREQUENCY OF OCCURRENCE OF CONSONANTS

Table 6-4 contains the percentages of occurrence of intended American English consonants in continuous speech. The information is from Shriberg and Kwiatkowski (1983), who summarized several studies of the frequency of consonant productions in natural speech. The studies they evaluated included data from children with normal and delayed speech development, as well as adults with normal speech.

A cumulative percentage of consonant occurrence is provided in the right-hand column of the table. Note that the sounds /n/, /t/, /s/, /r/, /d/, and /m/ cumulatively represent

TABLE 6-4   The Frequency of Occurrence of Individual English Consonants

SOUND	PERCENTAGE OF OCCURRENCE	CUMULATIVE PERCENTAGE
n	12.0	12.0
t	11.9	23.9
s	6.9	30.8
r	6.7	37.5
d	6.4	43.9
m	5.9	49.8
z	5.4	55.2
ð	5.3	60.5
l	5.3	65.8
k	5.1	70.9
w	4.9	75.8
h	4.4	80.2
b	3.3	83.5
p	3.1	86.6
g	3.1	89.7
f	2.1	91.8
ŋ	1.6	93.4
j	1.6	95.0
v	1.5	96.5
ʃ	0.9	97.4
θ	0.9	98.3
dʒ	0.6	98.9
tʃ	0.6	99.5
ʒ	<0.1	99.6

SPEECH SOUND DISORDERS

nearly one-half of the total consonants used. When misarticulated, these sounds will have a greater negative effect on speech than the less frequently occurring sounds such as /ʒ/, /tʃ/, /dʒ/, and /θ/.

DESCRIPTIVE FEATURES OF PHONEMES

Phonemes of the English language can be grouped and separated according to similar and dissimilar features. Sounds are most commonly described according to place of articulation, manner of articulation, and voicing, as shown in Table 6-5. When completing an assessment, take note of whether phoneme errors tend to occur within specific categories (e.g., errors of fricatives, errors of alveolars, errors of voicing).

TABLE 6-5   The Sounds of English Categorized by Place, Manner, and Voicing

	CONSONANTS PLACE OF ARTICULATION						
MANNER OF ARTICULATION	**BILABIAL**	**LABIODENTAL**	**DENTAL**	**ALVEOLAR**	**PALATAL**	**VELAR**	**GLOTTAL**
Stop	p*			t*		k*	
				d		g	
Fricative		f*	θ*	s*	ʃ*		h*
		v	θ	z	ʒ		
Affricate					tʃ*		
					dʒ		
Glide	w				j		
Liquid				l	r		
Nasal	m			n	ŋ		

	VOWELS PLACE OF ARTICULATION		
	FRONT	**CENTER**	**BACK**
High	i		u
	ɪ		ʊ
	e	ɜ	
			o
Mid	ɛ	ə ɚ	
		ʌ	ɔ
Low	æ		a

Unvoiced sounds are shown with an asterisk.

DISTINCTIVE FEATURES OF CONSONANTS

Individual sounds consist of unique and distinct features that, make each sound different from all other sounds. For example, /f/ and /v/ are two sounds that share four features (consonantal, anterior, continuant, strident) but differ by one feature (voicing), which makes them separate sounds. Clinicians often use distinctive features to identify error patterns. Once the patterns are identified, therapy focuses on training the features that will improve speech productions. The advantage of the distinctive features approach is its ability to target one or more specific features that will help improve more than one sound at the same time.

The following examples show several distinctive feature patterns:

Example One:

/t/ for /k/	(*tup* for *cup*)
/d/ for /g/	(*dumb* for *gum*)
/n/ for /ŋ/	(*lawn* for *long*)

The erred feature in this example is an *anterior* placement. Sounds are produced in front of the mouth instead of the back.

Example Two:

/d/ for /n/	(*dice* for *nice*)
/b/ for /m/	(*bake* for *make*)
/g/ for /ŋ/	(*lug* for *lung*)

The erred pattern involves *nasality*. Nonnasal sounds are substituted for nasal sounds.

Example Three:

/w/ for /f/	(*wine* for *fine*)
/l/ for /v/	(*lase* for *vase*)
/t/ for /s/	(*toap* for *soap*)

omissions of /s/, /ʃ/, /tʃ/, /ʒ/, and /dʒ/

Although these errors do not initially appear to be related, the missing distinctive feature in all the sounds is *stridency*.

Table 6-6 is based on Chomsky and Halle's (1968, 1991) listing of the distinctive features of English consonants. Definitions of each feature are also provided.

TABLE 6-6   Distinctive Features of English Consonants

	w	f	v	θ	ð	t	d	s	z	n	l	ʃ	ʒ	j	r	tʃ	dʒ	k	g	ŋ	h	p	b	m
Voiced	+	−	+	−	+	−	+	−	+	+	+	−	+	+	+	−	+	−	+	+	−	−	+	+
Consonantal	−	+	+	+	+	+	+	+	+	+	+	+	+	−	+	+	+	+	+	+	+	−	+	+
Anterior	+	+	+	+	+	+	+	+	+	+	+	−	−	−	−	−	−	−	−	−	−	+	+	+
Coronal	−	−	−	+	+	+	+	+	+	+	+	+	+	−	+	+	+	−	−	−	−	−	−	−
Continuant	+	+	+	+	+	−	−	+	+	−	+	+	+	+	+	−	−	−	−	−	+	−	−	−
High	−	−	−	−	−	−	−	−	−	−	−	+	+	+	−	+	+	+	+	+	−	−	−	−
Low	−	−	−	−	−	−	−	−	−	−	−	−	−	−	−	−	−	−	−	−	+	−	−	−
Back	−	−	−	−	−	−	−	−	−	−	−	−	−	−	−	−	−	+	+	+	−	−	−	−
Nasal	−	−	−	−	−	−	−	−	−	+	−	−	−	−	−	−	−	−	−	+	−	−	−	+
Strident	−	+	+	−	−	−	−	+	+	−	−	+	+	−	−	+	+	−	−	−	−	−	−	−
Vocalic	−	−	−	−	−	−	−	−	−	−	+	−	−	−	+	−	−	−	−	−	−	−	−	−
Round	+	−	−	−	−	−	−	−	−	−	−	−	−	−	−	−	−	−	−	−	−	−	−	−

Voiced: Produced with vocal fold vibration.
Consonantal: Produced with narrow constriction.
Anterior: Produced in the front region of the mouth, at the alveolar ridge, or forward.
Coronal: Produced by raising the blade of the tongue above the neutral position.
Continuant: Produced with partial obstruction of airflow.
High: Produced by raising the body of the tongue above the neutral position.
Low: Produced by lowering the body of the tongue below the neutral position.
Back: Produced in the back of the mouth with the body of the tongue retracted from the neutral position.
Nasal: Produced by lowering the velum to allow air to pass through the nasal cavity.
Strident: Produced with rapid airflow pressing against the teeth.
Vocalic: Produced without significant constriction and with voicing.
Round: Produced by rounding the lips.

PHONOLOGICAL PROCESSES

As stated previously, distinctive features refer to the characteristic features of individual sounds. Phonological processes, on the other hand, apply to larger segments that *include* individual sounds. Phonological processes describe what children do in the normal developmental process of speech to simplify standard adult productions. When a child uses many different processes or uses processes that are not commonly present during speech acquisition, intelligibility may be impaired.

The advantage of using a phonological processes approach when analyzing articulation is that the clinician can identify error patterns and then target those patterns to remediate more than one sound at a time. For example, if a child exhibits a *final consonant deletion* pattern, the clinician may choose to target final consonants in general rather than focus on only a few sounds in the final position. Many commonly used tests for evaluating phonological processes are listed earlier in this chapter under the heading "Formal Tests."

Different authorities describe numerous phonological processes. Consult the "Sources of Additional Information" at the end of this chapter for suggested sources. Descriptions and examples of 23 phonological processes are provided next. Refer to these descriptions or to the specific guidelines provided by the test used when evaluating clients with multiple articulation errors. Realize that some of the following examples may illustrate more than one process change.

Alveolarization

Substitution of an alveolar phoneme for a labial or linguadental phoneme:

/tæn/	for *pan*
/don/	for *bone*
/bæs/	for *bath*

Assimilation (Harmony)

Alteration of a consonant phoneme that is influenced by, and becomes more like, a surrounding phoneme:

/bɛb/	for *bed*
/dʌn/	for *gun*
/gɛnk/	for *thank*

Backing

Substitution of a more posteriorly produced phoneme for an anteriorly produced phoneme:

/kɑp/	for *top*
/bok/	for *boat*
/hup/	for *soup*

Cluster Reduction

Reduction of a cluster to a singleton:

/pen/	for *plane*
/tʌk/	for *truck*
/sip/	for *sleep*

Coalescence

Substitution of a single phoneme that is different from two adjacent target phonemes yet takes on features of the target:

/fok/	for *smoke*
/tufe/	for *Tuesday*
/læθ/	for *last*

Deaffrication

Substitution of a fricative for an affricate phoneme:

/ʃɪp/	for *chip*
/peʒ/	for *page*
/ʃiz/	for *cheese*

Denasalization

Substitution of a homorganic stop (similar place of articulation) for a nasal phoneme:

/do/	for *no*
/bæd/	for *man*
/sɪg/	for *sing*

Depalatalization

Substitution of an alveolar fricative or affricate for a palatal fricative or affricate:

/dʒu/	for *cue*
/wats/	for *wash*
/fɪs/	for *fish*

Diminutization

Addition of /i/ or consonant + /i/:

/lɛgi/	for *leg*
/hæti/	for *hat*
/maɪmi/	for *my*

Doubling

Repetition of a word:

/gogo/	for *go*
/dædæ/	for *dad*
/mimi/	for *me*

Epenthesis

Insertion of a new phoneme:

/bəlu/	for *blue*
/sθop/	for *soap*
/kləlɚ/	for *color*

Final Consonant Deletion

Deletion of the final consonant:

/kʌ/	for *cup*
/dɑ/	for *doll*
/pu/	for *pool*

Fronting

Substitution of a more anteriorly produced phoneme:

/su/	for *shoe*
/frɔd/	for *frog*
/tændɪ/	for *candy*

Gliding

Substitution of a glide for a liquid:

/pwey/	for *play*
/wʌn/	for *run*
/jɛwo/	for *yellow*

Initial Consonant Deletion

Deletion of the initial singleton consonant:

/ʌp/	for *cup*
/æn/	for *man*
/ul/	for *pool*

Labialization

Substitution of a labial phoneme for a phoneme produced with the tip of the tongue:

/bɔg/	for *dog*
/hæf/	for *hat*
/fʌn/	for *sun*

Metathesis (Spoonerism)

Transposition of two phonemes:

/bəskɛtɪ/	for *spaghetti*
/faʊlə/	for *flower*
/lɪkstɪp/	for *lipstick*

Reduplication

Repetition of a complete or incomplete syllable:

/wɑwɑ/	for *water*
/dɑdɑ/	for *dog*
/wæwæ/	for *wagon*

Stopping

Substitution of a stop for a fricative or affricate:

/top/	for *soap*
/kæt/	for *catch*
/pʌdl/	for *puzzle*

Stridency Deletion

Omission of a strident or the substitution of a nonstrident consonant:

/op/	for *soap*
/wʌn/	for *fun*
/kɪθ/	for *kiss*

Unstressed Syllable Deletion

Deletion of an unstressed syllable:

/gɛdɪ/	for *spaghetti*
/markwev/	for *microwave*
/nænə/	for *banana*

Voicing or Devoicing

Alteration in voicing influenced by a surrounding phoneme:

/dʒɑp/	for *job*
/beg/	for *bake*
/gʌp/	for *cup*

Vocalization (Vowelization)

Substitution of a vowel for a liquid phoneme in the final position:

/kʌvʊ/	for *cover*
/pipo/	for *people*
/hɛə/	for *hair*

Most phonological processes are seen in normal speech acquisition. The most common processes that occur in normal speech are unstressed syllable deletion, final consonant deletion, gliding, and cluster reduction. Note that some children never produce certain processes. Children typically outgrow all phonological processes and produce correct adult targets

TABLE 6-7   Developmental Norms for Phonological Processes

AGE OUTGROWN	PHONOLOGICAL PROCESS
Gone by age 3	Denasalization
	Doubling
	Assimilation
	Diminutization
	Reduplication
	Prevocalic voicing
	Final consonant devoicing
	Stopping /f/ and /s/
Gone by age 4	Final consonant deletion
	Fronting
	Consonant assimilation
	Unstressed syllable deletion
	Cluster reduction
	Deaffrication
	Stopping /v/ and /z/
Gone by age 5	Alveolarization
	Depalatalization
	Stopping /ʃ/, /tʃ/, /dʒ/, /θ/, and /ð/**
Gone by age 6	Gliding
	Labialization
Gone by age 8	Epenthesis

by age 8. Table 6-7 presents developmental norms for phonological processes in normally developing children. Keep in mind that some children may be diagnosed with a phonological disorder even if certain phonological processes identified are considered within normal expectations for their age. This can occur when many processes are present and intelligibility is significantly impaired.

Form 6-3, "Phonological Processes Worksheet," is a worksheet for identifying phonological processes elicited during connected speech or on a formal test. An inventory of phonological processes is most valuable when working with children who have poor speech intelligibility due to multiple articulation errors. For children with only a few errors, use Form 6-1, "Comparison of Sound Errors from an Articulation Test and Connected Speech."

CHILDHOOD APRAXIA OF SPEECH

Childhood apraxia of speech (CAS) is a motor speech disorder. A child with CAS has difficulty sequencing sounds, syllables, and words for speech even though there is no muscle weakness, paralysis, or other physical limitation. Its etiology is usually unknown, although in some cases it is secondary to a genetic disorder or acquired from a stroke or brain injury. It is similar to acquired apraxia of speech (AOS; presented in Chapter 14) in that oral-motor programming for speech is impaired. What makes CAS different from AOS, however, is the significant negative impact it has on linguistic and phonologic development. It is not a disorder a child will outgrow, and severe cases can have a potentially devastating impact on oral communication.

Published tests for the diagnosis of apraxia of speech include:

- *Apraxia Battery for Adults* (ABA-2) (Dabul, 2000)
- *Quick Assessment for Apraxia of Speech* (Tanner & Culbertson, 1999)

Differential diagnosis is challenging because behaviors associated with CAS are also associated with other communicative disorders. These may include dysarthria, speech delay, fluency disorder, expressive and receptive language impairment, literacy disorder, and phonological impairment. This is complicated by the fact that CAS often co-occurs with one or more of these other communicative disorders. Behaviors associated with CAS vary from one child to another, and also vary within the same child as the child matures.

Table 6-8 presents behaviors and characteristics that are associated with CAS. It is relevant to note that not all professionals are in agreement about symptoms of CAS, and some behaviors are considered characteristic even though they have not been validated through controlled studies.

Although currently there are no distinguishing features that completely differentiate CAS from other childhood speech disorders, there are behaviors that are especially characteristic of CAS. An American Speech-Language-Hearing Association (ASHA) ad hoc committee identified the following three segmental and suprasegmental features of CAS:

1. Inconsistent errors on consonants and vowels in repeated productions of syllables or words

2. Lengthened and disrupted coarticulatory transitions between sounds and syllables

3. Inappropriate prosody, especially in the realization of lexical or phrasal stress (ASHA, 2007a)

The same committee stressed that clinicians should focus on differentiating CAS from other similar disorders during an assessment. Evaluate all aspects of speech that may be affected, with particular emphasis on:

- Automatic versus volitional actions
- Single postures versus sequences of postures
- Simple contexts versus more complex or novel contexts
- Repetitions of the same stimuli versus repetitions of varying stimuli
- Tasks for which responses can be judged after auditory versus visual cues, auditory versus tactile cues, visual versus tactile cues, or which combinations (e.g., auditory and visual) seem to produce the best results.
- Fluidity, rate, and accuracy of speech in relationship to one another
- Performance of tasks in multiple contexts (e.g., spontaneous speech, imitation, elicited speech, discourse, utterances of varying lengths, etc.) (ASHA, 2007a)
- Impaired auditory comprehension

TABLE 6-8   Communicative Behaviors Associated with Childhood Apraxia of Speech

Nonspeech Motor Behaviors	General awkwardness or clumsiness Impaired volitional oral movements Mild delays in motor development Mildly low muscle tone Hyper- or hyposensitivity in the oral area Oral apraxia
Speech Motor Behaviors	Difficulty with repetitions of syllables and diadochokinesis Slow speech development Multiple speech sound errors Reduced intelligibility Reduced phonetic or phonemic inventories Reduced vowel inventory Vowel errors Inconsistency of errors Increased errors in longer or more complex syllable and word shapes Errors in the ordering of sounds (migration and metathesis), syllables, morphemes, or even words Groping Persistent or frequent regression Differences in performance of automatic versus volitional activities
Prosodic Characteristics	Excessive-equal stress of syllables Staccato speech (syllable segregation) Variations in rate, including prolonged sounds and prolonged pauses between sounds, syllables, or words Reduced range of pitch or variable pitch Reduced range of loudness or variable loudness Monotone Monoloud Variable nasal resonance
Speech Perception Characteristics	Reduced auditory perception Reduced auditory discrimination Reduced auditory memory
Language Characteristics	Significant language deficits Morphologic omissions Deficits in expressive and receptive language, with expressive consistently lagging behind receptive language Family history of language impairment
Metalinguistics/Literacy Characteristics	Reduced phonological awareness Difficulty with word identification Poor spelling Increased self-awareness of speech production limitations (metalinguistic awareness)

Source: Adapted from American-Speech-Language-Hearing Association (2007).

- Impaired verbal expression
- Presence of paraphasias
- Perseveration
- Agrammatism, or grammatical errors
- Nonfluent speech or nonmeaningful fluent speech
- Impaired prosodic features of speech
- Difficulty repeating words, phrases, and sentences

Materials provided in other sections of this text may be helpful for completing portions of the assessment. Consider using Form 14-2, "Checklists for Limb, Oral, and Verbal Apraxia" or Form 14-3, "Identifying Apraxia," and adapt as needed. Published assessments include:

- *The Apraxia Profile* (Hickman, 1997)
- *Kaufman Speech Praxis Test for Children (KSPT)* (Kaufman, 1995)
- *Screening Test for Developmental Apraxia of Speech (STDAS-2)* (Blakeley, 2000)
- *Verbal Dyspraxia Profile* (Jelm, 2001)

CONCLUDING COMMENTS

Various assessment materials and procedures were presented in this chapter. These ranged from articulation screening to administration of formal articulation tests, and from obtaining speech samples to assessing stimulability. The resource materials included normative data, distinctive features, and phonological processes. Some of the resources in Chapter 5 are also useful for assessing disorders of articulation and phonological processes.

SOURCES OF ADDITIONAL INFORMATION

Print Sources

Bauman-Waengler, J. (2011). *Articulatory and phonological impairments: A clinical focus* (4th ed.). Needham Heights, MA: Allyn & Bacon.

Bleile, K. M. (2004). *Manual of articulation and phonological disorders* (2nd ed.). Clifton Park, NY: Cengage Learning.

Downing, R. S., & Chamberlain, C. E. (2006). *The source for childhood apraxia of speech*. East Moline, IL: Linguisystems.

Lowe, R. J. (2010). *Workbook for the identification of phonological processes and distinctive features* (4th ed.). Austin, TX: Pro-ed.

Pena-Brooks, A., & Hedge, M. N. (2007). *Assessment and treatment of articulation and phonological disorders in children* (2nd ed.). Austin, TX: Pro-ed.

Electronic Sources

American Speech-Language Hearing Association:
http://www.asha.org

"Articulation Test Center" app by Little Bee Speech

"Phonological Process Finder" app by Home-Speech-Home.com

"Sunny Articulation Phonology Test" app by Smarty Ears

Form 6-1.

Comparison of Sound Errors from an Articulation Test and Connected Speech

Name: _____ Age: _____ Date: _____

Examiner's Name: _____

Instructions: Compare speech errors identified during an articulation test and connected speech. Here are recommended ways to mark errors:

Omission:	use a dash (—) or write *omit*
Distortion:	use diacritics; describe the error; or use a D or write *dist* and indicate severity with 1 (mild), 2 (moderate), or 3 (severe). For example, D^3 is a severe distortion.
Substitution:	transcribe the error
Addition:	transcribe the error
Stimulable:	use a check (✓) or a plus (+); if the error is improved but not perfectly correct, mark an upward arrow (↑) or describe the nature of the improvement.
Not Stimulable:	use NS (not stimulable) or zero (0)

Then summarize your findings to identify error patterns.

	Articulation Test Errors			Connected Speech Errors		
Sound	**Initial**	**Medial**	**Final**	**Initial**	**Medial**	**Final**
p	_____	_____	_____	_____	_____	_____
b	_____	_____	_____	_____	_____	_____
t	_____	_____	_____	_____	_____	_____
d	_____	_____	_____	_____	_____	_____
k	_____	_____	_____	_____	_____	_____
g	_____	_____	_____	_____	_____	_____
f	_____	_____	_____	_____	_____	_____
v	_____	_____	_____	_____	_____	_____
θ	_____	_____	_____	_____	_____	_____
ð	_____	_____	_____	_____	_____	_____
s	_____	_____	_____	_____	_____	_____
z	_____	_____	_____	_____	_____	_____
ʃ	_____	_____	_____	_____	_____	_____
ʒ	_____	_____	_____	_____	_____	_____
h	_____	_____	_____	_____	_____	_____
tʃ	_____	_____	_____	_____	_____	_____

(continues)

SPEECH SOUND DISORDERS

Form 6-1. continued

	Articulation Test Errors			**Connected Speech Errors**		
Sound	Initial	Medial	Final	Initial	Medial	Final
dʒ	_____	_____	_____	_____	_____	_____
w	_____	_____	_____	_____	_____	_____
j	_____	_____	_____	_____	_____	_____
l	_____	_____	_____	_____	_____	_____
r	_____	_____	_____	_____	_____	_____
m	_____	_____	_____	_____	_____	_____
n	_____	_____	_____	_____	_____	_____
ŋ	_____	_____	_____	_____	_____	_____
i	_____	_____	_____	_____	_____	_____
ɪ	_____	_____	_____	_____	_____	_____
e	_____	_____	_____	_____	_____	_____
ɛ	_____	_____	_____	_____	_____	_____
æ	_____	_____	_____	_____	_____	_____
ɝ	_____	_____	_____	_____	_____	_____
ɚ	_____	_____	_____	_____	_____	_____
ə	_____	_____	_____	_____	_____	_____
ʌ	_____	_____	_____	_____	_____	_____
u	_____	_____	_____	_____	_____	_____
ʊ	_____	_____	_____	_____	_____	_____
o	_____	_____	_____	_____	_____	_____
ɔ	_____	_____	_____	_____	_____	_____
ɑ	_____	_____	_____	_____	_____	_____

(continues)

Form 6-1. continued

Consistent Sound Errors:

Sounds Containing More Than One Error:

Patterns of Sound Errors:

Consistent Correct Sound Productions:

SPEECH SOUND DISORDERS

Form 6-2.

Sounds That Are Stimulable

Name: _____ Age: _____ Date: _____

Examiner's Name: _____

Instructions: Record all stimulable sounds under the appropriate category using a check (✓) or plus (+). If a sound is stimulable at the phrase level, indicate the number of syllables in the phrase. For example:

p   ✓   ✓   ✓   _____   3   3   _____

	Sound Level	Word Level Initial	Medial	Final	Phrase Level Initial	Medial	Final
p	_____	_____	_____	_____	_____	_____	_____
b	_____	_____	_____	_____	_____	_____	_____
t	_____	_____	_____	_____	_____	_____	_____
d	_____	_____	_____	_____	_____	_____	_____
k	_____	_____	_____	_____	_____	_____	_____
g	_____	_____	_____	_____	_____	_____	_____
f	_____	_____	_____	_____	_____	_____	_____
ʋ	_____	_____	_____	_____	_____	_____	_____
θ	_____	_____	_____	_____	_____	_____	_____
ð	_____	_____	_____	_____	_____	_____	_____
s	_____	_____	_____	_____	_____	_____	_____
z	_____	_____	_____	_____	_____	_____	_____
ʃ	_____	_____	_____	_____	_____	_____	_____
ʒ	_____	_____	_____	_____	_____	_____	_____
h	_____	_____	_____	_____	_____	_____	_____
tʃ	_____	_____	_____	_____	_____	_____	_____
dʒ	_____	_____	_____	_____	_____	_____	_____
w	_____	_____	_____	_____	_____	_____	_____
j	_____	_____	_____	_____	_____	_____	_____
l	_____	_____	_____	_____	_____	_____	_____
r	_____	_____	_____	_____	_____	_____	_____
m	_____	_____	_____	_____	_____	_____	_____
n	_____	_____	_____	_____	_____	_____	_____
ŋ	_____	_____	_____	_____	_____	_____	_____

(continues)

SPEECH SOUND DISORDERS

Form 6-2. continued

	Sound Level	**Word Level**	**Phrase Level**
i	_____	_____	_____
ɪ	_____	_____	_____
e	_____	_____	_____
ɛ	_____	_____	_____
æ	_____	_____	_____
ɝ	_____	_____	_____
ɚ	_____	_____	_____
ə	_____	_____	_____
ʌ	_____	_____	_____
u	_____	_____	_____
ʊ	_____	_____	_____
o	_____	_____	_____
ɔ	_____	_____	_____
ɑ	_____	_____	_____

Form 6-3.

Phonological Processes Worksheet

Name: _____ Age: _____ Date: _____

Examiner's Name: _____

Instructions: Record the child's exact articulatory productions and the intended target words. Then determine the phonological processes used for each error. If a process cannot be identified, leave the final column blank or write a question mark (?). Note which processes occur with the greatest frequency.

Child's Production	Intended Production	Phonological Process

(continues)

Form 6-3. continued

Child's Production	Intended Production	Phonological Process
_____	_____	_____
_____	_____	_____
_____	_____	_____
_____	_____	_____
_____	_____	_____
_____	_____	_____
_____	_____	_____
_____	_____	_____
_____	_____	_____
_____	_____	_____
_____	_____	_____
_____	_____	_____
_____	_____	_____
_____	_____	_____
_____	_____	_____
_____	_____	_____
_____	_____	_____
_____	_____	_____
_____	_____	_____
_____	_____	_____
_____	_____	_____

(continues)

Form 6-3. continued

Child's Production	Intended Production	Phonological Process
_____	_____	_____
_____	_____	_____
_____	_____	_____
_____	_____	_____
_____	_____	_____
_____	_____	_____
_____	_____	_____
_____	_____	_____
_____	_____	_____
_____	_____	_____
_____	_____	_____
_____	_____	_____
_____	_____	_____
_____	_____	_____

Comments:

SPEECH SOUND DISORDERS

Appendix 6-A.

The words and sentences provided in Table 6-9 are designed for assessing stimulability of misarticulated phonemes. Three words and sentences are provided for each phoneme in the initial, medial, and final positions. For each sound, the single words contain a front vowel, a central vowel, and a back vowel for assessing consonant productions in different contexts. The normative age data for individual phonemes in the left-hand column are from Prather, Hedrick, and Kern (1975), and reflect the age at which 75% of the children tested correctly produced the targeted sound in the initial and final positions. Initial position blends are included, following the singletons. The normative age data for blends are from Smit, Hand, Frelinger, Bernthal, and Byrd (1990), and reflect the age at which 75% of the children tested correctly produced the targeted sound in the initial position of words. (Refer to the "Developmental Norms for Phonemes and Blends" in the chapter for more information on the use of norms.) Three words (each containing a front, central, and back vowel when possible) and a short phrase or sentence are provided for each blend.

TABLE 6-9 Words and Phrases for Assessing Stimulability

AGE	SOUND	INITIAL	MEDIAL	FINAL
2;0	/p/	pin	happy	sleep
		person	puppy	cup
		pool	soapy	soup
		Pie is good.	The hippo is big.	Let's move up.
		Pete didn't go.	What happened?	I found my cap.
		Peggy is nice.	It was a super effort.	Get the soap.
2;0–8;0	/b/	bake	rabbit	grab
		bird	cupboard	tub
		boot	robin	knob
		Bill is very tall.	It's above the sink.	She has a robe.
		Buy some milk.	The robber is quiet.	He needs a job.
		Bacon is good.	The label was torn.	He hurt his rib.
2;0–8;0	/t/	tan	guitar	sat
		tough	attend	mutt
		tooth	hotel	got
		Tim went home.	The motel was full.	They were late.
		Taste this.	No details are known.	Here's the boot.
		Tony is nice.	The cartoon is funny.	It's a goat.
2;0–4;0	/d/	dim	ladder	need
		dump	muddy	word
		duty	soda	food
		Do they know?	He's hiding in there.	It's too loud.

continued on the next page

SPEECH SOUND DISORDERS

Table 6-9, continued from the previous page

AGE	SOUND	INITIAL	MEDIAL	FINAL
		Debbie went home.	The radio was loud.	Plant a seed.
		Dive right in.	The wedding is fun.	She has a braid.
2;0–4;0	/k/	cat	bacon	music
		cup	bucket	truck
		call	rocket	look
		Can I help you?	He's making a mess.	He saw a duck.
		Cake tastes good.	The pocket is full.	It is black.
		Cut it out.	He's looking for her.	They like steak.
2;0–4;0	/g/	give	tiger	fig
		gum	again	rug
		ghost	soggy	dog
		Go away.	Read the magazine.	He found a frog.
		Get some more.	The sugar is sweet.	Sit on the rug.
		Good job.	It is foggy outside.	They like to dig.
2;0–4;0	/f/	fish	safety	stiff
		fun	muffin	rough
		fall	coffee	goof
		Find the other one.	Go before dinner.	Slice the loaf.
		Feel this paper.	It was safer inside.	Don't laugh.
		Food is good.	The café was full.	He likes beef.
4;0	/v/	vase	beaver	have
		verdict	oven	curve
		vote	over	stove
		Visit him.	The movie was good.	They will arrive.
		Value your time.	It's a heavy box.	He wore a glove.
		Victory is sweet.	It's in the oval office.	He might move.
4;0	/θ/	thin	bathtub	math
		third	nothing	earth
		thought	author	tooth
		Think about it.	The athlete won.	I need a bath.
		Thank you.	Say something.	It's a myth.
		Thunder is loud.	The cathedral is big.	Tell the truth.
4;0	/ð/	that	feather	breathe
		there	mother	bathe
		those	bother	soothe
		These are old.	I would rather go.	He can breathe.
		They didn't like it.	The weather is hot.	It feels smooth.
		This is not right.	Her father is nice.	We sunbathe.

AGE	SOUND	INITIAL	MEDIAL	FINAL
3;0	/s/	sand	hassle	chase
		sunny	mercy	fuss
		soap	bossy	moose
		Sip lemonade.	Leave a message.	It's a mess.
		Surprises are fun.	They saw a castle.	She has a horse.
		Soup is good.	They are chasing us.	His dog is loose.
4;0	/z/	zip	easy	peas
		zero	cousin	does
		zone	closet	chose
		Zip the coat.	They will visit us.	Touch the toes.
		Zoo trips are fun.	The closet was full.	He likes cheese.
		Zebras are big.	The dessert was good.	Hear the noise.
3;0–8;0	/ʃ/	ship	special	fish
		shirt	brushes	rush
		show	bushy	push
		Shall we go?	The dishes are dry.	He used cash.
		Shoes get lost.	The ocean is near.	It is fresh.
		Shells are pretty.	The machine broke.	Make a wish.
4;0	/ʒ/		measure	luge
			version	rouge
			fusion	
			Bury the treasure.	
			Wear casual clothes.	
			His vision is good.	
2;0	/h/	hiss	behave	
		hut	rehearse	
		hop	forehead	
		Hurry for dinner.	The playhouse is large.	
		He is going.	Go unhook it.	
		Have you done it?	Look behind you.	
3;0–8;0	/tʃ/	cheese	matches	beach
		chunk	merchant	much
		choose	nachos	watch
		China is far away.	The ketchup spilled.	Sit on a couch.
		Chuck is a friend.	He is pitching.	Strike a match.
		Chew your food.	He's a natural.	She ate a peach.
4;0	/dʒ/	jeep	magic	age
		jug	budget	budge

continued on the next page

Table 6-9, continued from the previous page

AGE	SOUND	INITIAL	MEDIAL	FINAL
		joke	project	dodge
		Jets are fast.	The pigeon flew.	Turn the page.
		Jump the fence.	The pajamas are red.	Cross a bridge.
		Jelly is good.	It was a raging fire.	She likes fudge.
2;0–8;0	/w/	well	freeway	
		won	away	
		wood	mower	
		Winter is here.	The sidewalk is hot.	
		Wake up now.	The reward was paid.	
		Why did he do it?	He has a power saw.	
2;0–4;0	/j/	yell	kayak	
		yummy	royal	
		yacht	coyote	
		Yellow is bright.	The tortilla was warm.	
		Yogurt is good.	He is a loyal friend.	
		You can go now.	The lawyer called.	
3;0–4;0	/l/	leap	jelly	fell
		learn	color	pearl
		look	pillow	ball
		Linda went home.	She is silly.	It is full.
		Lay it on the table.	The palace was large.	We will.
		Let me see.	The jello was good.	Walk a mile.
3;0–4;0	/r/	rip	erase	steer
		run	carrot	hair
		row	borrow	car
		Rake the leaves.	The parade is today.	It was not far.
		Rub it in.	He is sorry about it.	He ate the pear.
		Ruth is nice.	Her earring was lost.	Go to the store.
2;0	/m/	make	hammer	same
		money	summer	hum
		moon	human	boom
		Meet me later.	It's lemon pie.	You're welcome.
		Mark is nice.	He's coming back.	Play the drum.
		My dog is brown.	Let Jimmy see it.	They like ham.
2;0	/n/	net	many	mean
		nothing	sunny	learn
		new	phony	soon

AGE	SOUND	INITIAL	MEDIAL	FINAL
2;0	/ŋ/	Never do that. Nancy said yes. Nobody was home.	He's a piano player. We cannot go. The bunny is white. finger hunger longer The singer is short. Put the hanger away. It's a jungle animal.	David is his son. Did you win? She has grown. ring hung song He was young. He was wrong. Play on a swing.

AGE	BLEND	WORD	PHRASE
5;0	/bl/	black blunt blue	a black shoe a blunt pencil the blue car
6;0	/br/	brave brush broke	the brave hero The brush fell. He broke it.
6;0	/dr/	drink drum draw	Don't drink it all. the drum beat Let's draw a picture.
6;0	/fr/	free front frog	set free in the front a big frog
5;6	/fl/	fly flurry float	a fly swatter the snow flurry a root beer float
4;6	/gl/	glad glove glue	a glad boy the glove box sticky as glue
6;0	/gr/	green grudge grow	the green tree hold a grudge They grow corn.
3;6	/kw/	quit quirk quad	Do not quit. a quirk of fate Meet in the quad.
5;6	/kl/	clam club closet	a clam bake the clubhouse the closet door

continued on the next page

SPEECH SOUND DISORDERS

Table 6-9, continued from the previous page

AGE	BLEND	WORD	PHRASE
5;6	/kr/	cry	Do not cry.
		crumb	the crumb cake
		cruise	a cruise liner
5;6	/pl/	place	first-place ribbon
		plum	the plum pudding
		plot	The plot thickened.
6;0	/pr/	price	The price was high.
		protect	He will protect us.
		prove	Can you prove it?
5;0	/sk/	sky	The sky is blue.
		scare	Don't scare me.
		scoop	a scoop of ice cream
8;0	/skr/	screen	a screen door
		scrub	He will scrub the sink.
		scroll	the scroll cards
7;0	/skw/	squeak	a loud sqeak
		squirt	a squirt of water
		squash	Eat the squash.
7;0	/sl/	slam	a slam dunk
		slush	The snow was slush.
		slow	She should slow down.
5;0	/sp/	spy	the secret spy
		spurt	a spurt of energy
		spoon	a soup spoon
7;0	/spl/	split	a banana split
		splurge	They splurged for it.
		splotch	the splotch of ink
8;0	/spr/	spray	a spray bottle
		sprung	They sprung up.
		sprout	an alfalfa sprout
5;0	/sm/	smell	a nice smell
		smug	a smug look
		smooth	baby-smooth skin
5;6	/sn/	snack	The snack was good.
		snuggle	a snuggle bear
		snow	the snow shovel

AGE	BLEND	WORD	PHRASE
5;0	/st/	stiff	a stiff shirt
		stunt	a tricky stunt
		stop	Don't stop yet.
8;0	/str/	stray	a stray dog
		struggle	a struggle to win
		strong	the strong man
5;6	/sw/	sweet	Candy is sweet.
		swirl	black and white swirl
		swan	a beautiful swan
3;6	/tw/	twins	They are twins.
		twirl	She can twirl.
		twelve	the twelve boys
5;6	/tr/	tray	the breakfast tray
		trumpet	a trumpet solo
		true	her true colors
7;0	/θr/	three	the three blind mice
		thrust	the initial thrust
		throw	Let's throw the ball.

Chapter 7

ASSESSMENT OF LANGUAGE IN CHILDREN

This chapter focuses on the evaluation of spoken language disorders, primarily developmental comprehension and expression of oral language. Disorders of written language are presented in Chapter 8, Assessment of Literacy. Language disorders that result from neurological damage—aphasia, right-hemisphere syndrome, and cognitive impairments due to dementia or traumatic brain injury—are addressed in Chapter 13.

OVERVIEW OF ASSESSMENT

History of the Client

    Procedures

        Written Case History

        Information-Gathering Interview

        Specific Questions to Ask About Language Development/Disorder

        Information from Other Professionals

    Contributing Factors

        Hearing Impairment

        Medical or Neurological Factors

        Maturation and Motor Development

        Intelligence, Sex, Birth Order, Motivation, and Levels of Concern

        Cognitive Abilities

Assessment of Language

    Procedures

        Screening

        Informal Tests

        Standardized Tests

        Language Sampling

    Areas to Assess

        Pragmatics

        Semantics

        Syntax

        Morphology

    Analysis

        Error Types

        Forms of Errors

        Consistency of Errors

        Contextual Differences

Orofacial Examination

Hearing Assessment

Determining the Diagnosis

Providing Information (written report, interview, etc.)

Assessment Approaches

Even though there are a multitude of resources for assessment, language pathology can sometimes be one of the most challenging disorders to evaluate. This is not surprising considering how varied and complex language really is. Consider these complicating factors:

- The development of language is influenced by other aspects of development such as cognition, motor development, and social development. Clinical conditions such as mental retardation, hearing impairment, various genetic syndromes, and autism also affect language.

- The components of language (i.e., pragmatic, semantic, syntactic, morphologic, and phonologic) do not occur in isolation; they are integrated with one another. In addition, assessment of these individual components does not provide information about a client's use of language holistically.

- Expectations of language performance change across time. What is normal at age 1 may be deviant at age 3.

- Speakers of any given language are not a homogeneous group. Individual experiences and abilities result in a broad definition of *normal* language.

- Because of individual variability, there is no "best" approach for the assessment of language with all clients.

Owens (2013) described two approaches for assessing language: the *psychometric approach* and the *descriptive approach*. The psychometric approach is a traditional language assessment approach with an emphasis on ranking individuals according to norms. Performance is summarized by using percentile ranks and standard scores. The use of standardized, norm-referenced tests is emphasized.

There are certain advantages of using a psychometric approach for the assessment of language. A broad content area is usually assessed with a high degree of objectivity, reliability, and validity. Norm-referenced tests also help determine whether a problem exists and help identify specific problem areas. There are also limitations of the psychometric approach. Norm-referenced tests often do not adequately assess the complex, multidimensional aspects of language, nor are they appropriate for many of the clients speech-language pathologists typically evaluate (i.e., profiles of the clients do not match the profiles of the sample group on which the norms are based).

The second approach, the descriptive approach, is an authentic assessment method with a focus on describing behaviors and comparing past performance to current performance. Spontaneous speech-language sampling and observation in naturalistic contexts is emphasized. Language is assessed in all of its richness and complexity. This approach allows clinicians to determine whether (and if yes, how) the presenting problems are affecting the client's day-to-day communicative interactions. This approach also has its limitations. Reliability and validity of the findings are dependent upon the level of expertise of the clinician and how representative the language samples obtained are. The speech-language pathologist must be truly expert in understanding and evaluating the complexities of language.

An integrated approach that combines aspects of both the psychometric and the descriptive approaches is the recommended assessment approach. The assessment is typically a work in progress, as findings in the earlier stages of the assessment inform later assessment choices. For example, the case history, caregiver interview responses, and direct observation of the child will likely guide the clinician toward certain formal tests that will yield the most beneficial objective data. Findings from formal assessments may guide the clinician to probe for and analyze specific aspects of language during language sampling.

Components of Language

When completing a language evaluation, it is important to understand the basic elements of language. The five components of language are defined below. Four of the five components are described in more detail later in this chapter. The phonologic component is described in greater detail in Chapter 6.

1. Semantic: refers to the meaning of language
2. Syntactic: refers to the rules of grammar
3. Morphologic: refers to units of meaning
   a. Free morphemes: units that can stand alone (most words)
   b. Bound morphemes: units that cannot stand alone; they must be attached to a free morpheme (e.g., *pre-*, *-ing*)
4. Pragmatic: refers to the social aspects of language (e.g., eye contact, turn-taking)
5. Phonologic: refers to speech sounds, sound patterns, and rules of sound organization

Cognition and Language

Cognition is not a component of language; however, cognition is intrinsically related to language and is worthy of mention in this chapter. A child's cognitive abilities affect language in all aspects. Mental processes for learning, remembering, and using knowledge are essential for normal language acquisition and use. During a language assessment, it is helpful to take note of the child's cognitive abilities, including his or her attention and focus, reasoning ability, perception, memory, organization of self and thoughts, and overall executive function. If concerns arise, further cognitive assessment may be warranted. Chapter 13, Assessment of Neurocognitive Disorders, provides more information about assessment of cognition.

Language Disorder Categories

There are several diagnostic categories of language disorders. In most cases, deficient language is not the only clinically significant feature of these conditions. We mention them here to provide a framework for understanding language disorders in a broad sense. This chapter is primarily concerned with the assessment and diagnosis of the first one, specific language impairment, although chapter materials can be modified to aid in the assessment of several of the other categories as well.

Specific language impairment (SLI)

A seemingly pure language impairment with no obvious cause or co-occurring condition. Children with SLI follow the same general sequence of language acquisition as normally developing children, although at an impaired rate.

Language-learning disability (LLD)

A condition characterized by difficulties in acquiring and using skills for listening, speaking, reading, writing, reasoning, or mathematics. It is believed to be caused by central nervous system dysfunction.

LANGUAGE IN CHILDREN

Autism spectrum disorder (ASD) or pervasive developmental disorder (PDD)

A disorder characterized by impairment in communication and social skills and stereotyped and restricted behavioral patterns. The assessment of clients with an autism spectrum disorder is discussed in Chapter 9.

Brain injury

A neurological condition that occurs after some type of insult to the brain, such as traumatic brain injury, stroke, tumor, convulsive disorder, infection, or congenital malformation. Brain injury as a result of traumatic brain injury or stroke is discussed in Chapter 13.

Mental retardation (MR)

A condition characterized by intellectual function that is significantly below normal. It usually is caused by a biological medical condition or syndrome.

Deafness

A state of having minimal to no hearing. Causes may be biological or environmental. The impact of deafness on language is profound.

SCREENING

In some settings, screening for language disorders may seem like an overwhelming task. All of the components of language need to be screened in both receptive and expressive contexts quickly and efficiently. The purpose of a screen is to determine whether an in-depth assessment is necessary. Various tests and scales are commercially available for screening purposes. These include:

- *Adolescent Language Screening Test* (Morgan & Guildford, 1984)
- *Boehm Test of Basic Concepts* (Boehm, 2001)
- *Clinical Evaluation of Language Fundamentals (CELF-4) Screening Test* (Semel, Wiig, & Secord, 2004)
- *Early Language Milestone Scale, 2nd ed. (ELM Scale-2)* (Coplan, 1993)
- *Fluharty Preschool Speech and Language Screening Test* (2nd ed.) (Fluharty, 2000)
- *Joliet 3-Minute Preschool Speech and Language Screen* (Kinzler, 1993)
- *Joliet 3-Minute Speech and Language Screen-Revised* (Kinzler & Johnson, 1993)
- *Kindergarten Language Screening Test* (Gauthier & Madison, 1998)

When selecting an appropriate screening tool, consider variables such as the amount of time necessary for administration and the areas of language that are sampled. Many clinicians develop their own informal screening instruments. Several items in this resource (such as Forms 7-3, "Assessment of Language Development"; 7-5, "Checklist for an Informal Assessment of Language"; 7-6, "Worksheet for Recording a Language Sample"; 7-9, "Assessment of Semantic Skills" and 7-10, "Assessment of Syntactic Skills") can be adapted for screening purposes.

ASSESSMENT OF EARLY LANGUAGE DEVELOPMENT

Babies are born with limited ability to communicate. By the time they reach their fifth birthdays, normally developing children achieve nearly adult-like communication skills. Their language growth is dramatic from one year to the next. Table 7-1 provides a general summary of the major milestones of language development in the first five years. For a more detailed listing, which also includes speech and motor development, see content in Chapter 18.

The first three years of life are extremely important for setting the foundation for later development; therefore intervention for very young children who are struggling is critical. Research has shown that language problems in the early years may persist well into the school years and will likely affect academic performance in all areas.

Traditional methods of assessment are not feasible with the youngest clients. Most toddlers will not attend to the static formal tests that are commonly used with older children. Instead, information gathered on a case history form, questionnaire, and through parent interview are

TABLE 7-1   Major Milestones of Language Acquisition in Children

AGE RANGE	TYPICAL LANGUAGE BEHAVIORS
0–1 mos.	Startle response to sound; quieted by human voice.
2–3 mos.	Cooing; production of some vowel sounds; response to speech; babbling.
4–6 mos.	Babbling strings of syllables; imitation of sounds; variations in pitch and loudness.
7–9 mos.	Comprehension of some words and simple requests; increased imitation of speech sounds; may say or imitate "mama" or dada."
10–12 mos.	Understanding of "No"; response to requests; response to own name; production of one or more words.
13–15 mos.	Production of 5 to 10 words, mostly nouns; appropriate pointing responses.
16–18 mos.	Following simple directions; production of two-word phrases; production of "I" and "mine."
2;0–2;6 yrs.	Response to some yes/no questions; naming of everyday objects; production of phrases and incomplete sentences; production of the present progressive, prepositions, regular plural, and negation "no" or "not."
3;0–3;6 yrs.	Production of three- to four-word sentences; production of the possessive morpheme, several forms of questions, negatives "can't" and "don't"; comprehension of "why," "who," "whose," and "how many"; and initial productions of most grammatical morphemes.
3;6–5;0 yrs.	Greater mastery of articles, different tense forms, copula, auxiliary, third-person singular, and other grammatical morphemes; production of grammatically complete sentences.

Source: *Introduction to Communicative Disorders* (3rd ed., p. 150), by M. N. Hegde, 2001, Austin, TX: Pro-Ed. Copyright 2001 by Pro-Ed.

primary sources of data. Interaction with the client is play-based, with the clinician manipulating the play situation just enough to test desired behaviors. The clinician's goal is to ask the right questions, observe the right behaviors, and administer the right tests in order to obtain valid findings that are an accurate reflection of the child's true abilities and disabilities. Testing in the child's natural environment using familiar toys, people, and routines is ideal.

The young child's parents are active participants in the assessment process. They are the best source of information about a child's history and present skill level. They can answer questions about what the child can and cannot do, describe the child's daily routine, report about the client's behavior in other environments and with other people, and validate or clarify the clinician's observations. It is helpful to ask the parent if behaviors observed during the session are typical or atypical. Parents can often interpret what they believe their child is trying to communicate. Parents can also be called on to administer test probes when the child is reluctant or shy. For example, the clinician might ask the parent to see if the child can identify certain objects in a picture book while parent and child read together.

An important consideration is parent–child interaction. Observing the child with a parent or very familiar caregiver can often provide the best and most representative language and behavioral samples. It is also enlightening to note the *parent's* communication style. It may become clear that a child is not developing within normal expectations because the parent model is deficient. Form 7-1, "Worksheet for Analyzing Child–Caregiver Interactions" is useful for analyzing the communicative behaviors of the child with the parent or other caregiver.

Because normal expectations vary significantly as babies mature to toddlers and then preschoolers, we have grouped the assessment for early intervention into three broad categories. When evaluating a nonverbal or preverbal child, note these communicative behaviors:

- Does the child use gestures or signs to communicate?
- Are there nonspeech vocalizations?
- Are there meaningful vocalizations?
- How does the child respond to verbal stimulation?
- Does the child use eye contact?
- Does the child use objects and toys appropriately?
- Can the child imitate words?
- Does the child attempt to spontaneously produce words?
- How does the child communicate intent?
- Does the child follow simple commands?
- Can the child point to named objects in a picture book or in the environment?

If the client is minimally verbal, consider all of the above and also include:

- Does the child name familiar objects?
- Can the child count or say the alphabet?
- Does the child use any word combinations?
- Does the child use simple grammatical morphemes (e.g., -ing, -s)?
- What is the child's mean length of utterance?
- Does the child understand words and simple phrases?
- Does the child take turns in conversation?

If the child speaks in short phrases, consider all of the above plus the following:

- Does the child respond to multiple-step commands?
- Does the child use appropriate syntax?
- Does the child use a variety of descriptive and objective words?
- Is the child difficult to understand?
- What phonological processes are noted?
- Does the child demonstrate appropriate back-and-forth communicative exchanges?

And if the child is conversational, consider all of the skills previously mentioned and also include the following:

- Does the child have narrative ability?
- Does the child understand humor?
- Can the child respond to complex commands?

In addition to the more obvious aspects of language, an assessment for early intervention should include an expanded focus. The clinician should also consider the child's language-learning aptitude in general. For example:

- What is the child's temperament?
- Is the child easily distracted?
- How determined is the child?
- What is the child's attention span?
- What are the child's coping behaviors?
- Does the child seek help when needed?
- Does the child visually focus on and track objects of interest?

Piaget's Stages of Early Cognitive Development

Early cognitive behaviors lay a foundation for the development of language. Part of our current understanding of intelligence comes from research by Jean Piaget. Piaget described four stages of cognitive development. These are summarized in Table 7-2. The sensorimotor stage is strongly correlated with the development of language and is summarized in Table 7-3. Of particular interest to speech-language pathologists is the development of the concepts defined in the following list because they, in particular, are related to the ability to comprehend and use language.

- Imitation: Acknowledgement of the existence of a behavior and the ability to repeat it.
- Deferred imitation: Imitation of a behavior following a lapse of time.
- Means-end: Production of a volitional act to achieve a desired goal.
- Object permanence: An understanding that an object exists even though it is not currently seen.
- Functional use of objects: The use of an object as it was intended to be used.
- Symbolic play: The use of an object to represent something else.

TABLE 7-2   Piaget's Stages of Cognitive Development

Sensorimotor stage (birth–2 years)	Uses senses and motor activities to understand reality
	Develops concepts or schemes through physical interaction with the environment
	Initially relies on reflexive actions; eventually gains understanding of volition
	Imitates behaviors
	Develops the ability to act in order to achieve a goal (means-end)
	Develops an understanding of object permanence
	Develops an ability to play with objects symbolically
Pre-operational stage (2–7 years)	Characterized by egocentricism
	Focuses on one dimension in problem solving
	Cannot adopt alternative viewpoints (think from another person's perspective)
	Develops an ability to categorize objects through direct comparisons
	Gradually refines word meanings
	Cannot reverse events
Concrete operational stage (7–11 years)	Onset of logical operations, although thinking remains concrete
	Cannot solve abstract or hypothetical problems
	Develops an ability to consider more than one dimension in problem solving
	Able to adopt alternative viewpoints
	Mentally categorizes objects without direct comparisons
	Can reverse events
Formal operational stage (11–18+ years)	No longer limited to concrete thinking
	Able to mentally generalize and think abstractly
	Understands analogies
	Uses complex forms of language, including metaphors and sarcasm
	Able to reason flexibly and verbally through complex problems
	Able to reason through hypothesis testing

TABLE 7-3   The Six Substages of Piaget's Sensorimotor Stage of Cognitive Development

STAGE	AGE (MONTHS)	CHARACTERISTICS
1. Reflexive	0–1	Egocentric
		Unable to differentiate self from objects
2. Primary circular reactions (repetition of spontaneous pleasant behaviors)	1–4	Repeats interesting actions
		Earliest acts of intent
		Earliest repetition of behaviors
		Follows objects with eyes until out of view
		Out of sight, out of mind
		Unable to differentiate self from objects
		Holds head up
		Smiles

STAGE	AGE (MONTHS)	CHARACTERISTICS
3. Secondary circular reactions	4–8	Deliberately repeats actions Actions achieve goals (means-end) Recognizes objects Imitates actions that are in current repertoire Anticipates new position of moving object Sees self as the cause of all events Increasing interest in the environment Combines existing schemes with new stimuli
4. Coordination of secondary circular reactions	8–12	More purposeful and deliberate behaviors Crawling, thus expansion of the environment Emerging knowledge of object permanence Looks for object where last seen Coordinates already existing schemata Applies known means to new ends Imitates actions that are not in current repertoire Realizes that objects can cause action Establishes goal prior to initiating activity Anticipates outcomes
5. Tertiary circular reactions	12–18	Invents new means to an end Walks Imitates behaviors that are markedly different from those in current repertoire Aware of object spatial relations Realizes that he or she is one of many objects in the environment Uses tools
6. Inventive abilities via mental combinations	18–24	Mentally represents self Able to invent own play activity; play becomes the primary learning realm Symbolic play Early language emerges Uses language rather than actions to construct and record experiences Defers imitation Aware of unseen movements Predicts cause–effect relationships Fully aware of object permanence

Late Talker vs. Language Disordered

Some children are "late bloomers" when it comes to verbal expression. It is sometimes difficult to determine which children will experience lasting language impairment and which will outgrow it. Form 7-2, "Language Development Survey" is a predictive tool for the identification of expressive language delay in toddlers. Children who have fewer than 50 expressive words or no word combinations at age 2 are at increased risk of long-term language concerns. Those children who do not catch up to their same-age peers by age 3 demonstrate a language delay that is likely to persist throughout the school years. Additional risk factors and developmental signs that help clinicians predict whether a child will or will not outgrow a language delay include:

- Family history of language disorders
- Medical conditions such as frequent ear infections, hearing loss, or medical syndromes
- Prematurity, especially with low birth weight
- Maternal drug abuse or alcohol consumption
- Poor nutrition
- Minimal use of gestural communication
- Poor eye contact
- Minimal smiling
- Reduced joint attention
- Lack of symbolic play
- Does not seem curious about surroundings or point out things of interest
- Delayed babbling
- Early phonological difficulties
- Limited and simplified syllable structures
- Limited phonetic inventories
- Frequent deletion of initial and final consonants
- Numerous vowel errors
- Substitution of /h/ or glottal consonants for other consonants
- Atypical error patterns
- Fewer than 50 expressive words and no word combinations at age 2

Children who are more likely to outgrow a language delay tend to demonstrate:

- Frequent and effective nonverbal communication
- Strong language comprehension
- Good articulatory accuracy
- Complexity of syllable structures
- Larger phonetic inventories
- Typical developmental error patterns

Form 7-3, "Assessment of Language Development," and Form 7-4, "Parent Question-naire for Early Language Development" are provided in this manual to aid in the assessment of very young children.

FORMAL LANGUAGE TESTING

There are literally hundred of formal language tests available for the assessment of language. Some commonly used formal tests, each with a brief summary of its focus and purpose, are listed in Table 7-4. A more comprehensive list can be found on the American Speech-Language-Hearing Association (ASHA) website. Access at http://www.asha.org/assessments.aspx or search for "Directory of Speech-Language Pathology Assessment Instruments" from the homepage.

With so many tests to choose from, it is sometimes difficult to select the most appropriate one. Each test is unique and useful in a different situation. There is no one test, or even set of tests, that is right for all children or all clinicians. Be thoughtful when selecting appropriate testing materials. Questions to consider include:

- How old is the client?
- What are the specific language concerns that need to be evaluated
- What is the client's ethnic background?
- How much time is available to administer the test?
- How well will the client be able to participate in testing?
- Is an insurance company, employer, or other agency requiring a certain test?

In all situations, administer only the most recent edition of a test. Also become familiar with each test's uses, strengths, and weaknesses. See Form 1-1, "Test Evaluation Form," in Chapter 1 for guidelines on evaluating formal assessment instruments.

INFORMAL ASSESSMENT

Informal assessment is an important component of a complete language evaluation. It allows the clinician to assess certain aspects of language more deeply than formal assessment allows, and it provides the opportunity to view a client's functional use of language in natural contexts. Relevant cognitive abilities can also be considered. In some situations, informal assessment data are the primary source of diagnostic information.

Informal tasks can be receptively or expressively based. They often require a certain amount of creativity on the part of the clinician to assess targeted behaviors. A small sampling of activities some clinicians use to assess language skills informally is presented in the following list. The techniques used will depend upon many things, including the age of the child, his or her current linguistic abilities, and the specific behaviors to be assessed.

- Ask the child to follow verbal commands.
- Ask the child to count, recite the alphabet, or perform other serial tasks.

TABLE 7-4   Several Formal Tests for the Assessment of Language

TEST	REFERENCE	ADMINISTRATION TIME (MINUTES)	AGE (YEARS; MONTH)	RECEPTIVE/ EXPRESSIVE	AREAS OF ASSESSMENT
Bankson Language Test (BLT-2)	Bankson (1990)	30	3;0–6;11	Expressive	Semantic, syntactic, pragmatic, morphologic
Battelle Developmental Inventory (BDI-2)	Newborg (2004)	60–120	birth–7;11	Both	Preverbal, early language, plus other domains
Bayley Scales of Infant and Toddler Development (Bayley-III)	Bayley (2005)	30–60	0;1–3;6	Both	Preverbal, early language, plus other domains
Boehm Test of Basic Concepts (Boehm-3)	Boehm (2001)	30–45	K–2nd	Receptive	Basic concepts, primarily semantic
Clinical Evaluation of Language Fundamentals (CELF-5)	Semel, Wiig, & Secord (2013)	30–60	5;0–21;11	Both	Semantic, syntactic, phonologic memory
Comprehensive Assessment of Spoken Language (CASL)	Carrow-Woolfolk (1999)	30–45	3;0–21;11	Both	Semantic, syntactic, supralinguistic, pragmatic
Comprehensive Receptive and Expressive Vocabulary Test (CREVT-3)	Wallace & Hammill (2013)	20–30	5;0–89;0	Both	Vocabulary
Evaluating Communicative Competence	Simon (1994)	45	9;0–17;0	Both	Pragmatic
Expressive One-Word Picture Vocabulary Test (EOWPVT)	Brownell (2000)	30–45	2;0–18;11	Expressive	Vocabulary
Expressive Vocabulary Test (EVT-2)	Williams (2007)	10–20	2;6–90+	Expressive	Vocabulary
Illinois Test of Psycholinguistic Abilities (ITPA-3)	Hammill, Mather, & Roberts (2001)	45–60	5;0–12;11	Expressive	Vocabulary, grammar, writing, phonologic, morphologic
Language Processing Test—Elementary (LPT-3: Elementary)	Richard & Hanner (2005)	35	5;0–11;11	Expressive	Semantic
Peabody Picture Vocabulary Test (PPVT-4)	Dunn & Dunn (2007)	10–15	2;6–90+	Receptive	Vocabulary
Preschool Language Scales (PLS-5)	Zimmerman, Steiner, & Pond (2011)	45–60	birth–7;11	Both	Preverbal, early language
Receptive-Expressive Emergent Language Test (REEL-3)	Bzoch, League, & Brown (2003)	20	0;0–3;11	Both	Preverbal, early language

TEST	REFERENCE	ADMINISTRATION TIME (MINUTES)	AGE (YEARS; MONTH)	RECEPTIVE/ EXPRESSIVE	AREAS OF ASSESSMENT
Receptive One-Word Picture Vocabulary Test (ROWPVT)	Brownell (2000)	15–20	2;0–18;11	Receptive	Vocabulary
Rossetti Infant -Toddler Language Scale	Rossetti (2006)	Varies	0;0–3;11	Both	Preverbal, early language
Test for Auditory Comprehension of Language (TACL-4)	Carrow-Woolfolk (2014)	20–30	3;0–12;11	Receptive	Vocabulary, grammar, syntax
Test for Examining Expressive Morphology (TEEM)	Shipley, Stone, & Sue (1983)	7	3;0–8;0	Expressive	Morphologic
Test of Adolescent and Adult Language (TOAL-4)	Hammill, Brown, Larsen, & Weiderholt (2007)	60–180	12;0–24;11	Both	Vocabulary, grammar, reading, writing
Test of Adolescent/Adult Word Finding (TAWF)	German (1989)	20–30	12;0–8;0	Expressive	Vocabulary
Test of Cognitive Skills (TCS/2)	CTB/McGraw Hill (1996)	50–55	6;8–18;0	Both	Verbal, nonverbal, memory
Test of Early Language Development (TELD-3)	Hresko, Reid, & Hammill (1999)	15	2:0–7:11	Both	Early language
Test of Expressive Language (TEXL)	Carrow-Woolfolk & Allen (2014)	20-30	3;0–12;11	Expressive	Vocabulary, morphemes, syntax
Test of Language Development—Intermediate (TOLD-I:3)	Hammill & Newcomer (1997)	30–60	8;0–12;11	Both	Semantic, syntactic, phonologic
Test of Language Development—Primary (TOLD-P:3)	Newcomer & Hammill (1997)	60	4;0–8;11	Both	Semantic, syntactic, phonologic
Test of Semantic Skills- Intermediate (TOSS-I)	Huisiugh, Bowers, LoGuiudice, & Orman (2003)	25-30	9;0–13;11	Both	Semantic
Test of Semantic Skills—Primary (TOSS-P)	Bowers, Huisingh, LoGiudice, & Orman (2002)	25–30	4;0–8;11	Both	Semantic
Test of Word Finding (TFW-2)	German (2000)	20–30	4;0–12;11	Expressive	Semantic
Utah Test of Language Development (UTLD-4)	Mecham (2003)	30–45	3;0–9;11	Expressive	Semantic, syntactic, morphologic, phonologic

- Ask the child to name objects or pictures. Ask the child to point to more than one of a named item. For example, "point to the *pencils*" (versus *pencil*).
- Ask the child to name items from a category, or identify a category when provided examples.
- Ask the child to describe similarities and differences of objects.
- Ask the child to place an object (e.g., a block) *over*, *under*, and *beside* the table (to sample basic prepositional understanding).
- Ask the child to describe a picture, recount an event, or tell a short story.
- Describe absurd situations and ask why they are absurd.
- Ask the child to explain how to play a game, such as Go Fish.
- Play Simon Says.
- Engage in role-playing activities. For example, pretend to serve food at a restaurant; then reverse roles.
- Ask the child to guide a blindfolded listener through a task, such as putting lids on pens.
- Present *what-if* scenarios and have the child offer solutions. For example, "What would happen if you forgot to bring your lunch to school?" or "What would you do if you found $100 in your backpack?"
- Play deductive "I'm thinking of . . ." games.

LANGUAGE SAMPLING AND ANALYSIS

Language sampling is a vital part of a complete evaluation of language. Specific procedures for collecting a language sample are described in Chapter 5. There are several aspects of collecting a language sample that are especially important for assessing language disorders:

- Collect a representative sample based on real conversation, not a contrived situation.
- Collect multiple samples.
- Vary the contexts and activities used to elicit the sample to assess different aspects of language.
- Ask others to interact with the client during the sample, such as a parent, a sibling, a friend, or a teacher. Children commonly vary their language use depending on the audience.
- Video-record the sample for later analysis.

Form 7-6, "Worksheet for Recording a Language Sample," is helpful for collecting data. The following guidelines are useful when transcribing the language sample:

- Transcribe the entire sample.
- Indicate the speaker for all utterances. For example, mark A for adult (or P for partner) and C for client or child. Create your own abbreviations as needed.
- Use phonetic symbols only to transcribe unintelligible or partially intelligible utterances. A dash (—) can also be used to indicate each unintelligible word. For example, "I want — —" indicates a four-word utterance with two unintelligible words.

- Capitalize only proper nouns and the pronoun *I*.
- Keep punctuation to a minimum.
- Indicate utterance endings with a slash (/).
- Number the client's utterances.
- Transcribe utterances consecutively from the recording. The first few utterances can be omitted because this could be considered a "warming-up" period.

A good language sample may provide the most useful information about a client's functional use of language. When analyzing the language sample, make observations about the following features of language:

- Form of language: Does the child primarily use single words, phrases, or sentences? Are the sentences of the subject-verb-object form exclusively? Are there mature negatives, interrogatives, and passive sentences? Does the child elaborate the noun or verb phrase? Is there evidence of embedding and conjoining?
- Understanding of semantic intent: Does the child respond appropriately to the various question forms (what, where, who, when, why, how)? Does the child confuse words from different semantic classes?
- Language use: Does the child display a range of illocutionary functions such as asking for information, help, and objects; replying; making statements; providing information? Does the child take conversational turns? Does the child introduce topics and maintain them through several turns? Does the child signal the status of the communication and make repairs?
- Rate of speaking: Is the rate inordinately slow or fast? Are there noticeable or lengthy pauses between the caregiver's and the child's turn? Are there noticeable or lengthy pauses between the child's adjacent utterances? Does the child use fillers frequently or pause before producing certain words? Are there frequent word substitutions?
- Sequencing: Does the child relate events in a sequential fashion based on the order of occurrence? Can the child discuss the recent past or recount stories? (Owens, 1995, p. 76)

The analysis of a language sample can be a very time-consuming endeavor. Computerized tools are helpful for analyzing samples efficiently. The clinician also benefits from having data stored electronically for future retrieval. Computer-based tools for the analysis of a language sample include:

- *Computerized Profiling* (Long, Fey, & Channell, 2006)
- *Systematic Analysis of Language Transcripts (SALT)* (Miller, 2012)
- *The CHILDES Project: Tools for Analyzing Talk* (MacWhinney, 2000)

ASSESSMENT OF MORPHOLOGIC SKILLS

Morphology is the study of how morphemes (the smallest units of meaning) are combined to form meaning. Free morphemes are words that can stand alone to convey meaning (e.g., *case* or *boy*), whereas bound morphemes (e.g., *-s* or *-ing*) are word segments that must be attached to a free morpheme to convey meaning. Grammatic morphemes are free or bound morphemes with little or no meaning when produced by themselves, such as articles (*a, the,* etc.), prepositions (*in, at,* etc.), and grammatical word segments (*-ing, -ed,* etc.).

Bound morphemes can be either derivational or inflectional. Derivational morphemes are those that change the meaning and grammatical class of a word (e.g., the verb *vote* to the noun *voter,* or the adjective *quick* to the adverb *quickly*). Inflectional morphemes are those that affect nuances of meaning, but not the basic meaning or grammatical class of a word (e.g., the noun *apple* still refers to the same fruit when an *-s* is added to form *apples*). An extensive list of bound morphemes is presented in Table 7-5. The clinician can use the information in this table to identify which features a client is using appropriately and which features are not used or have not yet been sampled.

TABLE 7-5   Derivational and Inflectional Morphemes

	SUFFIXES	
PREFIXES	**DERIVATIONAL**	**INFLECTIONAL**
a- (in, on, into, in a manner)	-able (ability, tendency, likelihood)	-ed (past)
bi- (twice, two)	-al (pertaining to, like, action, process)	-ing (at present)
de- (negative, descent, reversal)		-s (plural)
ex- (out of, from, thoroughly)	-ance (action, state)	-s (third-person marker)
inner- (reciprocal, between, together)	-ation (denoting action in a noun)	
	-en (used to form verbs from adjectives)	-'s (possession)
mis- (ill, negative, wrong)		
out- (extra, beyond, not)	-ence (action, state)	
over- (over)	-er (used as an agentive ending)	
post- (behind, after)	-est (superlative)	
pre- (to, before)	-ful (full, tending)	
pro- (in favor of)	-ible (ability, tendency, likelihood)	
re- (again, backward motion)	-ish (belonging to)	
semi- (half)	-ism (doctrine, state, practice)	
super- (superior)	-ist (one who does something)	
trans- (across, beyond)	-ity (used for abstract nouns)	
tri- (three)	-ive (tendency or connection)	
un- (not, reversal)	-ize (action, policy)	
under- (under)	-less (without)	
	-ly (used to form adverbs)	
	-ment (action, product, means, state)	
	-ness (quality, state)	
	-or (used as an agentive ending)	
	-ous (full of, having, like)	
	-y (inclined to)	

The "Assessment of Morphologic Features," Form 7-7, is provided to help identify the morphologic structures a client uses correctly and incorrectly. This is a challenging task because it is difficult at times to structure opportunities to produce the various target features. We recommend using the language sample to identify as many forms as possible, then using structured questions to elicit those forms that were not sampled through the language sample.

DETERMINING MEAN LENGTH OF UTTERANCE

The mean length of utterance (MLU) is the average number of morphemes (or words, as will be described later) that a client produces in an utterance. MLU provides important information about language development, and it is one indicator of a language delay or disorder. Generally, a normal child's chronological age (up to age 5) will correspond closely to his or her MLU. For example, a normally developing 4-year, 3-month-old child will often exhibit a MLU of approximately 4.3 (plus or minus a few tenths). This method of interpretation is very general and must, of course, be used with caution when diagnosing or ruling out language disorders. Remember, children develop language at varying rates.

Roger Brown's (1973) classic study of three preschool-age children—Adam, Eve, and Sarah—provided the foundation for much of our current understanding of the relationship between MLU and language development.

Although Brown's research was based on only three subjects, subsequent research has largely validated his early findings. MLU is considered to be a valid and reliable index of general language development. Brown's developmental stages are presented in Table 7-6. In addition to identifying stages of language development, Brown also identified a sequence of normal development for 14 grammatical morphemes. His findings are based on 90% mastery of each morpheme. His sequence of morphologic development is presented in Table 7-7.

TABLE 7-6   Brown's Stages of Language Development

STAGE	AGE	MLU	LANGUAGE DEVELOPMENT
I	12–26 mos. (1;0–2;2 yrs)	1.0–2.0	First words. Linear simple sentences.
II	27–30 mos. (2;3–2;6 yrs)	2.0–2.5	Linear simple sentences with emergence of grammatical morphemes.
III	31–34 mos. (2;7–2;10 yrs)	2.5–3.0	Noun phrases and auxiliary verbs. Emergence of different sentence modalities (e.g., questions, negatives, imperatives).
IV	35–40 mos. (2;11–3;4 yrs)	3.0–3.75	Emergence of complex sentences. Embedding of sentence elements.
V	41–46 mos. (3;5–3;10 yrs)	3.75–4.5	Compound sentences.

Source: Brown (1973).

TABLE 7-7   Order of Acquisition of Brown's 14 Grammatical Morphemes

STAGE	AGE (MONTHS)	MORPHEMES	EXAMPLE
II	27–30	Present progressive -ing	She's cry*ing*.
		Preposition in	Ball *in* box.
		Preposition on	Dog *on* bed.
		Plural -s	My toy*s*.
		Irregular past tense	I *ran*.
III	31–34	Possessive -'s	Daddy*'s* shoe.
		Uncontractible copula be	He *was* sad.
III–IV	31–46	Articles a, the, an	*The* cat ate *a* rat.
V	41–46	Regular past tense -ed	He jump*ed* up.
		Regular third-person singular -s	Daddy drive*s* fast.
		Irregular third-person singular	We *did* it.
		Uncontractible auxiliary	Mommy *was* sleeping.
		Contractible copula be	She*'s* funny. They *are* funny.
		Contractible auxiliary	He*'s* eating. They *are* eating.

Source: Brown (1973).

Using a larger number of subjects, Miller and Chapman (1981) conducted a study in which MLUs from conversational speech samples were compared with children's chronological ages. Their findings are presented in Table 7-8. The table outlines predicted MLUs and standard deviations (SDs) for children 18 months through 5 years of age. The sample group in Miller and Chapman's study consisted of 123 middle- to upper-class midwestern children in Madison, Wisconsin. As with any normative data, use caution when applying the information to children who are dissimilar to the population studied.

Before calculating MLU, it is important to obtain a sizeable speech-language sample. The more utterances sampled, the more accurate the MLU findings will be. (Information on obtaining speech samples can be found in Chapter 5.) After transcribing the sample, the clinician may use the following guidelines for counting morphemes per utterance (based on Brown, 1973; Lund & Duchan, 1993).

Count as one morpheme:

- Grammatical morphemes that are whole words (nouns, verbs, articles, prepositions)
- Auxiliaries (e.g., *is, will, have, must, would*)
- Diminutives (e.g., *mommy, doggy*)
- Catenatives (e.g., *wanna, gonna*)
- Uninflected lexical morphemes (e.g., *run, fall*)
- Inflections (possessive -*'s*, plural -*s*, third-person singular -*s*, regular past-tense -*ed*, progressive -*ing*)
- Irregular past tense (e.g., *did, was, got, went*)

TABLE 7-8   Developmental Norms for Mean Length of Utterance

AGE (YR.;MO.)	PREDICTED MLU	PREDICTED MLU, 1 SD (MIDDLE 68%)	PREDICTED MLU, 2 SDs (MIDDLE 95%)
1;6	1.31	0.99–1.64	0.66–1.96
1;9	1.62	1.23–2.01	0.85–2.39
2;0	1.92	1.47–2.37	1.02–2.82
2;3	2.23	1.72–2.74	1.21–3.25
2;6	2.54	1.97–3.11	1.40–3.68
2;9	2.85	2.22–3.48	1.58–4.12
3;0	3.16	2.47–3.85	1.77–4.55
3;3	3.47	2.71–4.23	1.96-4.98
3;6	3.78	2.96–4.60	2.15–5.41
3;9	4.09	3.21–4.97	2.33–5.85
4;0	4.40	3.46–5.34	2.52–6.28
4;3	4.71	3.71–5.71	2.71–6.71
4;6	5.02	3.96–6.08	2.90–7.15
4;9	5.32	4.20–6.45	3.07–7.57
5;0	5.63	4.44–6.82	3.26–8.00

(SD is standard deviation.)
Source: Adapted from "The Relation Between Age and Mean Length of Utterance in Morphemes," by J. F. Miller and R. Chapman, 1981, *Journal of Speech and Hearing Research*, 24, 154–161. Copyright 1981 by the American Speech-Language-Hearing Association. Reprinted with permission.

- Contractions (e.g., *I'll, can't*) only if individual segments do not occur elsewhere in the sample. If either of the constituent parts of the contraction occur elsewhere, the contraction is counted as two morphemes.
- Plurals that do not occur in singular form (e.g., *us, clothes*)
- Gerunds and participles that are not part of a verb phrase (e.g., She was *tired. Swimming* is fun.)
- Stuttered words (e.g., *My, my, my . . .*)
- Compound words (e.g., *birthday, see-saw, belly-button*)
- Single words or phrases (e.g., *Hi. No. Yeah.*)
- Proper names
- Ritualized reduplications (e.g., quack-quack, choo-choo)

Count as more than one morpheme:

- Inflected forms: regular and irregular plural nouns, possessive nouns, third-person singular verbs, present participle and past participle when part of the verb phrase, regular past-tense verbs, reflexive pronouns, comparative and superlative adverbs, adjectives

- Contractions only when one or both of the constituent parts occurs separately elsewhere in the sample (e.g., *It's* if *it* or *is* occurs elsewhere)
- Repeated words only if the word is produced for emphasis (e.g., *No, no, no!* is counted as three morphemes)

Do not count:

- Partial utterances
- Imitations that immediately follow a model utterance
- Elliptical answers to questions
- Unintelligible utterances
- Rote passages (e.g., nursery rhymes, songs)
- False starts and reformations
- Noises, unless they are meaningfully integrated into an utterance (e.g., She went *kkkhhh.*)
- Fillers (e.g., *um, oh, you know*)
- Counting, sequences, or other enumerations (e.g., *cow, dog, pig, horse*)

After the morphemes in each utterance are counted, the MLU can be calculated. The traditional method of calculating MLU is to divide the number of morphemes by the number of utterances. For example:

$$\frac{150 \text{ morphemes}}{50 \text{ utterances}} = 3.0 \text{ MLU}$$

Many clinicians also calculate the MLU for words by dividing the number of words by the number of utterances. This calculation does *not* reflect the use of bound morphemes (e.g., *-ing, -ed, -s*); therefore, the MLU for words will always be equal to or smaller than the MLU for morphemes. For example, the same 100-word sample might have:

$$\frac{100 \text{ words}}{50 \text{ utterances}} = 2.0 \text{ MLU-words}$$

$$\frac{120 \text{ morphemes}}{50 \text{ utterances}} = 2.0 \text{ MLU-morphemes}$$

MLU is a gross but reasonably accurate index of grammatical development up to four to five morphemes (Brown, 1973). It is considered gross because the MLU is a general measure that tells us nothing about specific forms or structures used. However, the use of both free and bound morphemes is needed for utterance lengths to increase.

ASSESSMENT OF PRAGMATIC SKILLS

Pragmatics is the study of the use of language in communicative interactions. Pragmatic behaviors are situationally and environmentally specific; therefore, it is helpful to assess pragmatic skills in a variety of situations. Form 7-8, "Assessment of Pragmatic Skills," allows the clinician to assess 15 pragmatic behaviors in a semistructured manner. Several suggestions are provided for each behavior for eliciting pragmatic responses.

ASSESSMENT OF SEMANTIC SKILLS

Semantics is the study of language meaning, which can be expressed verbally, vocally, and gesturally. Meaning is complex and strongly influenced by context. Word definitions, syntactic structures, environmental situations, speaker relationships, pragmatic behaviors, and suprasegmental aspects of language intertwine to give language its meaning. Imagine greeting a friend by saying *starch* instead of *hi*. Even though the friend knows what the word *starch* means, it would have no meaning in such a social context.

Assessing semantic skills is difficult because of this inherent complexity and also due to a lack of normative standards. In general, when assessing semantic skills, look for *variety*. The more mature the speaker, the greater the range of words and word types the speaker should exhibit. Children with semantic language disorders usually demonstrate limited vocabularies and difficulty integrating semantic information with other aspects of language, particularly grammar.

Some clinicians evaluate language according to semantic relations. The most common semantic relations are presented in Table 7-9. When categorizing a language sample according to semantic relations, note the range of semantic categories used by the client. A limited range would indicate a possible language disorder.

TABLE 7-9   Common Semantic Relations

RELATION	EXAMPLE
Nomination	This book
Nonexistence	No shoe
Agent + object	Mommy book
Agent + action	Daddy work (daddy is working)
Action + object	Read book
Nonexistence	No book
Action + indirect object	Kiss mommy
Recurrence	More juice
Cessation	All done
Action + locative	Go outside
Entity + locative	Daddy here
Possessor + possession	Daddy phone (daddy's phone)
Attribution	Big boat
Agent + action + object	Mommy tie shoe
Agent + action + locative	Daddy go outside
Rejection	No juice (I don't want juice)
Denial	Not tired
Instrumental	Cut knife (Cut with a knife)
Notice	Hi mommy

Form 7-9, "Assessment of Semantic Skills," is a worksheet for the informal assessment of semantic abilities. The clinician may also want to use other materials in this book, such as "Pictures," "Narratives," or "Conversation Starters for Eliciting a Language Sample" (see Chapter 5). Playing games such as Simon Says, telling jokes, and looking through picture books may also be helpful. While conversing with the child, try using words inappropriately or making nonsense remarks and note the child's response. When assessing semantic skills, note the following:

- Number of different words
- Unusual use of words
- Incorrect word substitutions
- Overgeneralizations
- Undergeneralizations
- Frequent use of empty words such as *thing* or *that*
- Word-finding problems, such as circumlocutions, repetitions, and frequent pauses
- Types of words (e.g., function, prepositions, negatives, descriptive)
- Excessive use of pronouns
- Frequent use of routinized expressions such as *you know*
- Unusual sentence formulations
- Difficulty with word comprehension
- Difficulty with sentence comprehension
- Poor understanding of nonliteral forms (e.g., idioms, metaphors, proverbs)
- Poor understanding of common slang terms

ASSESSMENT OF SYNTACTIC SKILLS

Syntax refers to sentence structure. Our English language is based on many syntactic structures, making syntax a difficult area to assess. A solid understanding of the basic syntactic elements of language is necessary before any type of analysis can be completed. The various parts of speech are summarized in the following list. For more in-depth study, consult a book on English grammar and form.

There are eight major parts of speech:

- Noun: A word that represents a person, place, or thing (e.g., *flower, family, anger*)
- Pronoun: A word that takes the place of a noun (e.g., *I, it, this, which*)
- Adjective: A word that modifies a noun or pronoun, usually by description (e.g., *happy, long, difficult*)
- Verb: A word that indicates action or a state of being (e.g., *run, make, have, am*)
- Adverb: A word that modifies a verb, adjective, or another adverb by answering the question *how? when? where? why?* or *to what extent?* (e.g., *badly, loudly, well*)
- Preposition: A word that shows the relationship of the noun or pronoun to some other word in the sentence (e.g., *in, by, with, throughout*)

- Conjunction: A word that joins a phrase, clause, sentence, or other words together (e.g., *and, but, because, or*)
- Interjection: A stand-alone word that expresses emotion (e.g., *ouch, oh, yeah, bravo*)

These foundational parts of speech are combined into units. The most basic units are phrases and clauses. Phrases are groups of related words that do not contain both a subject and a predicate. These include:

- Noun phrase: A group of words that acts as a noun (*That book* is funny. *Going to the zoo* was the highlight. *The boy in the middle* is David.)
- Verb phrase: A group of words that acts as a verb (The project *will be finished* soon. Good mothers *discipline with love and patience*.)
- Prepositional phrase: A group of words that acts as a preposition (the girl *in front*, a tree *in the park*)
- Adjective phrase: A group of words that modifies a noun or pronoun (*Tired from the long day*, he fell asleep. The girl *with the long hair*)

Clauses are groups of related words that have both a subject and a predicate. There are two types:

- Main clause or independent clause: A grammatically complete unit that can stand alone and make sense (*She went to the store*, and *she bought same cookies. The ball rolled away* and landed under the table.)
- Subordinate clause or dependent clause: A unit that cannot stand alone and make sense without being joined to a main clause (*Because it is late*, I must leave now. Sarah wrote *that you were coming*.)

Clauses and phrases are combined to form sentences. Sentences are generally classified according to structure or function. There are four basic sentence structures:

- Simple sentence: A sentence that contains one main clause (*He is old. Why are you doing that?*)
- Compound sentence: A sentence that contains two or more related main clauses (*Mommy made the cake and daddy made the punch. You like green; I like blue.*)
- Complex sentence: A sentence that has one main clause and one or more subordinate clauses (*Even though it was late, <u>mom let us stay up to watch the fireworks</u>. After we went home, <u>we fell asleep quickly</u> just as you said we would.* [main clauses are underlined])
- Compound-complex sentence: A sentence that has two or more main clauses and one or more subordinate clauses (*Because the weather was nice, <u>the children played and I planted flowers</u>. If it's heads, <u>you win</u>; if it's tails, <u>I win</u>.* [main clauses are underlined]).

Sentence classification according to function is as follows:

- Declarative: A sentence that states a fact or makes an assertion (*I am going now. You're late.*)
- Interrogative: A sentence that asks a question (*What happened? Whose is it?*)
- Imperative: A sentence that gives a command or makes a request. The subject "you" is often understood and not expressed (*Go away! Please give this to your teacher.*).
- Exclamatory: A sentence that conveys a strong feeling. In some cases, the subject is understood without being expressed (*How thoughtful! We were so surprised!*).

The most predominant and basic order of words in a sentence is subject-verb-object (S-V-O) word order (*I went home. The children are playing soccer.*) This is an *active sentence* format in which the subject performs an action. Normally developing speakers learn to rearrange the subject/verb/object elements. For example, a *passive sentence* is based on an object-verb-subject format (*The boy was bit by a dog. The crops were destroyed by the rain.*)

The most significant strides in semantic aspects of language development are made during the first 5 years of life. Table 7-10 outlines the developmental stages of early syntactic acquisition. The more complex forms just described continue to be learned well into the elementary and middle school years.

In the preceding section on assessment of semantic skills, it was stated that variety is one of the best indicators of a child's language abilities. The same is true when analyzing semantic features of language. Look for a variety of word types, phrases, clauses, and sentence

TABLE 7-10 Developmental Stages in Early Syntactic Acquisition

STAGE	DEVELOPMENTAL FEATURES	MLU
I	*Semantic roles and syntactic relations:* Characterized by thematic relationships among multiple single words and by true word combinations (agent + action, action + object, agent + object, action + locative, entity + locative, possessor + possession, entity + attribute, demonstrative + entity)	1.0–2.0
II	*Modulated relations:* Characterized by the emerging use of grammatical morphemes (present progressive, plural -s, *in*)	2.0–2.5
III	*Modalities of simple sentences:* Characterized by the emergence of simple clauses and further acquisition of grammatical morphemes (possessive, *on*)	2.4–3.25
IV	*Advanced sentence modalities (embedding):* Characterized by multiple-clause utterances formed with connectives (e.g., *and*), or through complementation (e.g., "I wanna [want to] . . .") or relativization (e.g., *that*)	3.25–3.75
V	*Categorization (coordination):* Characterized by further differentiation of words within word classes (mass/count noun, transitive/intransitive, verbs, pronouns, prepositions) and acquisition of grammatical morphemes (articles, irregular past, regular past, contractile copula "be," regular third-person singular)	3.75–4.0+
VI (V+)	*Complex structures:* Characterized by further acquisition of grammatical morphemes (contractible auxiliary "be," uncontractible copula "be," irregular third-person singular, uncontractible auxiliary "be"), complex structures and sentence transformations, and ability to deal with structural ambiguities	4.0+

Source: *Language Assessment and Intervention for the Learning Disabled* (2nd ed., p. 297), by E. H. Wiig and E. Semel, 1984, Columbus, OH: Merrill. Copyright 1984 by Merrill. Reprinted with permission.

types. Also look for patterns of correct usage and incorrect usage. Children with language impairments are likely to demonstrate:

- Simple, less elaborate noun phrases
- Shorter utterances
- Limited range of sentence types
- Overreliance on the S-V-O sentence structure
- Lack of sentence complexity
- Confusion with pronoun references
- Misinterpretations of passive sentences

Form 7-10, "Assessment of Syntactic Skills," is a worksheet for identifying syntactic features utterance by utterance. There are also computerized programs that are particularly helpful for evaluating syntactic elements of language. Several were listed earlier in this chapter in the section as language sampling and analysis.

MAKING A DIAGNOSIS

In each subsection of this chapter, criteria for diagnosing the particular element of language addressed are provided. There are also some general guidelines that are helpful for making an appropriate diagnosis. A child with a language disorder will typically demonstrate one or more of the following deficiencies:

- Delayed onset of language
- Limited amount of language
- Deficiencies in syntactic, semantic, and morphologic components
- Deficient cognitive skills
- Academic problems
- Limited language comprehension
- Poor listening skills
- Limited conversational skills
- Limited ability to narrate experiences
- A general inappropriate use of language

CONCLUDING COMMENTS

Spoken language is complex, varied, and often challenging to evaluate. A combination of formal and informal assessment measures usually provides the most complete diagnostic information. For children who are still in the early developmental stages of language, parental input and involvement is particularly important. A representative language sample is valuable for understanding a client's functional use of language, including pragmatic, semantic, syntactic, and morphologic components.

SOURCES OF ADDITIONAL INFORMATION

Print Sources

Bernstein, D. K., & Tiegerman-Farber, E. (2008). *Language and communication disorders in children* (6th ed.). Needham Heights, MA: Allyn & Bacon.

Hughes, D., McGillivray, L., & Schmidek, M. (1997). *Guide to narrative language: Procedures for assessment.* Eau Claire, WI: Thinking Publications.

McLaughlin, S. (2006). *Introduction to language development.* (2nd ed.). Clifton Park, NY: Cengage Learning.

Owens, R. E. (2013). *Language disorders: A functional approach to assessment and intervention* (6th ed.). San Antonio, TX: Pearson.

Vinson, B. P. (2012). *Language disorders across the lifespan* (3rd ed.). Clifton Park, NY: Cengage Learning

Electronic Sources

American Speech-Language-Hearing Association:
http://www.asha.org

Speech-Language_Therapy Dot Com:
http://www.speech-language-therapy.com

"Common Care Early Language Screener" app by Smarty Ears

Form 7-1.

Worksheet for Analyzing Child–Caregiver Interactions

Child: _____   DOB: _____

Caregiver: _____   Relationship to Child: _____

Date: _____   Location: _____

Instructions: Use the questions below to analyze child–caregiver interactions. Include as much detail as possible.

Child Behaviors

In general, how does the child interact with the caregiver?

Does the child make eye contact with the caregiver?

With you, the clinician?

What gestures does the child use?

Facial expressions?

Does the child seem to understand words?

Sentences?

Conversation?

(continues)

Form 7-1. continued

What words does the child understand?

Sentences?

What kinds of instructions is the child able to follow?

Does the child answer simple questions?

Transcribe spontaneous vocalizations?

Words:

Multiword utterances:

How does the child respond to you, the clinician (e.g., nonverbal, withdrawn, answers questions)?

How does the child express wants?

Frustration?

Happiness?

(continues)

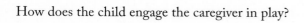

Form 7-1. continued

Can you make inferences about communicative intent?

What toys or objects is the child most interested in?

How does the child engage the caregiver in play?

What can be noted about the quality of the child's play?

Does the child demonstrate knowledge of the following cognitive concepts:

Immediate imitation?

Deferred imitation?

Means-end?

Object permanence?

Functional use of objects?

Symbolic play with objects?

(continues)

LANGUAGE
IN CHILDREN

Form 7-1. continued

Describe any antisocial behaviors observed.

Caregiver Behaviors

In general, how does the caregiver interact with the child?

How do the caregiver's communication patterns differ from typical child-directed speech?

Voice:

Fluency:

Syntactic aspects:

Semantic aspects:

Phonologic aspects:

Pragmatic aspects:

Describe the caregiver's eye contact with the child.

(continues)

Form 7-1. continued

Describe the caregiver's use of gestures.

Facial expressions?

What does the caregiver talk about most?

What types of questions does the caregiver ask the child?

Does the caregiver use pauses to allow the child to respond?

Does the caregiver repeat salient words and concepts?

Does the caregiver talk about things that are immediately present or visible?

(continues)

LANGUAGE
IN CHILDREN

Form 7-1. continued

Does the caregiver talk about things that are not immediately present or visible?

How does the caregiver engage the child in play?

What can be noted about how the caregiver plays with the child?

Do the caregiver and child exhibit joint attention?

How well does the caregiver interpret nonverbal communications?

Unintelligible verbal communications?

(continues)

Form 7-1. continued

What does the caregiver do when the child does not respond to a question or command?

How effectively does the caregiver expand on what the child has said?

What behaviors does the caregiver demonstrate that may be conducive to language development?

What behaviors does the caregiver demonstrate that may *not* be conducive to language development?

LANGUAGE
IN CHILDREN

Form 7-2.

Language Development Survey

Child's Name: _____   Birth Date: _____ Age: _____

Parent's Name: _____   Date: _____

Instructions: Please circle each word your child says spontaneously (not imitating). Do not include words your child understands but does not say. It's all right to count words that aren't pronounced clearly.

FOODS

apple
banana
bread
butter
cake
candy
cereal
cheese
chips
coffee
cookie
crackers
drink
egg
food
grapes
gum
hamburger
hot dog
ice cream
juice
meat
milk
orange
pizza
pop
pretzel
raisins
soda

soup
spaghetti
toast
water
_____
_____
_____

TOYS

ball
balloon
blocks
book
bubble
crayons
doll
present
slide
swing
teddy bear
_____
_____
_____

OUTDOORS

flower
house
moon
rain
sidewalk

snow
star
street
sun
tree
_____
_____
_____

ANIMALS

bear
bee
bird
bug
bunny
cat
chicken
cow
dog
duck
elephant
fish
frog
horse
monkey
pig
puppy
snake
tiger
turkey

turtle
_____
_____
_____

BODY PARTS

arm
belly
bottom
chin
ear
elbow
eye
face
finger
foot
hair
hand
knee
leg
mouth
neck
nose
teeth
thumb
toe
tummy
_____
_____
_____

PLACES

church
home
hospital
library
McDonalds
park
school
store
zoo
_____
_____
_____

ACTIONS

bath
breakfast
bring
catch
clap
close
come
cough
cut
dance
dinner
eat
feed
finish
fix

(continues)

Adapted from "The Language Development Survey: A Screening Tool for Delayed Language in Toddlers," by L. Rescorla, 1989, *Journal of Speech and Hearing Disorders, 54*, pp. 587–599. Copyright by the American Speech-Language Hearing Association. Reprinted with permission.

LANGUAGE IN CHILDREN

Form 7-2. continued

get
give
go
have
help
hit
hug
jump
kick
kiss
knock
look
love
lunch
make
nap
outside
patty-cake
peek-a-boo
pee-pee
poo-poo
push
read
ride
run
see
show
sing
sit
sleep
stop
take
throw
tickle
walk
want
wash
_____
_____
_____

HOUSEHOLD

bathtub
bed
blanket
bottle
bowl
chair
clock
crib
cup
door
floor
fork
glass
knife
light
mirror
phone
pillow
plate
potty
radio
room
sink
soap
sofa
spoon
stairs
table
towel
trash
TV
window
_____
_____
_____
_____

PERSONAL

bath

brush
comb
glasses
key
money
paper
pen
pencil
penny
tissue
toothbrush
umbrella
watch
_____
_____
_____

PEOPLE

aunt
baby
boy
brother
daddy
doctor
girl
grandma
grandpa
lady
man
mommy
own name
pet name
uncle
_____
_____
_____

CLOTHES

belt
boots

coat
diaper
dress
gloves
hat
jacket
mittens
pajamas
pants
shirt
shoes
slippers
sneakers
socks
sweater
_____
_____
_____
_____

VEHICLES

bike
boat
bus
car
motorbike
plane
stroller
train
truck
_____
_____
_____

MODIFIERS

all done
all gone
all right
bad
big

black
blue
broken
clean
cold
dark
dirty
down
good
happy
heavy
hot
hungry
little
mine
more
open
pretty
red
shut
stinky
that
this
tired
up
wet
white
yellow
yucky
yummy
_____
_____
_____

OTHERS

A,B,C, etc.
animal sounds
away
boo-boo
bye-bye

(continues)

Form 7-2. continued

curse words	night-night	thank you	yes	_____
here	no	there	you	_____
hi/hello	off	under	1, 2, 3, etc.	_____
in	on	welcome	TV/movie	_____
me	out	what	character names	_____
meow	please	where	_____	_____
my	'scuse me	why	_____	
myself	shut up	woof-woof	_____	

Does your child combine two or more words in phrases? (e.g., *more cookie*, *car bye-bye*, etc.)

yes _____ no _____

Please list below **three** of your child's longest and best sentences or phrases:

1. _____

2. _____

3. _____

LANGUAGE IN CHILDREN

Form 7-3.

Assessment of Language Development

Name: _____ Age: _____ Date: _____

Examiner's Name: _____

Instructions: Mark a plus (+) or a check (✔) if the child *does* exhibit the behavior, a minus (−) or a zero (0) if the child *does not* exhibit the behavior, and an *S* if the child exhibits the behavior *sometimes*. This form can be used during informal observation or completed by a parent or knowledgeable caregiver. Because children develop at different rates, avoid using strict application of the age approximations. The time intervals are provided only as a general guideline for age appropriateness.

0–6 Months

_____ Frequently coos, gurgles, and makes pleasure sounds

_____ Uses a different cry to express different needs

_____ Smiles when spoken to

_____ Recognizes voices

_____ Localizes to sound

_____ Listens to speech

_____ Uses the phonemes /b/, /p/, and /m/ in babbling

_____ Uses sounds or gestures to indicate wants

_____ Responds to *no* and changes in tone of voice

7–12 Months

_____ Understands *no* and *hot*

_____ Responds to simple requests

_____ Understands and responds to own name

_____ Recognizes words for common items (e.g., cup, shoe, juice)

_____ Babbles using long and short groups of sounds

_____ Uses a large variety of sounds in babbling

_____ Imitates some adult speech sounds and intonation patterns

_____ Uses speech sounds rather than only crying to get attention

_____ Listens when spoken to

_____ Uses sound approximations

_____ Begins to change babbling to jargon

(continues)

Form 7-3. continued

7–12 Months (continued)

_____ Uses speech intentionally for the first time

_____ Uses nouns almost exclusively

_____ Has an expressive vocabulary of one to three words

_____ Uses characteristic gestures or vocalizations to express wants

13–18 Months

_____ Imitates individual words

_____ Uses adult-like intonation patterns

_____ Uses echolalia and jargon

_____ Omits some initial consonants and almost all final consonants

_____ Produces mostly unintelligible speech

_____ Follows simple commands

_____ Receptively identifies one to three body parts

_____ Has an expressive vocabulary of 3 to 20 or more words (mostly nouns)

_____ Combines gestures and vocalization

_____ Makes requests for more of desired items

19–24 Months

_____ Uses words more frequently than jargon

_____ Has an expressive vocabulary of 50 to 100 or more words

_____ Has a receptive vocabulary of 300 or more words

_____ Starts to combine nouns with verbs and nouns with adjectives

_____ Begins to use pronouns

_____ Maintains unstable voice control

_____ Uses appropriate intonation for questions

_____ Is approximately 25–50% intelligible to strangers

_____ Asks and answers "What's that?" questions

_____ Enjoys listening to stories

_____ Knows five body parts

_____ Accurately names a few familiar objects

_____ Understands basic categories (e.g., toys, food)

_____ Points to pictures in a book when named

(continues)

Form 7-3. continued

2–3 Years

_____ Speech is 50–75% intelligible

_____ Understands *one* and *all*

_____ Verbalizes toilet needs (before, during, or after act)

_____ Requests items by name

_____ Identifies several body parts

_____ Follows two-part commands

_____ Asks one- to two-word questions

_____ Uses two- to four-word phrases

_____ Uses words that are general in context

_____ Continues use of echolalia when difficulties in speech are encountered

_____ Has a receptive vocabulary of 500 to 900 or more words

_____ Has an expressive vocabulary of 50 to 250 or more words

_____ Exhibits multiple grammatical errors

_____ Understands most things said to him or her

_____ Frequently exhibits repetitions—especially starters, "I," and first syllables

_____ Increases range of pitch

_____ Uses vowels correctly

_____ Consistently uses initial consonants (although some are misarticulated)

_____ Frequently omits medial consonants

_____ Frequently omits or substitutes final consonants

_____ Uses auxiliary *is* including the contracted form

_____ Uses some regular past-tense verbs, possessive morphemes, pronouns, and imperatives

_____ Maintains topic over several conversational turns

3–4 Years

_____ Understands object functions

_____ Understands opposites (stop-go, in-out, big-little)

_____ Follows two- and three-part commands

_____ Produces simple verbal analogies

_____ Uses language to express emotion

_____ Uses four to five words in sentences

(continues)

LANGUAGE IN CHILDREN

Form 7-3. continued

3–4 Years (continued)

_____ Repeats 6- to 13-syllable sentences accurately

_____ May continue to use echolalia

_____ Uses nouns and verbs most frequently

_____ Is conscious of past and future

_____ Has a receptive vocabulary of 1200 to 2000 or more words

_____ Has an expressive vocabulary of 800 to 1500 or more words

_____ May repeat self often, exhibiting blocks, disturbed breathing, and facial grimaces during speech

_____ Increases speech rate

_____ Speech is approximately 80% intelligible

_____ Appropriately uses *is, are,* and *am* in sentences

_____ Tells two events in chronological order

_____ Engages in long conversations

_____ Sentence grammar improves, although some errors still persist

_____ Uses some contractions, irregular plurals, future-tense verbs, and conjunctions

_____ Consistently uses regular plurals, possessives, and simple past-tense verbs

_____ Uses an increasing number of compound or complex sentences

4–5 Years

_____ Imitatively counts to five

_____ Continues understanding of spatial concepts

_____ Has a receptive vocabulary of 10,000 or more words

_____ Counts to 10 by rote

_____ Listens to short, simple stories and can answer questions about them

_____ Answers questions about function

_____ Uses adult-like grammar most of the time

_____ Grammatical errors primarily in irregular forms, reflexive pronouns, adverbial suffixes, and comparative/superlative inflections

_____ Has an expressive vocabulary of 900 to 2000 or more words

_____ Uses sentences of four to eight words

_____ Answers complex two-part questions

_____ Asks for word definitions

_____ Speaks at a rate of approximately 186 words per minute

_____ Reduces total number of repetitions

(continues)

Form 7-3. continued

4–5 Years (continued)

_____ Significantly reduces number of persistent sound omissions and substitutions

_____ Frequently omits medial consonants

_____ Speech is usually intelligible to strangers even though some articulation errors may persist

_____ Accurately tells about experiences at school, at friends' homes, etc.

5–6 Years

_____ Follows instructions given to a group

_____ Asks *how* questions

_____ Uses past tense and future tense appropriately

_____ Uses conjunctions

_____ Has a receptive vocabulary of approximately 13,000 words

_____ Sequentially names days of the week

_____ Counts to 30 by rote

_____ Continues to drastically increase vocabulary

_____ Uses sentence length of four to six words

_____ Reverses sounds occasionally

_____ Exchanges information and asks questions

_____ Uses sentences with details

_____ Accurately relays a story

_____ Sings entire songs and recites nursery rhymes

_____ Communicates easily with adults and other children

_____ Uses appropriate grammar in most cases

6–7 Years

_____ Understands *left* and *right*

_____ Uses increasingly more complex descriptions

_____ Engages in conversations

_____ Has a receptive vocabulary of approximately 20,000 words

_____ Uses a sentence length of approximately six words

_____ Understands most concepts of time

_____ Counts to 100 by rote

_____ Uses most morphologic markers appropriately

_____ Uses passive voice appropriately

Form 7-4.

Parent Questionnaire for Early Language Development

Child's Name: _____ DOB: _____ Date: _____

Parent's Name: _____ Relationship to Child: _____

Number of People Living in Child's Home: _____

Age and Gender of Siblings: _____

Instructions: Answer each question with as much detail as possible. Add any additional information you may think relevant after each question.

Yes No

☐ ☐ Do you understand your child's nonverbal communication (e.g., pointing, fussing)? Describe nonverbal techniques used:

_____

☐ ☐ Do you understand your child's verbal communication? If no, why not? _____

☐ ☐ Does your child attend daycare or preschool? If yes, number of hours/week: _____

_____

Number of other children _____ Number of tearchers _____

☐ ☐ Does your child make speech sounds? Please describe: _____

_____

☐ ☐ Does your child use any words? Please list: _____

_____

☐ ☐ Does your child combine words? Please list: _____

_____

☐ ☐ Does your child imitate facial expressions?

☐ ☐ Does your child imitate speech sounds?

☐ ☐ Does your child imitate behaviors he or she observed at an earlier time (not immediately following the model)?

☐ ☐ Can your child point to common objects when you name them (e.g., using picture books)?

☐ ☐ Does your child understand you when you talk to him or her?

☐ ☐ Does your child answer simple questions?

☐ ☐ Does your child respond to simple commands (e.g., "Get your cup.")?

(continues)

LANGUAGE IN CHILDREN

Form 7-4. continued

Yes	No	
☐	☐	Does your child make eye contact with you?
☐	☐	Does your child smile?
☐	☐	Does your child play well with others?
☐	☐	Does your child play well alone?
☐	☐	Does your child seem to understand the functions of objects (e.g., a cup is for drinking)?
☐	☐	Does your child ask questions?

How does your child get your attention?

How does your child communicate wants and needs?

With whom does your child spend a majority of the day?

What kinds of play activities does your child engage in?

Describe a typical day (include details):

Form 7-5.

Checklist for an Informal Assessment of Language

Name: _____ Age: _____ Date: _____

Examiner's Name: _____

Instructions: Mark a plus (+) or a check (✔) if the child does exhibit the behavior, a minus (−) or a zero (0) if the child does not exhibit the behavior, and an *S* if the child exhibits the behavior *sometimes*. Make comments about what the child does on the right-hand side of the form. If a specific behavior is not assessed, leave the line blank. This form can be used during informal observation or completed by a parent or knowledgeable caregiver.

_____ The child takes turns during communication _____
_____

_____ The child enjoys playing with other children _____
_____

_____ The child enjoys playing with his or her parents _____
_____

_____ The child enjoys playing with his or her siblings _____
_____

_____ The child usually plays alone _____
_____

_____ The child plays silently _____
_____

_____ The child talks during play activities _____
_____

_____ The child acts out common activities (e.g., plays house, plays store) _____
_____

_____ The child uses play objects that are similar (in size, looks, etc.) to the true objects (e.g., a saucepan for a drum) _____
_____

_____ The child uses play objects in a realistic manner (e.g., uses a toy dump truck in the way intended)
_____

_____ The child looks at picture books page by page from front to back _____
_____

(continues)

Form 7-5. continued

———————— The child explores a variety of toys and does not repeatedly use the same item(s) ————————
——

———————— The child uses coordinated motor movements ————————————————————
——

———————— The child uses complete sentences during play ————————————————————
——

———————— The child asks questions during play ————————————————————————————
——

———————— The child answers questions during play ————————————————————————
——

———————— The child responds to requests ————————————————————————————————
——

———————— The child primarily uses gestures to communicate ————————————————————
——

———————— The child uses gestures and speech to communicate ————————————————————
——

———————— The child looks at the listener when speaking ————————————————————————
——

———————— The child uses appropriate vocabulary words ————————————————————————
——

———————— The child relates real life experiences during conversation ————————————————
——

———————— The child usually communicates in phrases of greater than two words ————————————
——

———————— The child usually communicates in phrases of greater than three words ————————————
——

———————— The child usually communicates in phrases of greater than four words ————————————
——

———————— The child initiates conversations or activities ————————————————————————
——

———————— The child dominates conversations ————————————————————————————————
——

(continues)

Form 7-5. continued

_____ The child is able to follow conversational shifts _____

_____

_____ The child uses simple sentences _____

_____

_____ The child uses complex sentences _____

_____

_____ The child uses the correct word order when speaking _____

_____

_____ The child uses plurals (e.g., *boys, animals*) _____

_____

_____ The child uses more than one verb tense (e.g., present, past, future) _____

_____

_____ The child uses pronouns (e.g., *he, she, I*) _____

_____

_____ The child uses articles (e.g., *the, an, a*) _____

_____

_____ The child uses the verbs *is* and *are* _____

_____

_____ The child uses prepositions (e.g., *on, in, under, beside*) _____

_____

_____ The child varies his or her communication depending on the listener _____

_____

_____ The child has good reading skills _____

_____

_____ The child has good writing skills _____

_____

_____ The child is able to follow the story line of a TV show _____

_____

(continues)

LANGUAGE IN CHILDREN

Form 7-5. continued

How does the child's language differ from that of other children the same age?

How does the child's language differ from that of an adult?

Form 7-6.

Worksheet for Recording a Language Sample

Name: _____ Age: _____ Date: _____

Examiner's Name: _____

Setting: _____

Conversational Partner(s): _____

Instructions: List the utterance number in the first column and the speaker (C = child; A = adult) in the second column. The third column is for recording each utterance.

#	C/A	Utterance
_____	_____	_____
_____	_____	_____
_____	_____	_____
_____	_____	_____
_____	_____	_____
_____	_____	_____
_____	_____	_____
_____	_____	_____
_____	_____	_____
_____	_____	_____
_____	_____	_____
_____	_____	_____
_____	_____	_____
_____	_____	_____
_____	_____	_____
_____	_____	_____
_____	_____	_____
_____	_____	_____
_____	_____	_____
_____	_____	_____
_____	_____	_____

(continues)

LANGUAGE IN CHILDREN

Form 7-6. continued

#	C/A	Utterance

Form 7-7.

Assessment of Morphologic Features

Name: _____ Age: _____ Date: _____

Examiner's Name: _____

Instructions: Analyze your client's language sample or ask structured questions to assess morphologic features. Mark a plus (+) or a check (✓) if the client is correct and a minus (−) or a zero (0) if incorrect. Make additional comments on the right-hand side.

Plurals

_____ /z/ as in *trees* _____

_____ /s/ as in *books* _____

_____ /vz/ as in *wolves* _____

_____ /əz/ as in *dishes* _____

_____ irregular such as *feet* _____

Possessive

_____ /z/ as in *boy's* _____

_____ /s/ as in *cat's* _____

_____ /əz/ as in *mouse's* _____

Articles

_____ a _____

_____ the _____

Present Progressive Tense

_____ /ɪŋ/ as in *eating* _____

Past Tense

_____ /d/ as in *spilled* _____

_____ /t/ as in *dropped* _____

_____ /əd/ as in *melted* _____

_____ irregular such as *broke* _____

(continues)

LANGUAGE IN CHILDREN

Form 7-7. continued

Third-Person Singular

_____ /z/ as in *move**s*** _____

_____ /s/ as in *walk**s*** _____

_____ /əz/ as in *push**es*** _____

Comparatives/Superlatives

_____ /ɚ/ as in *soft**er*** _____

_____ /əst/ as in *small**est*** _____

_____ irregular such as *best* _____

Negation

_____ /ʌn/ as in ***un**happy* _____

_____ not as in *not now* _____

Reflexive Pronouns

_____ /sɛlvz/ as in *them**selves*** _____

_____ /sɛlf/ as in *my**self*** _____

Prepositions

_____ in _____

_____ on _____

_____ under _____

_____ behind _____

_____ beside _____

_____ between _____

_____ in front _____

Form 7-8.

Assessment of Pragmatic Skills

Name: _____ Age: _____ Date: _____

Examiner's Name: _____

Instructions: Use activities such as those suggested in the right-hand column to elicit the desired pragmatic behaviors. Mark a plus (+) or a check (✔) if the response is correct or appropriate and a minus (−) or a zero (0) if the response is incorrect, not present, or inappropriate.

Pragmatic Behavior	Sample Activities
_____ Respond to greetings	Observe the client's response when you say, "Hi! How are you?"
	Put your hand out to shake hands.
_____ Make requests	Ask the client to draw a circle but don't immediately provide a pencil.
	Ask "What would you say to your mom if you were in the grocery store and wanted a candy bar?"
_____ Describe events	Ask the client what he or she did this morning.
	Ask the client to tell you about a holiday or a special occasion.
_____ Take turns	Ask the client to alternately count or recite the alphabet with you (e.g., you say *a*, client says *b*, you say *c*, client says *d*).
	Take turns telling one to two lines of *The Three Bears* or another children's story.
_____ Follow commands	Ask the client to turn his or her paper over and draw a happy face or a square.
	Say to the client, "Touch your ears, then clap your hands twice."
_____ Make eye contact	Consider whether the client has maintained normal eye contact during other parts of this assessment.
	Ask the client to tell you his or her address or phone number.
_____ Repeat	Ask the client to repeat the following sentences: Michael is 7 years old. The oven door was open. She got a new book for her birthday.
_____ Attend to tasks	Consider how the client has attended to this assessment.
	Ask the client to describe a picture you provide.

(continues)

Form 7-8. continued

Pragmatic Behavior	**Sample Activities**
_____ Maintain topic	Ask the client to tell you about a recent movie or TV show he or she has watched.
	Ask the client to describe a hotdog.
_____ Role-play	Ask the client to be the "teacher" for a while and give you things to complete.
	Pretend you are in a fast-food restaurant. Tell the client to be the cashier while you pretend to be the customer.
_____ Sequence actions	Ask the client to describe the steps involved in making the bed, buying groceries, or writing a letter.
	Ask the client to describe how to make a hamburger or salad, or prepare breakfast.
_____ Define words	Ask the client to define words such as
	scissors
	kitchen
	computer
_____ Categorize	Ask the client if the following words are days or months:
	Sunday
	June
	April
	Wednesday
	Ask the client to name several farm animals, foods, or sports.
_____ Understand object functions	Ask the client to show you how to use scissors.
	Ask what a ruler is used for.
_____ Initiate activity or dialogue	Place an odd-looking object on the table and see if the client asks what it is.
	Observe the client with his or her parents, teacher, or with other children.

Form 7-9.

Assessment of Semantic Skills

Name: _____ Age: _____ Date: _____

Examiner's Name: _____

Instructions: Use the following questions or tasks to assess semantic skills. Record child responses and your observations in the spaces provided.

Point to a variety of objects in the room and have the child name them. Record your results here.

Tell a short story and ask the child to tell it back to you. Record your findings here.

Ask the child to define the following words. Also probe for additional information such as word category, description, function, shape, etc.

Pumpkin:

Train:

President:

(continues)

Form 7-9. continued

Turquoise:

Language:

Ask the child to name the opposite of each word.

Hot:

Before:

Open:

Dark:

Uncle:

Winter:

Ask the child to provide a word that means the same as:

Big:

Begin:

Terrific:

Afraid:

Delicious:

Ask the child, "What do these words have in common?"

Water, orange juice, milk:

Rain, snow, sunshine:

Starfish, whale, octopus:

New Mexico, Hawaii, Montana:

Stamp, pen, stationery:

(continues)

Form 7-9. continued

Ask the child to name three to five members of each category.

Colors:

Animals:

Vegetables:

Cities in (your state):

Feelings:

Ask the child to explain the following phrases:

Go for it:

Look before you leap:

Better late than never:

Don't cry over spilled milk:

He is like a tiger:

(continues)

LANGUAGE
IN CHILDREN

Form 7-9. continued

Ask the child to finish each phrase.

Red, white, and _____

Bacon and _____

Salt and _____

Shoes and _____

Dollars and _____

Ask the child to describe how these word pairs are similar and how they are different.

A basketball and a beachball:

A snake and an elephant:

A necklace and a watch:

Popcorn and potato chips:

A television and a computer:

Form 7-10.

Assessment of Syntactic Skills

Child: _____ Age: _____

Examiner's Name: _____ Date: _____

Instructions: Check each syntactic structure present for each utterance recorded in the language sample.

	Parts of Speech							Phrases				Clauses		Sentences								
Utterance	Noun	Pronoun	Adjective	Verb	Adverb	Preposition	Conjunction	Interjection	Noun	Verb	Prepositional	Adjective	Main	Subordinate	Simple	Compound	Complex	Compound-Complex	Active	Passive	Declarative	Imperative	Interrogative	Negative

(continues)

		Parts of Speech							Phrases				Clauses			Sentences							
Utterance		Noun	Pronoun	Adjective	Verb	Adverb	Preposition	Conjunction	Interjection	Noun	Verb	Prepositional	Adjective	Main	Subordinate	Simple	Compound	Complex	Compound-Complex	Active	Passive	Declarative	Imperative	Interrogative	Negative

Form 7-10. continued

Chapter 8

ASSESSMENT OF LITERACY

Literacy is commonly defined as an ability to read and write.[1] There is a strong reciprocal relationship between expressive language and literacy. Many of the same linguistic skills are necessary for the acquisition and functional use of both oral and written language, with additional higher-level skills required for written language. This chapter is an extension of the preceding chapter, as both chapters address issues of language assessment. Chapter 7 focused primarily on the assessment of nonwritten language. This chapter will provide resources for evaluating and diagnosing written language disorders.

OVERVIEW OF ASSESSMENT

History of the Client

    Procedures

        Written Case History
        Information-Gathering Interview
        Information from Other Professionals

    Contributing Factors

        Oral Language Impairment
        Hearing Impairment
        Visual Impairment
        Medical or Neurological Factors
        Family History of Literacy Deficit
        Maturation and Motor Development
        Intelligence, Sex, Birth Order, Motivation, and Levels of Concern

Assessment of Oral Language

Assessment of Literacy

    Procedures

        Screening
        Sampling
        Informal Tests
        Standardized Tests

    Areas to Assess

        Phonemic Awareness
        Phonemic Decoding
        Word Fluency
        Reading Fluency
        Reading Comprehension
        Narrative Schema Knowledge
        Writing
        Spelling

---

[1]   The Workforce Investment Act of 1998 defines literacy as "an individual's ability to read, write, and speak in English [or other language for non-English speakers], compute and solve problems at levels of proficiency necessary to function on the job, in the family of the individual and in society" (National Institute for Literacy, 2006). This text adheres to the more common definition, which is limited to reading and writing, even though technically it is less accurate.

Analysis

    Error Types

    Form of Errors

    Consistency of Errors

    Basis of Errors

    Contextual Differences

    Academic Benchmarks

Orofacial Examination

Hearing Assessment

Vision Assessment

Determining the Diagnosis

Providing Information (written report, interview, etc.)

Role of the Speech-Language Pathologist

Historically, speech-language pathologists have been involved in the diagnosis and treatment of receptive and expressive aspects of language; that is, listening, comprehension, and speaking. More recently, we have become important members of the interdisciplinary team that serves clients with developmental reading and writing disabilities. Other members of the team include teachers, reading specialists, and other special educators. Because of their training in language acquisition, speech-language pathologists are able to identify literacy problems and also explain *why* problems exist. Specific roles and responsibilities of speech-language pathologists are:

- Prevention of written language problems

- Identification of clients with, or at risk for, literacy problems

- Assessment of reading and writing as they relate to spoken communication and academic (or professional) achievement

- Intervention for reading and writing deficits

- Other roles, including advocating for effective literacy practices, advancing the knowledge base, and assisting teachers, families, and students (American Speech-Language-Hearing Association, 2002)

NORMAL READING AND WRITING DEVELOPMENT

The development of reading precedes the development of writing in much the same way auditory comprehension precedes verbal expression; the former lays the foundation for the latter. The development of all aspects of language begins at birth. The following developmental progression highlights milestones for reading and writing in a normally developing child (data from American Speech-Language Hearing Association, 2009; Chall, 1983, 1996; Gentry, 2004).

Birth–2 Years
Reading

- From birth, a child is exposed to print (e.g., on household items, billboards, books, etc.).

- Child accumulates knowledge about letters, words, and books.

3 Years

Reading

- Metalinguistic knowledge develops (i.e., knowledge that language consists of discrete phonemes, words, phrases, and sentences).
- Phonological awareness develops (i.e., awareness that words are made up of sound segments).
- Knowledge of the alphabetic principle begins (i.e., letters in English represent speech sounds).
- Child recognizes words that rhyme (e.g., *hat, rat*) and words that begin with the same sound (e.g., *big ball*).
- Print awareness develops; child understands that print has meaning and structure (e.g., moves from left to right, top to bottom; words are separated by space). Child recognizes trademark logos (e.g., McDonald's®) and the child's own name.

Writing

- Child scribbles, but with no discernable letters.
- Some scribble shows basic knowledge of conventional rules of writing; scribble may occur in lines, may flow from left to right and top to bottom, and may show some conventional spacing.

4 Years

Reading

- Phonemic awareness develops (i.e., awareness that words are made up of specific units of sounds that have distinct features).
- Child says words that rhyme (e.g., *dog, frog*) and words that begin with the same sound (e.g., *cup, cap*).
- Child segments a sentence into separate words (e.g., *The boy jumped* is segmented to *the-boy-jumped*).
- Child counts the number of syllables in words.

Writing

- Writing resembles standard letters and words.
- Child must interpret his or her writing for others.

5 Years (Kindergarten)

Reading

- Child knows when words do not rhyme (e.g., *hog* does not rhyme with *hat*).
- Child recites and names letters of the alphabet and numbers 1–10.
- Child identifies the first sound of a spoken word and separates it from the rime (the first vowel and any following vowels and consonants of a syllable) (e.g., *dog* begins with *d*).
- Child blends the beginning sound with the remaining sounds of a word.
- Child segments multisyllabic words into syllables (e.g., *elephant* is *el-e-phant*).
- Child reads some familiar words by sight.

Writing

- Child knows basic conventional rules of writing; scribble may occur in lines, may flow from left to right and top to bottom, and may show spacing between words.
- Child writes a few meaningful words, usually common nouns and the child's own name.
- Most upper- and lowercase letters are written legibly.

6 Years (First Grade)

Reading

- Phonetic decoding and blending develops; child isolates sounds in short words (e.g., *cat* is *c-a-t*) and can blend two to three sounds to form words (e.g., *b-a-t* is *bat*).
- Child makes up rhymes.
- Child associates sounds with alphabetic symbols (i.e., sound–symbol association).
- Child segments a final consonant from the rest of the word (e.g., separates *bi-* from *-g* in *big*).
- Simple words are sounded out when reading.
- Child matches spoken word with print.
- Child has a sight vocabulary of 100 words.
- Child reads and comprehends grade-level material.

Writing

- Child shows knowledge of the relationship between letters and sounds.
- Mostly uppercase letters are used.
- Child writes strings of letters (not words) with no spacing.
- Only one or some letters in a word are written, usually the first consonant, to represent a whole word or syllable.
- Invented spellings are typical; initial and final consonants are present, although vowels may be omitted.
- Begins sentences with a capital letter and ends sentences with a period.
- Subject matter of writing usually expresses feelings, personal ideas, and memories.
- Sentences are short and simple.
- Grammatical errors are common (e.g., verb tense, regular and irregular plurals).

7 Years (Second Grade)

Reading

- Child counts the number of phonemes in a word.
- Child uses phonetic strategies and orthographic processing (learned spelling patterns and sight words) to read new words.
- Child rereads and self-corrects as needed.
- Contextual clues for comprehension are used (e.g., pictures, titles, headings, etc.).
- Questions are answered by locating information in written material.
- Child has good comprehension of basic story elements.
- Child retells a story.
- Child reads spontaneously.

Writing

- Phonetic spellings decrease and traditional spellings increase; spelling rules are applied more frequently.
- Child correctly uses upper- and lowercase letters, space between words, and basic punctuation.
- Writing is legible.
- Child writes simple fiction and nonfiction based on a model and using a variety of sentence types.
- Writing is organized with a beginning, middle, and end.
- Familiar words are correctly spelled.
- Morphologic structures in the spelling system are better internalized.

8 Years (Third Grade)

Reading

- Basic phonetic patterns are mastered.
- Child segments and deletes consonant clusters.
- Maturing experience with sound–symbol associations allows decoding of more unfamiliar words.
- Child uses word analysis skills when reading.
- Child uses language content and schema knowledge to aid in comprehension.
- What will happen in a story is predicted.
- Child uses reading materials to learn about new topics.
- Child reads grade-level books fluently.

Writing

- Conventional spellings are used primarily, and a dictionary is used to learn new or correct spellings.
- Vowels are used correctly most of the time.
- Letters are transposed in less-frequently-used words.
- Child writes narratives, letters, and simple expository reports.
- Sentence lengths increase and include more complex forms.

9 Years (Fourth Grade)

Reading

- Decoding skills are fully automatic, enabling fluent reading.
- Child reads for pleasure and to learn.
- Child reads and understands a variety of literature types (e.g., fiction, nonfiction, historical fiction, poetry).
- Written instructions are followed.
- Child takes brief notes and uses reference materials.

- Child makes inferences from text.
- Content of text is paraphrased.

Writing

- Child recognizes misspellings and can correctly spell unfamiliar words by using orthographic knowledge.
- Conventions and exceptions in spelling rules are known.
- Child uses narrative and expository writing.
- Child organizes writing by using a beginning, middle, and end to convey a central idea.
- Own work is edited for grammar, punctuation, and spelling.

10 Years (Fifth Grade)

Reading

- Child reads a variety of literary forms.
- Character and plot development is described.
- Child describes characteristics of poetry.
- Lengthier and more complex text is comprehended.

Writing

- Child writes for a variety of purposes using a variety of sentence structures.
- Vocabulary is used effectively.
- Child revises and edits own writing.

11–18 Years (6th–12th Grade)

Reading

- Child reads for learning and entertainment.
- Child becomes a more mature, critical reader.
- Reading skills are applied to obtain new knowledge and specific information.

Writing

- Child writes sentences that are longer than spoken sentences and more linguistically complex.
- Expository writing is used to provide explanations and descriptions.

19+ Years (College)

Reading

- Materials are read for inquiry, critical analysis, and entertainment.
- New ideas are integrated into an existing knowledge base.

Writing

- Persuasive text is written.

Much of our current knowledge of reading and writing development is based on the work of psychologist Jeanne Chall. She was an advocate of phonics-based reading instruction and described reading as a developmental process. It is now widely accepted that children *learn to read* through third grade; from then on, they *read to learn*. Beginning in fourth grade, students face more complex sentence structures, abstract concepts, and advanced vocabulary. A person who has not mastered the basics of reading is likely to experience significant challenges throughout his or her lifetime academically and professionally.

DESCRIPTIONS AND CATEGORIES OF READING DISABILITIES

There are three main categories of reading disability: dyslexia, language-based learning disability (LLD), and hyperlexia. Descriptions and features of each category are as follows:

- *Developmental dyslexia* is also called *specific reading disability*. Dyslexia is genetically based and is caused by atypical neurological development (Shaywitz, 2003). Children with dyslexia are sometimes considered "unexpected reading failures" because they appear to be developing normally until they start trying to read. The primary symptom of dyslexia is poor phonemic awareness. A child with dyslexia will perform normally on receptive/expressive language tests, but poorly on reading tests.
- *Language-based learning disability (LLD)* is a more generalized language disability that includes deficiencies in all areas of language. A child with an LLD will perform poorly on both receptive/expressive language tests and reading tests.
- *Hyperlexia* is an ability to read words significantly above age expectations but without comprehension of what is read. It can be a symptom of autism.

There are certain behaviors and characteristics that children with a reading disability may demonstrate. These include:

- Poor phonemic awareness
- Poor word recognition
- Difficulty with orthographic processing
- Difficulty with phonetic decoding of new words
- Difficulty attaching meaning to words, phrases, and sentences
- Difficulty with grammar, including knowledge of regular and irregular morphemes and knowledge of various sentence structures
- Difficulty processing complex sentences
- Overreliance on contextual cues, sometimes guessing instead of decoding
- Lack of interest in literature; frustration instead of pleasure
- Reduced speaking rate and increased pausing during speaking
- Limited vocabulary
- Poor comprehension of stories
- Poor social skills

ASSESSMENT OF EARLY LITERACY

Preschool-age children with oral language deficits are at high risk of developing written language deficits in their school years. Deficits in oral language, phonological awareness, print awareness, and metalinguistics that are identified and remediated early can significantly increase a child's potential for academic success later in life. Speech-language pathologists in the preschool environment are often best able to identify children at risk for future literacy problems.

Early indicators of reading disability include:

- Family history of reading disability
- First word not produced until after 15 months of age
- Words not combined until after 24 months of age
- Difficulty pronouncing words past 6 years of age
- Poor memory for, and awareness of, rhymes during preschool years
- Inability to segment words into syllables before age 5 (Naremore, Densmore, & Harman, 2001; Shaywitz, 2003)

Children in pre-kindergarten and kindergarten should be screened for phonological awareness skills to predict the later development of a reading disability. Evaluate children on measures of the child's:

- Phonemic awareness
- Rapid naming of letters, numbers, and objects
- Print awareness (Goldsworthy, 2003)

Form 8-1, "Checklist of Early Literacy Skills," can be completed by a child's parent, teacher, resource specialist, speech-language pathologist, or other person involved in a child's care. Sections of Form 8-2, "Assessment of Phonemic Awareness," are also appropriate for evaluating early literacy.

ASSESSMENT OF READING

When testing for a reading disorder, evaluate all aspects of language, with a particular emphasis on the child's:

- Phonological awareness
- Word fluency
- Narrative schema knowledge

Clients with a reading disability are most likely to show struggle in one or more of these three areas. When evaluating older children, measures of writing skills are also important considerations. A referral to an audiologist for an assessment of hearing may be necessary to rule out hearing loss or (central) auditory processing disorder. A vision screen or evaluation may also be necessary to rule out visual deficiencies.

Phonological Awareness

The most distinguishing feature of a reading disability is poor phonological awareness. The child has difficulty identifying and blending together individual phonemes in words. Vinson (2001, 2007) recommends these considerations when assessing phonemic knowledge:

- Phonetic segmentation (sound differentiation): Can the child count phonemes in a word? Pronounce individual sounds? Delete or add sounds to words? Relocate phonemes in words?
- Phoneme synthesis (sound blending): Can the child blend sounds that are presented in isolation to form a word?
- Sound comparison: Can the child compare the sounds of different words (e.g., *Which words begin with the same sound: cat, tap, cap?*)

Clinical expectations of phonemic awareness vary depending upon a child's age. Table 8-1 presents a progression of phonemic awareness benchmarks for children ages 3 through 8. This information can be helpful in the diagnostic process to discern whether a child's skills are developmentally normal or if there is cause for concern.

TABLE 8-1   Phonemic Awareness Benchmarks

AGE OF DEVELOPMENT	PHONEMIC AWARENESS SKILLS
3 years	• Familiar with known nursery rhymes (e.g., *Jack and Jill*). • Recognizes alliteration (e.g., the words *my milk* begin with same first sound) • Recognizes words that rhyme (e.g., *cat* and *bat*)
4 years	• Segments a sentence into separate words • Segments multisyllabic words into syllables (e.g., *cowboy* has two parts, *cow* and *boy*) • Says words that rhyme
5 years	• Counts the number of syllables in words • Segments the beginning sound (onset) from the rest of a word (rime) (*b-at*) • Blends the beginning sound with the rest of a word • Identifies a word that does not rhyme with a target (e.g., *dog* does not rhyme with *jam* and *ham*)
6 years	• Makes up rhymes • Matches initial consonants in words (e.g., *big* and *boy* begin with same first sound) • Blends two or three phonemes to make a word (e.g., phonemes /k/ /æ/ /t/ form the word *cat*) • Segments initial consonant blends from the rest of the word (e.g., divides *trick* into *tr-* and *-ick*) • Segments the final consonant from the rest of the word (e.g., divides *make* into *ma-* and *-ke*)

AGE OF DEVELOPMENT	PHONEMIC AWARENESS SKILLS
7 years	• Counts the number of phonemes in a word • Blends isolated phonemes to form words • Segments phonemes within words • Spells phonetically • Adds phonemes to, or deletes phonemes from, words
8 years	• Relocates phonemes in a word to make a new word (e.g., moves *t* in *tar* to the end to make *art*) • Segments consonant clusters • Deletes consonant clusters

Sources: Goldsworthy (2003); Justice (2006); Naremore, Densmore, and Harman (2001).

Form 8-2, "Assessment of Phonemic Awareness," is an informal assessment for evaluating phonemic knowledge. There are also many commercially available tests for the evaluation of phonemic awareness and other aspects of literacy. Table 8-2 lists several commonly used tests. Age and grade ranges are provided, as well as assessment features of each test.

Word Fluency

Another strong indicator of a reading disability is word fluency, also called rapid naming skills. Word fluency is an ability to name symbols, words, or pictures rapidly. This discriminating skill is based on speed, not accuracy. Poor readers are usually able to name symbols, words, and pictures accurately, but they are characteristically slower than skilled readers.

An effective method of evaluating word fluency is to prepare index cards with letters, numbers, pictures, or words. The prompts on the cards will depend upon the age and abilities of the child; some children cannot be expected to read words but can be expected to name pictures, numbers, or letters. Present each card separately and take note of the amount of time taken by the child to name the prompt. Delay or struggle is symptomatic of reading difficulty.

Standardized assessments are also helpful for objectively evaluating word fluency. See Table 8-2 for a list of formal tests.

Reading Fluency

Reading fluency may be assessed in children who can read short paragraphs or longer reading passages. It is a measure of the average number of words the student correctly reads per minute. Poor reading fluency indicates possible problems with phonemic awareness, decoding skills, comprehension, or vocabulary. To determine word fluency for oral reading:

1. Count the number of correctly read words in a passage.
2. Multiply that number by 60.
3. Determine the number of seconds taken to read the passage.
4. Divide the number obtained in Step 2 by the number obtained in Step 3.

TABLE 8-2   Standardized Tests for the Assessment of Literacy

TEST	REFERENCE	AGE	GRADE	AREAS OF ASSESSMENT
Assessment of Literacy and Language (ALL)	Lombardino, Lieberman, & Brown (2005)	3;0–6;0	Preschool–1st grade	Phonological awareness; listening and language comprehension; syntax; semantics; phonics; print concepts
Comprehensive Test of Phonological Processing (CTOPP-2)	Wagner, Torgesen, & Rashotte (2009)	5;0–24;11	Kindergarten–postgraduate	Phonemic awareness; rapid naming; short-term phonologic memory
Gray Diagnostic Reading Tests (GDRT-2)	Bryant, Wiederholt, & Bryant (2004)	6;0–13;11	1st–8th grade	Letter/word naming; phonetic analysis; reading and listening vocabulary; meaningful reading; phonemic awareness
Gray Oral Reading Tests (GORT-4)	Wiederholt & Bryant (2001)	6;0–18;11	1st–12th grade	Speaking rate; accuracy; fluency; comprehension of oral reading
Gray Silent Reading Tests (GSRT)	Wiederholt & Blalock (2000)	7;0–25;11	2nd grade–postgraduate	Silent reading comprehension
Lindamood Auditory Conceptualization Test (LAC-3)	Lindamood & Lindamood (2004)	5;0–8;11	Kindergarten–3rd grade	Phonemic awareness
Phonological Awareness and Reading Profile—Intermediate	Salter & Robertson (2001)	8;0–14;11	3rd grade–9th grade	Phonemic awareness; fluency; spelling
Phonological Awareness Profile	Robertson & Salter (1995)	5;0–8;11	Kindergarten–3rd grade	Phonemic awareness
Test of Auditory Processing Skills (TAPS-3)	Martin & Brownell (2005)	4;0–18;11	Preschool–12th grade	Phonemic awareness; auditory memory; auditory cohesion
Test of Phonological Awareness Skills (TOPAS)	Newcomer & Barenbaum (2003)	5;0–10;11	Kindergarten–5th grade	Phonemic awareness
Test of Phonological Awareness-Second Edition: Plus (TOPA-2+)	Torgesen & Bryant (2004)	5;0–8;11	Kindergarten–3rd grade	Phonemic awareness
Test of Silent Contextual Reading Fluency (TOSCRF)	Hammill, Wiederholt, & Allen (2006)	7;0–18;11	2nd–12th grade	Word fluency

TEST	REFERENCE	AGE	GRADE	AREAS OF ASSESSMENT
Test of Silent Word Reading Fluency (TOSWRF)	Mather, Hammill, Allen, & Roberts (2004)	6;6–17;11	1st–11th grade	Screening tool for word fluency
Test of Word Reading Efficiency (TOWRE)	Torgesen, Wagner, & Rashotte (2009)	6;0–24;11	1st grade–postgraduate	Rapid reading of sight words; phonetic decoding
The Phonological Awareness Test-2	Robertson & Salter (2007)	5;0–9;11	Kindergarten–4th grade	Phonemic awareness; spelling
Woodcock-Johnson III Complete	Woodcock, McGrew, & Mather (2001)	2;0–90+	Preschool–postgraduate	Phonemic awareness; rapid naming; auditory memory; spelling
Woodcock Reading Mastery Test (WRMT-R/NU)	Woodcock (1998)	5;0–75+	Kindergarten–postgraduate	Reading readiness; word identification; word attack; comprehension
Word Identification and Spelling Test (WIST)	Wilson & Felton (2004)	7;0–18;11	2nd–12th grade	Word identification; spelling; sound–symbol knowledge

For example, if a student reads 407 words in 4 minutes, 25 seconds, that student's reading rate is 47 words per minute. Step-by-step, that is:

1. 407 words in the passage
2. $407 \times 60 = 24{,}420$
3. 4:25 minutes taken to read the passage = 265 seconds
4. $24{,}420 \div 265 = 92$ words correctly read per minute

A minimum of two unrehearsed samples should be obtained for calculating reading fluency. Table 8-3 summarizes reading fluency norms for students in grades 1–8, assessed at different times during the academic year. It is based on the extensive research of Hasbrouck and Tindal (2006). They recommend a fluency-building program for students who score 10 or more words below their grade level's 50th percentile, as shown in the table. Review their research for additional normative data.

Narrative Schema Knowledge

Another important component of a literacy assessment is evaluation of narrative schema knowledge, which is knowledge of story structure. Children with poor narrative schema knowledge also demonstrate poor linguistic complexity and reading comprehension (Naremore, Densmore, & Harman, 2001). Narrative production requires an ability to simultaneously sequence events, use appropriate vocabulary, follow rules of sentence structure, and

TABLE 8-3   50th Percentile Oral Reading Fluency Norms

GRADE	FALL	WINTER	SPRING
1st	—	23	53
2nd	51	72	89
3rd	71	92	107
4th	94	112	123
5th	110	127	139
6th	127	140	150
7th	128	136	150
8th	133	146	151

Source: Summarized from Hasbrouck and Tindal (2006).

present a story in a cohesive and logical fashion. Stein and Glenn (1979) labeled the essential and binding elements of a story the *story grammar*. Their elements are:

- Setting: introduction of main characters, time, place, and context
- Initiating event: the situation or event that sets up the conflict
- Internal response: the characters' plan or response to the initiating event
- Attempt: actions taken toward resolution of the conflict
- Consequences: success or failure of the attempt; resolution
- Reaction: characters' reaction to the resolution (feelings, actions)

Even simple narratives contain most, if not all, of these elements. As children mature, they are able to manipulate story grammars to weave multiple events and more complex layers into a single story.

There are different strategies for assessing narrative schema knowledge. The age and ability of the client will dictate the most appropriate method. One strategy is to read a short story to the client and ask comprehension questions. For example:

- Who was in the story?
- Where did the story take place?
- What was the problem in the story?
- How was the problem solved?
- What happened in the end?
- Did you like the story?
- What did you like/not like about it?
- What would you have done if you were (main character)?

- What would have happened if (change a key element of the story)?
- What is the title of the story?
- If you were to give this story a new title, what would it be?
- Who wrote this story?

Another strategy is to ask the client to retell a known story. Ask the client to tell the story of *Goldilocks and the Three Bears*, *Charlotte's Web*, or another popular children's tale. Or using one of the narratives with pictures located in Chapter 5 (see Figures 5-6 and 5-7), read the story to the client and then ask the client to retell the story. The pictures can be used to aid in retelling, or removed to assess the child's memory and comprehension of the story without visual cues. Telling stories from wordless picture books is also useful for assessing narrative schema knowledge.

More-capable clients may be able to make up a story or share a story from their lives. Use prompts such as:

- Make up a story about an alien coming to our school.
- Make up a story about winning a million dollars.
- Make up a story about meeting George Washington.
- Tell me about hitting a home run at your baseball game.
- Tell me an adventure you had with your pet.
- Tell me a story about something that happened to you when you were younger.

Regardless of the method used to elicit the narrative sample, analyze the narrative in these areas:

- Knowledge of story elements: Is it organized with a beginning, middle, and end? Is the setting clear? Does it have character and plot development? Does it contain conflict and resolution? Does is make sense? If a story was read to the client, can the client answer questions about the basic elements of the story?
- Comprehension of the story:
  - Literal comprehension: Does the client know the central theme of the story? Can the client paraphrase the story? Can the client identify the main characters? Can the client answer questions about the story?
  - Inferred comprehension: Can the client infer character thoughts, emotions or motivations? Can the client connect the story to personal experiences?
- Linguistic complexity of the narrative: Did the client use a variety of sentence types, including simple and complex sentences? Was the vocabulary appropriate?

Form 8-3, "Worksheet for Narrative Analysis," is provided to help with narrative assessment. Other commercially available materials for evaluating narrative knowledge include:

- *Assessment of Narrative Skills: What's the Story?* (Apel & Masterson, 1998)
- *Test of Narrative Language* (Gillam & Pearson, 2004)
- *Dynamic Assessment and Intervention: Improving Children's Narrative Abilities* (Miller, Gillam, & Pena, 2001)

Informal Reading Inventories

An informal reading inventory (IRI) is a useful diagnostic tool for assessing reading ability and comprehension of grade-level material. IRIs enable the clinician to evaluate the student using authentic classroom-like resources, thus providing information about how well the student is able to read and understand academic literature.

IRIs generally consist of grade-level word lists and reading passages. The clinician can obtain appropriate grade-level materials from teachers, or use books with publisher-rated reading levels. The word lists are used to assess word recognition and fluency. The reading passages are used to assess reading fluency, story schema knowledge, comprehension, and frustration level. The student may read passages orally and/or silently, or, to assess listening ability, the clinician may read passages to the student. After each passage, the clinician asks 5–10 comprehension questions, including simple questions based on knowledge and more difficult questions based on inference. Reading accuracy is the percentage of correctly read words.

Findings are often categorized according to the following three levels:

1. Independent: The student can read the material independently. Reading accuracy is 97–100%. Comprehension is excellent (90% or higher).

2. Instructional: The student can read the material with a typical amount of classroom help. Reading accuracy is 94–96%. Comprehension is satisfactory (75%).

3. Frustrational: The student has difficulty reading the material in a classroom setting. Reading accuracy is below 94%. Comprehension is poor (below 50%).

Form 8-4, "Informal Reading Inventory," is a worksheet for recording informal reading inventory findings.

ASSESSMENT OF WRITING

Writing is, in general, the most complex form of language. In many cases, a child's language difficulties are most pronounced in his or her writing. Children with oral expressive language problems are likely to demonstrate writing deficiencies such as spelling errors, syntactic and semantic errors, morphologic errors, omissions of words or word endings, and general content incongruities. Often, individuals with reading disabilities do not know how to edit or revise written materials, their own or another's, because they do not have functional knowledge of high-level language strategies.

Writing takes different forms depending on the audience and the writer's purpose. Evaluation of narrative, expository, and persuasive forms will be described later in this chapter. In general, however, assessment for all types of writing should focus on:

- Productivity: How many sentences are there? How many clauses? How many different ideas are presented? How many words are there altogether?

- Complexity: How many different clause types are there? How complex are they? How many words per sentence or clause? How many grammatically correct sentences?

- Appropriateness for audience and topic: Is the form appropriate for the topic? Is it written well for the intended audience?
- Cohesiveness: Is it organized well? Does it make sense?
- Mechanics: Are words spelled correctly? Is punctuation correct? Are capital letters used?
- Analytic aspects: Does the writing have the intended effect? How successfully can the writer revise and edit his or her work?

Form 8-5, "Worksheet for Analyzing a Writing Sample," is useful for analyzing a variety of written productions. It may be helpful to obtain samples of a client's writing from his or her teacher. The teacher can also provide additional information about the client's typical writing skills and grade-level academic benchmarks.

There are several commercially available tests for the assessment of writing skills. These include:

- *OWLS Written Expression (WE) Scale* (Carrow-Woolfolk, 1996)
- *Test of Early Written Language (TEWL-2)* (Hresko, Herron, & Peak, 1996)
- *Test of Written Language (TOWL-3)* (Hammill & Larsen, 1996)
- *Wechsler Individual Achievement Test (WIAT-II)* (Wechsler, 2001)

More specific analysis of writing takes different forms depending on the audience and the purpose of the writing. The following sections describe assessment of narrative writing, expository writing, and persuasive writing. Assessment of spelling is also described.

Assessment of Narrative Writing

Narrative writing tells a story or shares an experience. It can be fiction or nonfiction, and content is often from personal experience. The elements of a narrative were described earlier in this chapter in the section on narrative schema knowledge. The assessment of narrative writing is similar to the assessment of oral narrative except that, obviously, the written narrative is recorded on paper. Analyze written narrative in the same way as oral narrative with additional attention paid to writing mechanics. Also, compare a client's written narratives to oral narratives. Analyze similarities and differences in these areas:

- In what general ways is the language similar or different?
- Does the child use vocabulary in speaking that is not used in writing?
- What word forms are used in writing as opposed to speaking?
- In which sample is sentence complexity greater?
- What is the average number of words per sentence or clause in each sample?
- Which sample has a greater variety of clause types?
- Is there variation in presentation or audience considerations?

Form 8-3, "Worksheet for Narrative Analysis," can be used for analyzing written and oral narratives. The above questions are more easily answered if the form is used to analyze both sample types.

Assessment of Expository Writing

Expository writing is a more advanced form of writing. It is nonfiction essay writing and its purpose is to explain, describe, or inform. Personal feelings or opinions should not be included. Expository writing adheres to a three-part format:

1. The thesis statement is presented in the opening paragraph.
2. Supporting paragraphs each present a different central idea that lends credence to the thesis. All sentences within each supporting paragraph factually relate to the paragraph's central idea. Transition words and phrases are important for helping the reader to follow the writer's logic.
3. The concluding paragraph restates the thesis. New material is not introduced. Students are expected to use expository writing in the upper-elementary grades all the way through high school and college. Students with writing deficits of expository form are at risk for significant academic and life-long struggles. Form 8-6, "Worksheet for Expository Writing Analysis," is provided to help evaluate expository writing.

Assessment of Persuasive Writing

The most advanced form of writing is persuasive writing. Its purpose is to convince the reader that a particular point of view is valid and correct. It includes personal opinion, supported by factual information. The format of a persuasive essay is as follows:

1. The opening paragraph contains the topic sentence, which is a statement of a position, not fact.
2. The supporting paragraphs present specific evidence, examples, or statistics to support the position statement. Each sentence should clearly and logically relate to the sentence before it and to the topic sentence. Statements of transition are important so that the reader can follow the writer's logic.
3. The concluding paragraph restates the topic sentence and the most compelling supportive evidence. New material is not introduced.

Form 8-7, "Worksheet for Persuasive Writing Analysis," is provided to help evaluate persuasive writing.

Assessment of Spelling

Evaluating spelling proficiency can provide valuable diagnostic information about phonological awareness and language in general. When a student is struggling with spelling, it is helpful to determine why. Spelling ability may provide insight into other types of knowledge necessary for written communication. Poor spelling may reveal weaknesses in one or more of the following linguistic components:

- Phonemic awareness
- Orthographic knowledge
- Semantic knowledge
- Morphologic knowledge

Poor spelling may also be a possible indicator of a hearing deficit or auditory processing disorder. Table 8-4 presents expectations for spelling at different ages and stages of development.

TABLE 8-4   Spelling Benchmarks

STAGE	AGE	CHARACTERISTICS
Precommunicative Spellers	3–5 years	• Scribble; no discernable letters • The child interprets the scribble • Some scribble shows basic knowledge of conventional rules of writing: scribble may occur in lines, may flow from left to right and top to bottom, and may show some conventional spacing
Semiphonetic Spellers	5–6 years	• Child shows early knowledge of the relationship between letters and sounds • Child uses mostly uppercase letters • Child often writes in strings of letters (not words) with no spacing • Child writes only one or some letters in a word, usually the first consonant, to represent a whole word or syllable
Phonetic Spellers	6–7 years	• Child can phonetically map out most words; initial and final consonants are present, although vowels may not be • Words are often not recognizable, but can be deciphered using rules of phonetics • Child uses upper- and lowercase letters • Child uses space between words • Child correctly spells words he or she knows
Transitional Spellers	7–8 years	• Child uses less phonetic spelling and more conventional spelling • Vowels used are correct more often • Child transposes letters in less-frequently-used words
Conventional Spellers	8+ years	• Child knows conventional spelling for most familiar words • Child often knows when words don't look right • Child can often correctly figure out how to spell unfamiliar words by using orthographic knowledge • Child has knowledge of conventions and exceptions in spelling rules

Source: Adapted from Gentry (2004).

Commercially available assessments for spelling include the following:

- *Spelling Performance Evaluation for Language and Literacy (SPELL)* (Masterson, Apel, & Wasowicz, 2002). This is a software assessment tool that analyzes spelling errors and recommends objectives for treatment.
- *Test of Written Spelling (TWS-4)* (Larsen, Hammill, & Moats, 1999)
- *Word Identification and Spelling Test (WIST)* (Wilson & Felton, 2004)

MULTICULTURAL CONSIDERATIONS

Cultural-linguistic background must be taken into consideration during an assessment of literacy. Narrative conventions vary across cultures. Standards of reading and writing in American English are not necessarily the same, or even similar, in other languages. Clients who come from homes in which English is not the primary language frequently develop problems with written language. English may not be spoken in the home or, if spoken, it may not be a good model for oral and written English development. Some children may be from lower-income homes where the parents are not highly educated; the children may not be exposed to literature that facilitates the development of reading and writing.

Keep in mind that academic language ability, referred to as *cognitive academic language proficiency* (CALP), develops slower than social language proficiency, referred to as *basic interpersonal communication skills* (BICS), among individuals learning English as a second language. CALP and BICS are described in more detail in Chapter 2. A student's level of progress on the continuum of second-language acquisition needs to be considered when assessing reading and writing aptitude.

Speech-language pathologists working with multicultural children often find it beneficial to address the needs of both the child and the child's family. In many communities, family literacy programs exist that are designed specifically to help parents improve their own literacy skills and promote the literacy of their children. Information about local family literacy programs and other resources may be found by contacting the following organizations:

- County Offices of Education
- State Directors of Adult Education
- The National Center for Family Literacy
- U.S. Department of Education Division of Adult Education and Literacy Clearinghouse

CONCLUDING COMMENTS

Oral language provides the foundation for the development of reading and writing. Children with oral language problems frequently develop disorders of literacy. Speech-language pathologists are able to use their knowledge of language development, phonology, and morphologic, syntactic, semantic, and pragmatic systems to diagnose or predict language-based reading and writing disorders.

SOURCES OF ADDITIONAL INFORMATION

Print Sources

Goldsworthy, C. (2003). *Developmental reading disabilities: A language-based treatment approach* (2nd ed.). Clifton Park, NY: Cengage Learning.

Gunning, T. G. (2013). *Assessing and correcting reading and writing difficulties* (5th ed.). San Antonia, TX: Pearson.

Hegde, M. N., & Maul, C. A. (2006). *Language disorders in children: An evidence-based approach to assessment and treatment.* Boston: Allyn & Bacon.

Naremore, R. C., Densmore, A. E., & Harman, D. R. (2001). *Assessment and treatment of school-age language disorders: A resource manual.* Clifton Park, NY: Cengage Learning.

Vinson, B. P. (2012). *Language disorders across the lifespan* (3rd ed.). Clifton Park, NY: Cengage Learning.

Electronic Sources

American Speech-Language-Hearing Association (ASHA):
http://www.asha.org

International Reading Association:
http://www.reading.org

National Reading Panel:
http://www.nationalreadingpanel.org

The International Dyslexia Association:
http://www.interdys.org

Form 8-1.

Checklist of Early Literacy Skills

Name: _____ DOB: _____

School: _____ Date: _____

Teacher: _____

Instructions: Circle Y (yes) or N (no) for each question. Additional comments are helpful and can be written on the right-hand side of the page.

Y N 1. Can the child identify the front of a book? _____

Y N 2. Can the child identify the back of a book? _____

Y N 3. In general, does the child show an interest in books? _____

Y N 4. Does the child enjoy being read to? _____

Y N 5. Does the child have a favorite book? _____

Y N 6. Does the child notice print in his or her environment
       (e.g., business signs, household items)? _____

Y N 7. Does the child seem to understand that pictures
       in a book can tell a story? _____

Y N 8. Does the child seem to understand that adults read
       printed text when reading stories aloud? _____

Y N 9. Does the child seem to know that reading occurs
       from the top of the page to the bottom? _____

Y N 10. Does the child seem to know that reading occurs
       from left to right? _____

Y N 11. Does the child pretend to read? _____

Y N 12. Does the child make up stories? _____

Y N 13. Does the child ask and/or answer questions
       about a story? _____

Y N 14. Can the child predict events in a story using
       illustrations or already known facts? _____

Y N 15. Does the child recognize his or her name in print? _____

Y N 16. Does the child pretend to write? Please describe. _____

(continues)

Form 8-1. continued

Y N 17. Does the child use real letters when writing? _____

Y N 18. Does the child attempt to write real words,
          even if misspelled? _____

Y N 19. Does the child attempt to copy words? _____

Y N 20. Can the child write his or her first name? _____

Y N 21. Can the child name *some, most,* or *all* (circle one)
          letters of the alphabet? _____

Y N 22. Does the child visually identify *some, most,* or
          all (circle one) letters of the alphabet? _____

Y N 23. Does the child recognize simple rhymes
          (e.g., "Funny, honey . . . that rhymes!")? _____

Y N 24. Can the child make a rhyme? _____

Y N 25. Can the child tell a simple story with a
          beginning, middle, and end? _____

Y N 26. Can the child identify words with the same
          beginning sound (e.g., *ball, boy, bat*)? _____

Y N 27. Can the child clap the number of syllables
          in a multi-syllabic word (e.g., clap three times
          for *elephant*)? _____

Y N 28. Does the child know that letters have
          uppercase and lowercase forms? _____

Y N 29. Does the child understand short stories
          that are told, not read? _____

Y N 30. Does the child understand and participate
          in simple conversation? _____

Y N 31. Does the child's vocabulary seem appropriate
          for his or her age? _____

Y N 32. Does the child ask questions? _____

Y N 33. Does the child verbally express feelings,
          opinions, ideas, needs? _____

Y N 34. Does the child pronounce words clearly? _____

Y N 35. Does the child's language seem
          age-appropriate to you? _____

(continues)

Form 8-1. continued

Y   N   36.   Can the child tell you beginning sounds
of words (e.g., *popcorn* begins with *p*)? _____

Y   N   37.   Does the child know the beginning sound
of his or her name? _____

Y   N   38.   Does the child recognize common words
from his or her environment
(e.g., McDonald's®, FisherPrice®)? _____

Y   N   39.   Does the child seem to recognize that printed
alphabetic letters are visually different from
one another? _____

Y   N   40.   Can the child attend to small group activities
that seem appropriate for his or her age? _____

Y   N   41.   Does the child initiate play with others
by using language (e.g., "Do you want to
play with me?")? _____

Y   N   42.   Does the child seem spatially aware
(i.e., understand up, down, top, bottom,
across, right, left, etc.)? _____

Y   N   43.   Does the child use visual cues to "read"? _____

Y   N   44.   Does the child play computer games?
If yes, list games. _____

Y   N   45.   Can the child recognize sounds in
the environment (e.g., car door closing,
piano playing)? _____

Person completing form: _____

Relationship to client: _____

Signed: _____ Date: _____

Form 8-2.

Assessment of Phonemic Awareness

Name: _____   DOB: _____

School: _____   Grade: _____

Teacher: _____   Date: _____

Instructions: Ask the child to tell you which word does not rhyme with the others.

Examples: sit, hop, mop → sit
       my, high, go → go

can, man, hit	son, sew, one
win, up, thin	make, lake, jump
hot, seed, need	book, take, look
bring, sing, fill	hop, mop, step
when, won, then	mow, see, bee

Instructions: Ask the child to provide a word that rhymes. Nonsense words are acceptable as long as the rule is followed.

Examples: fan → man
       leap → reap

bell	shoe
cat	toe
run	book
star	free
make	cry

Instructions: Ask the child whether the following word sets start with the same sound or different sounds.

Examples: hit, hat
       vote, fun

see, zoo	cat, car
gate, girl	fan, vase
kite, goat	tooth, dog
ball, pail	that, this
find, foot	jump, chat

(continues)

Form 8-2. continued

Instructions: Ask the child to change the last sound to make a new word. Nonsense words are acceptable as long as the rule is followed.

Examples: hit → him

mop → mock

fan	cheese
rug	moon
tin	nice
boat	drape
lake	song

Instructions: Ask the child to make a word by putting the sounds together.

Examples: (*make*) /m/ /e/ /k/ → make

(*laugh*) /l/ /æ/ /f/ → laugh

(*jam*) /dʒ/ /æ/ /m/	(*sneeze*) /s/ /n/ /i/ /z/
(*hop*) /h/ /ɑ/ /p/	(*sunshine*) /s/ /ə/ /n/ /ʃ/ /aɪ/ /n/
(*good*) /g/ /ʊ/ /d/	(*stamp*) /s/ /t/ /æ/ /m/ /p/
(*baby*) /b/ /e/ /b/ /ɪ/	(*plate*) /p/ /l/ /e/ /t/
(*sausage*) /s/ /ɑ/ /s/ /u/ /dʒ/	(*travel*) /t/ /r/ /æ/ /v/ /l/

Instructions: Ask the child to separate the sounds in the following words.

Examples: dog → /d/ /ɑ/ /g/

bake → /b/ /e/ /k/

pot	ticket
man	blue
run	step
soup	truck
paper	frog

Instructions: Ask the child to name the words that begin with the same sound.

Examples: pop, pan, sit → pop, pan

soap, move, sand → soap, sand

far, hop, fan	dig, goat, dog
mouse, bat, bin	yellow, yo-yo, green
tooth, sun, time	mister, money, dollar
dog, game, dad	jump, vacation, violin
cup, computer, desk	plate, pray, straight

(continues)

Form 8-2. continued

Instructions: Ask the child to combine the following syllables to make a word. Be sure to put space between each syllable as you present the stimulus.

Examples: pop-corn → popcorn
           mon-key → monkey

hot-dog	Po-ke-mon
cow-boy	pi-a-no
sea-shell	De-cem-ber
pa-per	el-e-va-tor
trac-tor	im-po-ssi-ble

Instructions: Ask the child to divide the following words into syllables.

Examples: window → win-dow
           elephant → el-e-phant

garden	orchestra
sandwich	paperweight
summer	rhinocerous
popsicle	macaroni
cranberry	television

Form 8-3.

Worksheet for Narrative Analysis

Name: _____ DOB: _____

School: _____ Grade: _____

Teacher: _____ Date: _____

Instructions: Elicit a narrative sample. Answer the following questions.

How was the sample elicited (e.g., retelling of someone else's story; child-invented story)? Picture prompts used? Yes or No?

Who are the main characters?

What is the setting?

What is the conflict or problem?

List initiating events (that set up the conflict).

List internal responses (character responses to initiating events).

List attempts to resolve conflict.

(continues)

Form 8-3. continued

What is the resolution?

What is the reaction to the resolution?

Is there a conclusion? Is it logical?

Is vocabulary appropriate for the story? Yes or No? List essential vocabulary.

Is sentence structure acceptable? Yes or No? If no, describe.

How many words per sentence?

What clause types are used?

Are embedded clauses used? Yes or No? If yes, describe depth.

Do elements of the story tie together?

(continues)

Form 8-3. continued

Is there a clear beginning, middle, and end?

Does the story make sense?

For written narrative analysis include:

Describe spelling strategies.

Is correct punctuation and capitalization used?

Did the writer edit and proofread the original draft? Yes or No? If yes, comment on the quality of edits/revisions.

Other observations:

Form 8-4.

Informal Reading Inventory

Name: _____ DOB: _____

School: _____ Grade: _____

Teacher: _____ Date: _____

Passage: _____ Reading Level: _____ # Words: _____

Reading fluency: _____

Reading accuracy: _____

Observations (e.g., decoding strategies, phonemic knowledge, unknown vocabulary, self-corrections, etc.):

Literal Comprehension (who, what, where, when):

Inferential Comprehension (why, how):

Frustration Level:

Form 8-5.

Worksheet for Analyzing a Writing Sample

Name: _____ DOB: _____

School: _____ Grade: _____

Teacher: _____ Date: _____

Part I

Instructions: Ask the student to transcribe the following sentence on a clean sheet of manuscript paper. You may have the student write it without a visual prompt, or you may provide a sample of the sentence for the student to copy.

Purple flying monkeys always make me laugh.

Take note of these aspects of the student's writing:

Does the student hold the pencil properly?

Does the student apply appropriate pressure?

Is the transcription oriented appropriately on the paper?

Does the student write from left to right?

Is there appropriate spacing between words?

(continues)

Form 8-5. continued

Are letters formed accurately?

Is the writing legible?

If errors were made, did the student self-correct?

Does the student's visual-motor integration seem appropriate?

If the student did not use a visual prompt:
Did the student accurately transcribe the sentence?

Are all words spelled correctly?

If the student copied from a sample:
Did the student copy the sentence correctly?

Does the student's visual memory seem appropriate?

(continues)

Form 8-5. continued

Part II

Instructions: Obtain a typical writing sample from the student's teacher, or ask the student to write a sample. Use this worksheet to evaluate and analyze the writing sample.

Is the sample legible?

Is there a framework or a plan that holds everything together?

Is there a beginning, middle, and end?

Are you able to follow the text?

Is there an appropriate sense of audience?

Is tense consistent throughout?

Are there transitions between paragraphs or ideas?

Is the vocabulary appropriate considering the student's age/grade?

(continues)

Form 8-5. continued

Is there a variety of words and word-types used?

Are grammatical rules followed?

Are there complex sentences?

Are phrase structure rules followed?

Is there noun–verb agreement?

Is punctuation used correctly?

Are all words spelled correctly?

Is capitalization used correctly?

(continues)

Form 8-5. continued

Are paragraphs separated appropriately?

How many sentences or phrases are there altogether?

What is the average number of words per sentence or phrase?

Did the student edit and proofread the original draft? Yes or No? If yes, comment on the quality of edits/revisions.

Other observations:

Form 8-6.

Worksheet for Expository Writing Analysis

Name: _____ DOB: _____

School: _____ Grade: _____

Teacher: _____ Date: _____

Instructions: Obtain a sample of expository writing. Answer the following questions.

What was the assignment (basic instructions to student)?

Who is the intended audience?

What is the main thesis of the essay?

Is the thesis narrow enough so that the body of the paper can support it?

Is the thesis presented in the introductory paragraph?

What are the central supporting ideas?

Do the supporting paragraphs each contain a single central idea that supports the thesis?

(continues)

Form 8-6. continued

Do the supporting paragraphs contain extraneous information that does not support the central idea of the paragraph?

Are transitions appropriately used? List transitions used.

Is the thesis restated in the concluding paragraph?

Which main points are restated in the concluding paragraph?

Does the concluding paragraph contain new information?

Is the essay based on facts, not personal opinion or feeling?

Is the essay clear and well organized?

Is the vocabulary appropriate? Yes or No? List essential vocabulary.

Is a variety of words used?

(continues)

Form 8-6. continued

Is sentence structure acceptable? Yes or No? If no, describe.

How many words per sentence?

What clause types are used?

Are embedded clauses used? Yes or No? If yes, describe depth.

Does the essay make sense?

Are there spelling errors? Yes or No? If yes, describe.

Is correct punctuation and capitalization used?

Did the writer edit and proofread the original draft? Yes or No? If yes, comment on the quality of edits/revisions.

Other observations:

Form 8-7.

Worksheet for Persuasive Writing Analysis

Name: _____ DOB: _____

School: _____ Grade: _____

Teacher: _____ Date: _____

Instructions: Obtain a sample of persuasive writing. Answer the following questions.

What was the assignment (basic instructions to student)?

Who is the intended audience?

What is the main thesis of the essay?

Is the thesis a debatable statement of position?

Is the thesis presented in the introductory paragraph?

What are the central supporting ideas?

Are the supporting ideas based on fact?

Do the supporting paragraphs contain evidence, examples, and statistics that support the thesis?

(continues)

Form 8-7. continued

Do the supporting paragraphs contain extraneous information that does not support the central idea of the paragraph?

Do the supporting paragraphs contain too much personal opinion?

Are transitions appropriately used? List transitions used.

Is the thesis restated in the concluding paragraph?

Which main points are restated in the concluding paragraph?

Does the concluding paragraph contain new information?

Is the essay clear and well organized?

Is the vocabulary appropriate? Yes or No? List essential vocabulary.

Is a variety of words used?

(continues)

Form 8-7. continued

Is sentence structure acceptable? Yes or No? If no, describe.

How many words per sentence?

What clause types are used?

Are embedded clauses used? Yes or No? If yes, describe depth.

Does the essay make sense?

Are there spelling errors? Yes or No? If yes, describe.

Is correct punctuation and capitalization used?

Did the writer edit and proofread the original draft? Yes or No? If yes, comment on the quality of edits/revisions.

Other observations:

Form 8.7 continued

Is sentence structure acceptable? Yes or No? If no, describe.

How many words per sentence?

What clause types are used?

Are embedded clauses used? Yes or No? If yes, describe the depth.

Does the essay make sense?

Are there spelling errors? Yes or No? If yes, describe.

Is correct punctuation and capitalization used?

Did the writer edit and proofread the original draft? Yes or No? If yes, comment on the quality of the revisions.

Other observations.

Chapter 9

ASSESSMENT FOR AUTISM SPECTRUM DISORDER AND SOCIAL COMMUNICATION DISORDER

OVERVIEW OF ASSESSMENT

History of the Client

    Procedures

        Written Case History

        Information-Gathering Interview

        Information from Other Professionals

    Considerations

        Medical or Neurological Factors

        Age and Intelligence

        Situational Demands

Assessment of Social Communication

    Procedures

        Screening

        Consultation with Parents or Caregivers

        Consultation with Other Professionals

        Authentic Assessment

        Formal Testing

    Analysis

        Social Communication

        Restrictive and Repetitive Behaviors

        Theory of Mind

        Levels of Support

        Age of Onset

        Comorbid Conditions

Orofacial Examination

Speech and Language Assessment

Hearing Assessment

Determining the Diagnosis

Providing Information (written report, interview, etc.)

CHARACTERISTICS OF AUTISM SPECTRUM DISORDER

The *Diagnostic and Statistical Manual of Mental Disorders* (DSM), published by the American Psychiatric Association, is the authoritative resource for defining many deviant speech-language behaviors, including social communicative disorders and autism spectrum disorders. In the 5th edition of the DSM (DSM-5, 2013), the definition of autism spectrum disorder (ASD) was significantly redefined. The previous subcategories of autistic disorder—Asperger disorder, childhood disintegrative disorder, Rett syndrome, and pervasive developmental disorder not otherwise specified—are now replaced with a single diagnosis of autism spectrum disorder with varying degrees of severity. Most individuals with a pre-existing diagnosis are assigned the new DSM-5 diagnosis of ASD without need for reevaluation. The current definition of ASD is based on two areas of function: (1) social communication and (2) fixated interests and repetitive behaviors. A diagnosis of ASD requires evidence of deficits in both areas. A severity rating is then applied to each area based on the amount of support needed. Severity values are as follows:

- Level 1 — Requiring support
- Level 2 — Requiring substantial support
- Level 3 — Requiring very substantial support

A more complete summary of ASD symptoms is presented in Table 9-1. Severity guidelines are presented in Table 9-2.

TABLE 9-1. Diagnostic Criteria for Autism Spectrum Disorder

All five of these criteria must be present to positively diagnose ASD:

1. *Impaired Social Communication.* The individual has difficulties with social communication and interaction in multiple contexts that cannot be accounted for by general developmental delay, intellectual disability, or other condition. These difficulties are manifest by all three of the following symptoms:
   a. *Deficits in social-emotional reciprocity.* The individual demonstrates abnormal social approach, lack of social initiation or response, deficient back-and-forth communicative exchange, and/or limited sharing of interests, emotions, or affect.
   b. *Deficits in nonverbal communication used for social interaction.* The individual demonstrates poorly integrated verbal and nonverbal communication, abnormal eye contact and body language, poor knowledge and use of gestures, or lack of facial expression.
   c. *Deficits in developing, maintaining, and understanding relationships.* The individual does not adjust behaviors according to social context, demonstrates deficient imaginative play, has difficulty making friends, or altogether lacks interest in peers.
2. *Restricted and Repetitive Interests, Activities, and Behaviors.* The individual demonstrates at least two of the following four symptoms:
   a. *Stereotyped or repetitive speech, motor movements, or use of objects.* This may include abnormal motor behaviors such as rocking or spinning, echolalia, idiosyncratic phrases, or repetitive and unusual use of objects such as flipping, spinning, or lining up toys.
   b. *Inflexibility.* The individual is abnormally distressed by small changes in routine, has trouble with transitions, or expresses rigid patterns of thought. He or she may demonstrate ritualized verbal or nonverbal behavior, insist on the same driving routes or foods, or incessantly question changes to routine.
   c. *Abnormally restricted or fixated interests.* The individual demonstrates unusually strong attachments to or preoccupation with unusual objects, an extremely limited range of personal interests, or perseverative behavior.
   d. *Hyper- or hypoactive sensory behavior.* The individual may demonstrate extreme responses (overreaction or lack of response) to sensations such as pain, hot/cold temperatures, sounds, textures, or smells. He or she may be fascinated with lights or spinning objects.
3. The person's social communicative challenges have a negative impact on relationships, academic achievement, and/or occupational performance.
4. Onset of symptoms occurs in early childhood even if behaviors are not recognized until later when communication demands exceed abilities.
5. These behaviors cannot be accounted for by intellectual disability, developmental delay, or any other diagnosis.

SOCIAL COMMUNICATION DISORDER

TABLE 9-2. Autism Spectrum Disorder Severity Indicators

SEVERITY LEVEL	SOCIAL COMMUNICATION	FIXATED INTERESTS AND REPETITIVE BEHAVIORS
Level 1: Requires Support	• Noticeable deficits in verbal and nonverbal social communication skills without support • Difficulty initiating social interaction • Some atypical or unsuccessful responses to social bids from others • Reduced interest in social interactions	• Behaviors interfere with functioning in one or more contexts • Resists being redirected or interrupted
Level 2: Requires Substantial Support	• Marked deficits in verbal and nonverbal social communication skills even with support • Limited initiation of social interactions • Abnormal response to social bids from others	• Behaviors are apparent to casual observers • Behaviors interfere with functioning in multiple contexts • Some distress when rituals and routines are disrupted • Difficult to redirect from fixated interests
Level 3: Requires Very Substantial Support	• Severe deficits in verbal and nonverbal social communication skills • Limited to no initiation of social interactions • Minimal to no response to social bids from others	• Behaviors interfere significantly with functioning • Significant distress when rituals and routines are disrupted • Very difficult to redirect from fixated interests

It is important to note that ASD is separate from intellectual disability or other speech-language diagnosis; however, more than one diagnosis can co-occur in the same client. In order to accurately diagnose ASD, the client's social communication should be below what would be expected for his or her overall developmental level or other known diagnoses.

CHARACTERISTICS OF SOCIAL (PRAGMATIC) COMMUNICATION DISORDER

Some clients may seem to have difficulty with social communication, yet do not meet the requirements for a diagnosis of ASD. These clients may meet the criteria for social (pragmatic) communication disorder (SCD), a new diagnosis introduced in the DSM-5. Characteristics of SCD are:

• Difficulty with social verbal and nonverbal communication that cannot be accounted for by intellectual disability, specific language impairment, autism spectrum disorder, or other diagnosis.

- Difficulty acquiring and using spoken and written language. The individual may demonstrate difficulty following rules for conversation and storytelling, or may not understand nonliteral or ambiguous language.
- Inappropriate responses in conversation. The individual may have difficulty modifying communication according to changes in audience or context.
- The person's social communicative challenges have a negative impact on relationships, academic achievement, and/or occupational performance.
- Onset of symptoms occurs in early childhood even if behaviors are not recognized until later when communication demands exceed abilities.

EARLY INDICATORS OF AUTISM SPECTRUM DISORDER OR SOCIAL COMMUNICATION DISORDER

It is important to diagnose ASD or SCD as early as possible so that appropriate interventions can begin. Current research indicates that diagnoses before children are 3 years of age, when made by knowledgeable and experienced professionals, are stable; children do not outgrow the disorder. It is also worth noting that a positive diagnosis requires the presence of abnormal behaviors in early childhood, even if these behaviors are not clearly recognized until later in life. Many of the early indicators of ASD and SCD are listed below. In most cases, early signs have more to do with what a child does *not* do than what a child does do. Young children with autism often:

- Do not respond to social bids
- Do not smile responsively
- Do not reciprocate affection
- Use limited to no eye contact during interactions
- Do not imitate the actions of others (e.g., wave goodbye)
- Do not repeat behaviors that produce attention or laughter
- Show limited interest in other children
- Do not understand gestures or use gestures to communicate
- Do not engage in a broad repertoire of functional play activities
- Do not create simple play schemes or sequences with toys
- Do not engage in imaginative play
- Engage in repetitive play activities
- Demonstrate repetitive motor behaviors
- Respond inconsistently to sounds
- Show unusual visual interests (e.g., spinning objects, studying objects)

Although the behaviors in the previous list may or may not be early signs of ASD or SCD, the presence of the following behaviors are absolute indicators of a need for further evaluation:

- No warm smiles or joyful expressions by 6 months
- No back-and-forth communicative exchange of sounds, smiles, or other facial expressions by 9 months
- No babbling by 12 months

- No communicative gesturing by 12 months
- No single words by 16 months
- No meaningful two-word phrases by 24 months (some echolalic phrases may be present)
- Significant loss of any language or social skills at any age

The "Autism and Social Communication Disorder Screening Form," Form 9-1, is a parent questionnaire designed to identify young children who may have autism spectrum disorder or social communication disorder. Other screening tools for early identification include:

- *Modified Checklist for Autism in Toddlers-Revised with Follow Up (M-CHAT-R/F)* (Robins, Fein, & Barton, 2009) (Note: available online as free download for clinical use at www.m-chat.org)
- *Screening Tool for Autism in Two-Year-Olds* (Stone, Coonrod, & Ousley, 2000)
- *Social Communication Questionnaire* (Rutter, Bailey, Lord, & Berument, 2003)

SOCIAL COMMUNICATION

Social communication refers to the knowledge and use of language and pragmatics to interact with another person or group of people. There are many skills involved in effectively and naturally interacting with others. These include reciprocating experiences and emotions, understanding and using gestures and facial expressions, following rules of conversation, recognizing social cues and adjusting as needed, and using appropriate language and voice. A significant and central component of both autism spectrum disorder and social communication disorder is a client's deficient social communication. In order to assess a client's social communication skills, it is important to know normal developmental expectations. Table 9-3

TABLE 9-3.   Social Communication Benchmarks

Consider cultural and linguistic factors that may influence appropriateness and/or relevance of benchmarks.

AGE	BENCHMARK
Birth to 12 months	Prefers looking at human face and eyes
	Prefers listening to human voice
	Looks for source of voice
	Differentiates between tones of voice (e.g., angry, friendly)
	Smiles back at caregiver
	Follows caregiver's gaze
	Participates in vocal turn-taking with caregiver
	Vocalizes to get attention
	Demonstrates joint attention skills (sharing attention)
	Uses gestures to make requests and direct attention
	Plays simple interactive games, such as peek-a-boo

AGE	BENCHMARK
12–18 months	Brings objects to show caregivers
	Requests by pointing and vocalizing
	Solicits attention vocally
	Practices vocal inflection
	Says "bye" and other ritualized words
	Protests by shaking head, saying "no"
	Supplements gestures with verbal language
	Aware of social value of speech
	Responds to the speech of others with eye contact
	Demonstrates sympathy, empathy, and sharing nonverbally
18–24 months	Uses single words to express intention
	Uses single and paired words to command, indicate possession, express problems, and gain attention
	Uses *I, me, you, my,* and *mine*
	Participates in verbal turn-taking with limited number of turns
	Demonstrates simple topic control
	Interrupts at syntactic junctures or in response to prosodic cues
24–36 months	Engages in short dialogues
	Verbally introduces and changes topic
	Expresses emotion
	Begins to use language in imaginative way
	Relates own experiences
	Begins to provide descriptive detail to enhance listener understanding
	Uses attention-getting words
	Clarifies and asks for clarification
	Introduces and changes topics
	Uses some politeness terms or markers
	Begins to demonstrate some adaptation of speech to different listeners
3–4 years	Engages in longer dialogues
	Anticipates next turn at talking
	Terminates conversation
	Appropriately role-plays
	Uses fillers such as *yeah* and *okay* to acknowledge a partner's message
	Begins code-switching and uses simpler language when talking to very young children
	Uses more elliptical responses
	Requests permission
	Begins using language for fantasies, jokes, teasing
	Makes conversational repairs when not understood and corrects others
	Uses primitive narratives—events follow from central core/use of inferences in stories

continued on the next page

SOCIAL COMMUNICATION DISORDER

Table 9-3, continued from the previous page

AGE	BENCHMARK
4–5 years	Uses indirect requests
	Correctly uses deictic terms (e.g., *this, that, here, there*)
	Uses twice as many effective utterances as 3-year-olds to discuss emotions and feelings
	Uses narrative development characterized by unfocused chains—stories have sequence of events, but no central character or theme
	Develops basic understanding of theory of mind (ToM)
	Shifts topics rapidly
School-Age Years	Demonstrates increased understanding of ToM (e.g., reads body language, facial expressions, prosodic characteristics of language to predict behavior; takes the perspective of another and modifes language use accordingly)
	Provides assistance and demonstrates altruism
	Uses narrative development characterized by causally sequenced events using "story grammar"
	Demonstrates improved conversational skills (e.g., topic maintenance, repair, and increased number of turns)
	Extends topics of conversation
	Demonstrates refined social conventions
	Uses language for varied functions, including persuading and advancing opinion
Adulthood	Uses verbal and nonverbal language competently and flexibly
	Navigates multiple registers flexibly and fluidly
	Demonstrates refined understanding and use of nonverbal behavior

Source: American Speech-Language-Hearing Association, "Social Communication Benchmarks," no date, available at http://www.asha.org/uploadedFiles/ASHA/Practice_Portal/Clinical_Topics/Social_Communication_Disorders_in_School-Age_Children/Social-Communication-Benchmarks.pdf. Used with permission. As noted on the ASHA website, this table was developed based on information from Gard, Gilman, and Gorman (1993) and Russell (2007).

presents social communication benchmarks in normal development. When using this information, be sure to consider cultural and linguistic factors that may influence or negate the relevance of certain behaviors.

LANGUAGE CONCERNS

Even though language development and use are not identified as specific characteristics of autism or social communication disorder, clients with these disorders are likely to demonstrate certain patterns of language comprehension and expression. Several behaviors that are typical are listed below by category. Because of individual variability, not all of the behaviors will be seen in every client.

General Comprehension and Expression

- Difficulty with language comprehension
- High-pitched, monotonous speech
- Echolalia
- Stereotypic, meaningless speech
- Asocial monologues
- Preference for mechanical sounds over human voice
- Preoccupations
- Reduced interest in communication
- Errors in recognizing faces
- Poor use of environmental cues
- Poor response to commands

Pragmatic Behaviors

- Lack of responsiveness to others
- Difficulty with topic maintenance in conversation
- Use of only a few communication strategies
- Minimal use of gestural communication
- Lack of knowledge of speaker and listener roles
- Lack of eye contact
- Difficulty with topical shifts
- Preference for solitude
- Reluctance to be touched, hugged, or held

Semantic Patterns

- Slow acquisition of speech
- Word-finding difficulties
- Faster learning of concrete words than abstract words, particularly abstract words that refer to human relations or emotions
- Difficulty using correct names of other people
- Restricted use of word meanings (lack or word generalization)
- Poor categorization abilities
- Poor understanding of related words

Syntactic and Morphologic Patterns

- Reversal of pronouns
- Difficulties with morphologic inflections (plurals, possessives, verb tenses)
- Overuse of one or two basic sentence patterns
- Use of simple and short sentence structures

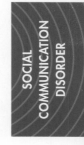

SOCIAL COMMUNICATION DISORDER

- Difficulty with word order
- Omission of grammatical morphemes

Phonologic Patterns

- Variable
- Some articulation disorders
- Delayed acquisition of speech sound production, although appropriate speech patterns develop over time
- Exaggerated articulation
- Difficulty with sound segmentation and knowledge of word boundaries

ASSESSMENT AND DIAGNOSIS

An authentic assessment approach is the most desirable approach for evaluating the speech and language skills of clients with autism spectrum disorder or social communicative disorder. Clinical judgments and decision are based primarily on case history information, consultations with other professionals who work with the client, clinical observations in multiple settings, play assessment, and communication and behavioral analysis. Traditional standardized tests may be used, but many have limitations. Most standardized tests do not evaluate the pragmatic deficits that are typical of these social disorders. Because these clients often perform better in structured environments, some may perform within normal expectations during formal testing even though they demonstrate functional communication deficits in nonstructured situations.

Specific strategies for assessing clients with ASD or SCD include:

- Interview teachers, parents, caregivers, and others who spend significant time with the client.
- Consult with other members of the multidisciplinary team. Review school records and medical records. Review cognitive assessment results obtained by a psychologist or psychiatrist.
- Rule out hearing problems, or determine the degree to which hearing problems are contributing to the overall behaviors.
- Obtain communication samples in a variety of settings. Include one-on-one settings and group settings.
- Assess the client during play situations
- Take note of inappropriate physical behaviors
- Consider the client's development of theory of mind

Theory of mind (ToM) is a person's ability to understand that people engage in mental processes, such as cognitive knowledge and emotion, separate from his or her own processes. More generally stated, it is an ability to "read another's mind." Individuals with ASD or SCD may have particular delays and deficits in the development of ToM. Normal developmental milestones of ToM are presented in Table 9-4.

TABLE 9-4   **Milestones of Metacognitive Knowledge ToM and Emotional Knowledge ToM in Normally Developing Children**

AGE OF MASTERY	ToM KNOWLEDGE
Metacognitive Knowledge	
3	Predict uncomplicated behaviors or situations (e.g., Mommy will get a puzzle out of the game closet, because that is where puzzles are stored.)
5	Understand that people can hold false beliefs (e.g., Mom thinks the cookie jar is full; she doesn't know I ate the cookies.)
7	Understand nested beliefs (e.g., "Mom thinks that Dad thinks . . .")
Emotional Knowledge	
5	Relate experiences in which they felt sad, happy, mad, scared, or surprised
7	Relate experiences in which they felt jealous, guilty, or embarrassed

Source: "Autism," by C. Westby and N. McKellar, in *The Survival Guide for School-Based Speech-Language Pathologists* (pp. 263–303), by E. P. Dodge (Ed.), 2000, Clifton Park, NY: Cengage Learning.

It is necessary to obtain samples of the client's communicative behaviors in a variety of clinical and extra-clinical situations. These suggestions may help to elicit certain targeted responses:

- Have the client assemble a simple puzzle. Before giving him or her the puzzle, remove one piece and replace it with a piece that is obviously from a different puzzle.
- Spin a top; when it stops spinning, hand it to the client.
- Place a desirable object out of the client's reach.
- Intentionally fall off your chair.
- When the client is engaged in something interesting, change the scene suddenly by taking away the interesting object and offering a new one.
- Place an object on the edge of a table where it might easily fall off.
- Open a jar of bubbles, blow a few, then close the jar and hand it to the client.
- Show pictures of people who are expressing different emotions. Ask what the people are feeling.
- Play a "let's pretend" game.
- Have the client make up a story. It may be helpful to offer an opening sentence (e.g., "Two brothers were lying in their beds, when suddenly they heard a loud noise").
- Have the client "read" a wordless, plot-based picture book. Ask the client to explain and predict events.
- Have the client interpret video stories that have music and sound effects, but no spoken words.

Form 9-2, "Behavioral Analysis Worksheet," is helpful for analyzing communicative behaviors in a variety of settings. A clinician, parent, teacher, or daycare provider can complete the form, or another person involved in the child's life. It is helpful to obtain information from a variety of settings using a different form to analyze each situation. It may also be helpful to video-record samples when possible. Audiotaped samples are less desirable because nonverbal aspects of communication are not recorded.

Form 9-3, "Assessment for Autism Spectrum Disorder," is provided to help clinicians assess clients with possible autism spectrum disorder. It is crucial to be thorough and thoughtful before making a positive diagnosis. Some behaviors may seem a bit "off" but may not justify a diagnosis of ASD. Consider the following:

- Are the behaviors clearly atypical?
- Can the behaviors be otherwise explained (e.g., physical, developmental, or intellectual explanation)?
- Do the behaviors occur regularly and in multiple settings? (This is not a determiner, but is an important consideration.)
- Are there multiple examples of a particular behavior?
- How persistent and frequent are the behaviors?
- Are there behaviors that occurred in the past but have since diminished or disappeared? (These are acceptable for positive diagnosis unless accounted for by normal development)

Clients who demonstrate atypical social behaviors but do not qualify for a diagnosis of ASD may qualify for a diagnosis of CSD. Form 9-4, "Assessment for Social (Pragmatic) Communication Disorder," is provided to help with this determination.

CONCLUDING COMMENTS

This chapter provided an overview of assessment procedures for autism spectrum disorder and social communication disorder. In some cases, behaviors of each condition are similar and overlap. However, these disorders are separate and distinct conditions. It is important to know the criteria for making an accurate diagnosis and thoroughly consider alternative diagnoses before assigning either diagnostic label to a client.

SOURCES OF ADDITIONAL INFORMATION

Print Sources

Janzen, J. E., & Zenko, C. B. (2012). *Understanding the nature of autism: A guide to the autism spectrum disorders* (3rd ed). Austin, TX: Pro-ed.

Luiselli, J. K. (2014). *Children and youth with autism spectrum disorder (ASD): Recent advances and innovations in assessment, education, and intervention.* New York: Oxford University Press.

Volkmar, F. R., Paul, R., Rogers, S. J., & Pelphrey, K. A. (Eds.). (2014). *Handbook of autism and pervasive developmental disorders, diagnosis, development, and brain mechanisms* (Vol. 1). Indianapolis, IN: Wiley.

Electronic Sources

Autism Society of America:
http://www.autism-society.org

Autism Speaks, Inc.:
http://www.autismspeaks.org

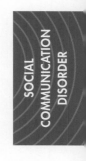

Volkmar, F. R., Paul, R., Rogers, S. J., & Pelphrey, K. A. (Eds.). (2014). Handbook of autism and pervasive developmental disorders: Diagnosis, development, and brain mechanisms (Vol. 1). Indianapolis, IN: Wiley.

Electronic Sources

Autism Society of America:
http://www.autism-society.org

Autism Speaks, Inc.:
http://www.autismspeaks.org

Form 9-1.

Autism and Social Communication Disorder Screening Form

Name: _____ DOB: _____

Informant's Name: _____

Informant's Relationship to Child: _____

Examiner's Name: _____

Date: _____

SOCIAL COMMUNICATION DISORDER

Instructions: Answer the following questions according to how your child usually behaves. If the behavior is rare (i.e., you've seen it once or twice), please answer as if the child does not do it.

Y N 1. Does your child respond to you when you call his or her name?

Y N 2. Does your child understand what others say?

Y N 3. When you smile at your child does he or she smile back?

Y N 4. Does your child imitate facial expressions?

Y N 5. Does your child make eye contact with you when you are interacting?

Y N 6. Does your child enjoy playing peek-a-boo or hide-and-seek?

Y N 7. Does your child engage in pretend play (e.g., take care of a doll or "cook" in the kitchen)?

Y N 8. Does your child enjoy many different types of play activities?

Y N 9. Does your child use gestures to communicate (e.g., wave goodbye or point to a desired object)?

Y N 10. Does your child seem to understand gestures used by others?

Y N 11. Does your child enjoy cuddling with you?

Y N 12. Does your child reciprocate affection, such as hugs and kisses?

Y N 13. Does your child repeat actions that make others laugh?

Y N 14. Does your child seem to enjoy playing with other children?

Y N 15. Does your child ever bring toys or objects to you to show you?

Y N 16. Does your child enjoy looking at picture books with you?

Y N 17. Does your child use toys appropriately (e.g., use a brush to brush a doll's hair or use blocks for building a tower)?

Y N 18. Does your child look at you to check your reactions to events or unfamiliar situations?

Y N 19. Would you say your child has an active imagination?

Y N 20. Does your child engage in unusual rocking behaviors?

Y N 21. Does your child engage in unusual finger movements?

(continues)

Form 9-1. continued

Y   N   22.   Does your child visually examine objects with an unusual fascination?

Y   N   23.   Is your child particularly interested in objects that spin?

Y   N   24.   Have you ever wondered if your child is deaf or hearing impaired?

Y   N   25.   Does your child prefer to play alone?

Y   N   26.   Has your child ever demonstrated a significant decline in any communicative ability (e.g., at one time talked with two- or three-word phrases and now does not)?

Y   N   27.   Does your child repeat phrases heard by others without using them meaningfully?

At what age did your child start babbling? _____

At what age did your child begin to use gestural communication (e.g., wave goodbye)? _____

At what age did your child produce his or her first word? _____

At what age did your child start combining words into two-word phrases? _____

Please list other comments, clarifications, or concerns:

Form 9-2.

Behavioral Analysis Worksheet

Name: _____

DOB: _____

Date: _____

Setting: _____

Number of People Present: _____

Relationships of People Present: _____

Person Completing Worksheet _____

Instructions: Use this form to analyze communicative behaviors from samples obtained in a variety of settings. Use a different form for each setting.

How does the child relate to others?

If the child gets hurt, how does he or she seek comfort?

How does the child express a desire for affection?

(continues)

Form 9-2. continued

How does the child respond when others attempt to engage the child in play or conversation?

Is echolalia present?

How does the child respond when the environment changes (e.g., someone walks in, sudden noise)?

How does the child communicate wants or needs?

How does the child express emotions?

Anger

Fear

(continues)

Form 9-2. continued

Frustration

Happiness

Sadness

Humor

Surprise

Does the child use toys in typical and appropriate ways?

(continues)

SOCIAL COMMUNICATION DISORDER

Form 9-2. continued

Does the child engage in pretend play?

Does the child appropriately anticipate and predict?

What communication strategies does the child use?

Does the child function better in one-on-one settings in comparison to group settings? If yes, in what ways?

Form 9-3.

Assessment for Autism Spectrum Disorder

Child's Name: _____ DOB: _____ Date: _____

Informant's Name: _____

Relationship to Child: _____

Instructions: Use this form to evaluate the child's behaviors in relationship to criteria for diagnosis of autism spectrum disorder per DSM-5. Note that a "yes" response is required for all prompts in sections 1, 3, 4, and 5, and at least two prompts in section 2 for positive diagnosis.

Section 1. Social Communication

Yes	No	Deficient social-emotional reciprocity. Possible behaviors:
☐	☐	Approaches social situations in unusual ways
☐	☐	Does not initiate social interaction
☐	☐	Does not reply when called on or spoken to
☐	☐	Has difficulty with back-and-forth communication
☐	☐	Does not share personal interests with others
☐	☐	Lack of joint attention
☐	☐	Speech is tangential or presented as one-sided monologue
☐	☐	Does not share social emotions (responsive smile, joy, achievement, concern for others)
☐	☐	Repels or indifferent to physical contact or affection
☐	☐	Other (describe):

Notes:

Yes	No	Deficient nonverbal communication. Possible behaviors:
☐	☐	Averts or avoids eye contact
☐	☐	Unusual body language such as turning away from listener
☐	☐	Does not use or understand gestures such as waving, nodding, or shaking head
☐	☐	Lack of facial expression
☐	☐	Limited ability to convey emotions via facial expression, gestures, or body language
☐	☐	Other (describe):

Notes:

Yes	No	Deficient ability to develop, maintain, and understand relationships. Possible behaviors:
☐	☐	Difficulty adjusting behaviors according to social context
☐	☐	Lack of theory of mind

(continues)

SOCIAL COMMUNICATION DISORDER

Form 9-3. continued

☐ ☐ Does not recognize other's disinterest in an activity
☐ ☐ Socially inappropriate questions or remarks
☐ ☐ Rarely or never engages in imaginative play
☐ ☐ Has difficulty making friends
☐ ☐ May be uninterested in making friends
☐ ☐ Unaware of being teased
☐ ☐ Does not recognize how his or her behaviors and comments affect others
☐ ☐ Lack of imaginative play
☐ ☐ Prefers to play alone
☐ ☐ Oblivious to peers or adults
☐ ☐ Other (describe):

Notes:

Severity:

Level 1: Deficits are noticeable to others but not severe; sometimes engages in social interactions, but is awkward and sometimes unsuccessful; has difficulty initiating

Level 2: Deficits are noticeable even with support; infrequent initiation of social interaction; abnormal responses to social bids from others

Level 3: Deficits are significant even with support; does not seem interested in initiating or engaging in social interaction

Notes:

Section 2. Restricted and Repetitive Interests, Activities, and Behaviors

For each prompt, determine if the behavior is clearly abnormal, in what contexts and situations the behavior occurs, and if the behavior can be explained by some other condition or factor.

Yes No Stereotyped or repetitive speech, motor movements, or use of objects. Possible behaviors:
☐ ☐ Echolalia
☐ ☐ Idiosyncratic phrases
☐ ☐ Use of formal speech
☐ ☐ Refers to self using own name
☐ ☐ Repetitively makes unusual vocalizations
☐ ☐ Abnormal motor behaviors such as rocking, spinning, clapping, etc.
☐ ☐ Abnormal body postures
☐ ☐ Tenses body, grimaces, or grinds teeth
☐ ☐ Uses toys and objects in nonconventional ways, such as waving or repeatedly dropping them

(continues)

Form 9-3. continued

☐ ☐   Lines up toys and objects
☐ ☐   Turns lights on and off repetitively
☐ ☐   Other (describe):

Notes:

Yes No   Inflexibility. Possible behaviors:
☐ ☐   Insists on following routine
☐ ☐   Overreaction to trivial changes in routine
☐ ☐   Difficulty with transitions
☐ ☐   Rigid patterns of thought
☐ ☐   Repeats questions about a single topic
☐ ☐   Maintains verbal rituals for self or others
☐ ☐   Maintains motor rituals for self or others
☐ ☐   Insists on same driving routes or foods
☐ ☐   Incessantly troubled by changes to routine
☐ ☐   Insists that rules be strictly followed
☐ ☐   Other (describe):

Notes:

Yes No   Abnormally restricted or fixated interests. Possible behaviors:
☐ ☐   Extreme attachments to or preoccupations with particular objects
☐ ☐   Limited range of personal interests
☐ ☐   Perseverates on same behaviors, objects, or topics
☐ ☐   Preoccupied with numbers, letters, and symbols
☐ ☐   Focuses on nonfunctional parts of objects
☐ ☐   Unusual and irrational fears
☐ ☐   Other (describe):

Notes:

Yes No   Hyper- or hypoactive sensory behavior. Possible behaviors:
☐ ☐   Overly sensitive to pain, hot or cold temperatures, sounds, textures, or smells
☐ ☐   Indifference to pain, hot or cold temperatures, sounds, textures, or smells
☐ ☐   Unusual licking, smelling, or touching of objects
☐ ☐   Does not like to touch certain objects
☐ ☐   Dislikes having hair or teeth brushed

(continues)

SOCIAL COMMUNICATION DISORDER

Form 9-3. continued

☐ ☐   Squints eyes

☐ ☐   Fascination with lights

☐ ☐   Fascination with spinning objects, doors opening/closing, fan movement

☐ ☐   Other (describe):

Notes:

Severity:

Level 1:   Behaviors interfere with functioning sometimes but not always; child can be redirected or interrupted but with some resistance

Level 2:   Behaviors are noticeable to outsiders and interfere with functioning in more than one setting; child shows noticeable distress when rituals and routines are disrupted; it is difficult to redirect the child from fixated interests

Level 3:   Behaviors significantly interfere with functioning; child shows significant distress when rituals and routines are disrupted; it is very difficult to redirect the child from fixated interests

Notes:

Section 3. Impact on Personal Life

Yes   No   Child's behaviors have a negative impact on his or her relationships, academic achievement, and/or occupational performance.

Notes:

Section 4. Onset of Symptoms

Yes   No   Some indicators of the child's behaviors were present in early childhood, whether or not they were identified in early childhood.

Notes:

Section 5. Other Conditions

Yes   No   Child's behaviors cannot be accounted for by another condition. Rule out:

☐ ☐   Intellectual disability disorder

☐ ☐   Developmental delay

☐ ☐   Language impairment

☐ ☐   Social (pragmatic) communicative disorder

☐ ☐   Other:

Notes:

Form 9-4.

Assessment for Social (Pragmatic) Communication Disorder

Child's Name: _____ DOB: _____ Date: _____

Informant's Name: _____

Relationship to Child: _____

Instructions: Use this form to evaluate the child's behaviors in relationship to criteria for diagnosis of social communicative disorder per DSM-5. Note that a "yes" response is required for all prompts in all sections for positive diagnosis.

Section 1. Verbal and Nonverbal Pragmatic Communication

Yes	No	Deficient use of communication for social purposes. Possible behaviors:
☐	☐	Has difficulty with social greetings
☐	☐	Avoids or averts eye contact
☐	☐	Has difficulty with back-and-forth communication
☐	☐	Lacks theory of mind
☐	☐	Lacks emotional expression
☐	☐	Does not understand or use gestural communication
☐	☐	Limited joint attention
☐	☐	Social behaviors are inappropriate for the setting and situation
☐	☐	Makes inappropriate requests or comments
☐	☐	Other (describe):

Notes:

Yes	No	Deficient modification of communication to match situation. Possible behaviors:
☐	☐	Vocal intensity does not match the environment (e.g., library voice, playground voice)
☐	☐	Does not modify communication according to audience (e.g., teacher, peer)
☐	☐	Language is formal and adult-like
☐	☐	Other (describe):

Notes:

Yes	No	Deficient use of conversational or storytelling rules. Possible behaviors:
☐	☐	Does not take turns in conversation
☐	☐	Does not initiate conversation
☐	☐	Does not rephrase when listener does not understand

(continues)

Form 9-4. continued

☐ ☐ Does not provide background information

☐ ☐ Does not use verbal or nonverbal signals to regulate interactions

☐ ☐ Difficulty understanding inference, humor, or ambiguous language

☐ ☐ Other (describe):

Notes:

Yes No Does not understand ambiguous or nonliteral language. Possible behaviors:

☐ ☐ Does not make inferences

☐ ☐ Does not understand idioms, metaphors, or multiple meanings that are dependent upon context for interpretation

☐ ☐ Does not understand nonliteral humor

☐ ☐ Other (describe):

Notes:

Section 2. Impact on Personal Life

Yes No Child's communicative deficits have a negative impact on his or her social relationships, academic achievement, and/or occupational performance.

Notes:

Section 3. Onset of Symptoms

Yes No Some indicators of the child's behaviors were present in early childhood, whether or not they were identified in early childhood.

Notes:

Section 4. Other Conditions

Yes No Child's behaviors cannot be accounted for by another condition. Rule out:

☐ ☐ Intellectual disability disorder

☐ ☐ Developmental delay

☐ ☐ Language impairment

☐ ☐ Autism spectrum disorder

☐ ☐ Other:

Notes:

Chapter 10

ASSESSMENT FOR AUGMENTATIVE OR ALTERNATIVE COMMUNICATION (AAC)

- ■ Overview of Assessment
- ■ Assessing Sensory and Motor Capabilities
- ■ Assessing Language and Cognitive Skills
- ■ Determining the Most Appropriate AAC System

  Apps for AAC

- ■ Concluding Comments
- ■ Sources of Additional Information
- ■ Chapter 10 Forms

OVERVIEW OF ASSESSMENT

History of the Client

    Procedures

        Written Case History
        Information-Getting Interview
        Information from Other Professionals

    Considerations

        Medical or Neurological Factors
        Age and Intelligence
        Situational Demands

Assessment of Social Communication

    Procedures

        Screening
        Consultation with Parents or Caregivers
        Consultation with Other Professionals
        Authentic Assessment
        Formal Testing

    Analysis

        Current Needs
        Sensory Skills
        Motor Skills
        Cognitive Abilities
        Language Abilities
        Appropriate AAC Options

Orofacial Examination

Speech and Language Assessment

Hearing Assessment

Determining the Diagnosis

Providing Information (written report, interview, etc.)

Some individuals are severely limited in their ability to communicate verbally, due to cognitive disabilities or physical impairments. These clients are often candidates for augmentative or alternative communication (AAC). AAC is a communication system that compensates for impairments and disabilities of clients with severe expressive communication disorders. There are a variety of AAC systems available, ranging from inexpensive, low-technology options such as sign language or communication boards, to costly, high-technology communication devices using synthesized speech output. An AAC system may be needed temporarily or permanently, depending on the client's individual abilities and prognosis.

Client conditions that may warrant use of an AAC device are not limited to but include the following:

- Severe aphasia
- Severe apraxia
- Intellectual disability
- Cerebral palsy
- Down syndrome
- Parkinson's disease
- Traumatic brain injury
- Amyotrophic lateral sclerosis
- Multiple sclerosis
- Autism spectrum disorder
- Alzheimer's disease
- Vocal surgery
- Intubation
- Limited English proficiency

A speech-language evaluation can determine whether AAC will be beneficial and what type of AAC system will be most appropriate for a client. When completing an evaluation of clients with a severe expressive impairment, the evaluation process needs to be modified to accommodate the client's language and physical limitations. The evaluation typically involves consulting a team of professionals, such as physicians, therapists, psychologists, social workers, and teachers, who can provide valuable information to help the clinician make the most appropriate assessment decisions. The assessment of clients for AAC generally includes four broad areas:

- Determining the client's communicative needs
- Assessing the client's sensory and motor abilities
- Assessing the client's language and cognitive abilities
- Predicting the most suitable AAC system

When determining the client's communicative needs, consider the client's current communication system, how effective that system is, what kind of success or failure the client has experienced with other systems, and what communicative situations and messages are typical for the client. This information can be gathered by interviewing the client as well as other caregivers who interact with the client regularly, especially parents and teachers. The assessment environment needs to be as natural as possible, mimicking what the client experiences during routine day-to-day activity. Glennen and DeCoste (1997) have devised an assessment worksheet that is helpful for evaluating a nonverbal client's communicative needs. We have adapted it and reprinted it in Form 10-1, "Augmentative and Alternative Communication Information and Needs Assessment."

ASSESSING SENSORY AND MOTOR CAPABILITIES

A client with limited verbal skills may have severe sensory or motor impairments that will need to be identified in order to make the most appropriate assessment decisions and AAC recommendations. It is important to modify test administrations to accommodate certain deficits, and to carefully consider the client's abilities and disabilities when selecting an AAC system. The specific sensory and motor abilities to consider are:

- positioning
- hearing
- visual tracking and scanning
- motor dexterity

During the assessment, position the client so that success in completing evaluative tasks is maximized. Pillows, wedges, foam rolls, or other support structures are sometimes helpful for achieving optimal positioning. Consider whether the client can position him- or herself or if restraints are needed. Also note whether the client is able to walk or is confined to a wheelchair. Various AAC systems accommodate a variety of user postures and positions.

The client's visual tracking and scanning abilities also need to be considered. Visual tracking refers to the ability to watch an object or person move through more than one visual plane, and visual scanning refers to the ability to look for and locate an object among several other objects. Both skills will have an impact on assessment administration and recommendations for AAC. Evaluate the client's ability to visually track vertically, horizontally, and diagonally in two directions. Evaluate the client's ability to visually scan words, objects, and symbols that may be used in an AAC system. Use a variety of stimulus items and include repeated trials. Also determine:

- Whether the client can visually focus on an object
- If the eyes move in a smooth, continuous motion
- If nystagmus (oscillating movement of the eyeball) is present
- Whether there are areas of visual neglect
- If the eyes move together
- At what rate the client tracks or scans (e.g., slowly, quickly, inconsistently)
- The distance from the face the item needs to be to successfully view it
- Where the client begins tracking or searching for objects (e.g., at midline, to the right, to the left, up, down)
- Whether there is an identifiable pattern of scanning
- The number of items the client is able to scan

Form 10-2, "Visual Scanning and Tracking Checklist," is provided to help evaluate a client's visual skills for the assessment for AAC.

Hearing acuity becomes particularly important if visual skills are deficient because many AAC devices have auditory scan features that clients with adequate hearing can access. Assessment of hearing is usually straightforward, and an audiologist with or without AAC experience can evaluate hearing abilities.

The evaluation process also includes a determination of the client's motor abilities and deficits and how they will impact the usefulness of various AAC systems. Specific considerations include:

- The primary medical diagnosis
- The presence of abnormal reflexes or tremor
- How easily and how much the client fatigues
- Loss of use of one or both hands

To use certain AAC systems, a client must be able to use some part of the body, preferably a hand, to produce voluntary, controlled, and consistent movements. If physical disability precludes the use of either hand, the head and chin, feet, knees, elbows, or other body part could possibly be used. Even controlled eye blinks or movements of the tongue have been used to access AAC devices.

ASSESSING LANGUAGE AND COGNITIVE SKILLS

The assessment of language and cognitive skills is important for determining current levels of expressive and receptive abilities, understanding how the client perceives the world, and accurately predicting the most suitable AAC system to maximize the client's communication. To determine cognitive levels, make observations about the client's abilities and deficits in the following areas:

- *Alertness*: Note whether the client is aware of his or her surroundings and if the client is oriented to time and space. The Rancho Los Amigos Levels of Cognitive Functioning (described in Chapter 13) is often used to assign or describe general levels of alertness.
- *Fatigue level*
- *Attention span*: Determine how long the client can attend to an activity or conversation.
- *Knowledge of "cause and effect"*: Note whether the client understands the concept that one behavior causes another, such as activating a switch causes a tape recorder to play music.
- *Symbolic representation skills*: Note whether the client recognizes symbols, such as pictures of common objects, and is able to correlate pictures with real objects. Also determine the client's reading and writing skills.
- *Memory skills*

Also important is knowledge of the client's receptive and expressive language abilities. Clearly, the method of assessing language will have to be modified to accommodate physical and verbal disabilities. For example, the clinician may need to allow the client to use eye gaze in place of pointing when administering certain tests. Client-specific stimulus activities may need to be created in order to elicit desired responses. For example, to assess the client's ability to follow simple or complex commands, present directives that the client is motorically capable of doing. Note whether comprehension occurs with verbal direction only or with verbal direction accompanied by gesture.

The Nonspeech Test for Receptive/Expressive Language (Huer, 1988) is an assessment tool designed specifically for evaluating the expressive and receptive language skills of nonverbal clients. Other commercially available tests that are not designed for this population but can be modified for such use include:

- *Boehm Test of Basic Concepts* (3rd ed.) (Boehm, 2001)
- *Peabody Picture Vocabulary Test* (4th ed.) (Dunn & Dunn, 2007)
- *Preschool Language Scale* (5th ed.) Auditory Comprehension Scale (Zimmerman, Steiner, & Evatt-Pond, 2011)
- *Receptive One-Word Picture Vocabulary Test* (4th ed.) (Brownell, 2010)
- *Test for Auditory Comprehension of Language* (4th ed.) (Carrow-Woolfolk, 2014)

Some of the assessment materials presented in Chapter 5, Assessment Procedures Common to Most Communicative Disorders, and Chapter 7, Assessment of Language in Children, in this resource manual can also be adapted.

The client's ability to identify objects and pictures will need to be known prior to administering certain language assessments. This will help determine whether incorrect responses are truly language based or simply due to physical limitations. The clinician can then proceed with more complex communicative tasks that will help in the selection of an appropriate AAC system based on the client's language, cognition, sensory skills, and motor skills. During the assessment, determine whether the client can associate icons with real objects and concepts, use multiple icons to convey a message (e.g., "I want" "to eat" "some cereal"), and recognize categories of icons, pictures, or objects. Also assess the client's ability to read and write. Take note of the size and position of the stimulus materials presented.

DETERMINING THE MOST APPROPRIATE AAC SYSTEM

Once the assessment information is gathered and evaluated, recommendations can be made regarding the type of AAC system that may be most appropriate to meet the client's needs. This is a complex decision, and the recommendation should be made by an individual, or team of individuals, with knowledge of and experience with the various types of AAC systems and devices available. Often, several options can be presented. Even with the most carefully considered decision, field testing will be necessary. Judgments should be made concerning:

- The appropriateness of the AAC system
- The client's proficiency in using the AAC system
- The client's progress in developing communication skills
- The proficiency of the client's communication partners in utilizing the AAC system

Types of AAC system options vary widely. For example, consider these AAC systems that range from free and simplistic to expensive and sophisticated:

- Body language, including gestures, mime, and sign language
- Pen and paper
- Communication boards or books

- Speech-generating machines
- iPads and tablets
- Computer devices

Apps for AAC

An iPad or other tablet can be a very desirable AAC device. These devices are relatively inexpensive and easy to transport, and the clinician can select apps appropriate to the client's current age and changing needs. Most apps are customizable, allowing the user to input the most relevant content, determine the complexity of the user experience, and add personal photos and messages. Some apps that are useful for AAC include:

- "AutisMate" by SpecialNeedsWare
- "GoTalk Now" by Attainment Company
- "LAMP Words for Life" by Prentke Romich Company
- "My First AAC" by NCSOFT
- "My Talk Tools" by 2nd Half Enterprises LLC
- "Predictable" by Therapy Box Limited
- "Proloquo2Go" by AssistiveWare
- "Sonoflex" by Tobii Technology
- "Speak for Yourself" by Speak for Yourself LLC
- "SPEAKall!" by SPEAK MODalities LLC
- "TouchChat" by Silver Kite
- "Verbally" by Intuary

For most clients, it is wise to make the iPad a dedicated communication device. Avoid using the same iPad for games, music, videos, or other entertainment, as these can be distracting for the user.

The selection of the most beneficial AAC system for a client is an ongoing process and is usually not completed during a single evaluation. There are many factors to consider, including the client's proficiency at using a particular system, the client's willingness to use it, and changes in the client's disability, needs, and maturation over time. Commercially available tests that are useful for initial evaluation and subsequent ongoing assessment include:

- *INteraction CHecklist for Augmentative Communication* (Bolton & Dashiell, 1998)
- *Lifespace Access Profile: Assistive Technology Assessment & Planning for Individuals with Severe or Multiple Disabilities* (Williams, Stemach, Wolfe, & Stanger, 1995)
- *Test of Aided-Communication Symbol Performance* (Bruno, 2010)

Probably the ultimate consideration in selecting AAC is the client's desire and willingness to use it. A recommended device may be seen as the answer to a client's communicative needs and have the enthusiastic support of the clinician, the client's family, teachers, and other communicative partners. However, if the client resists or rejects a device, it will serve as nothing more than a futile (and perhaps expensive) undertaking. Counseling, ongoing assessment, and alternative means of communication may need to be offered until an accepted system is found.

AUGMENTATIVE OR ALTERNATIVE COMMUNICATION

CONCLUDING COMMENTS

Augmentative or alternative communication may be indicated to improve the functional communication of severely impaired clients. This chapter provided an overview of assessment procedures and considerations for clients who may benefit from AAC. Selection of an AAC system is an ongoing process that must consider a client's current needs and abilities.

SOURCES OF ADDITIONAL INFORMATION

Print Sources

Beukelman, D. R., & Mirenda, P. (2013). *Augmentative and alternative communication: Supporting children and adults with complex communication needs* (4th ed.). Baltimore: Paul H. Brookes.

Green, J. (2014). *Assistive technology in special education: Resources for education, intervention, and rehabilitation* (2nd ed.). Waco, TX: Prufrock Press.

Hoge, D. R., & Newsome, C. A. (2002). *The source for augmentative and alternative communication.* East Moline, IL: Linguisystems.

Lancioni, G. E., & Singh, N. N. (Eds.). (2014). *Assistive technologies for people with diverse abilities.* New York: Springer.

Loncke, F. (2014). *Augmentative and alternative communication: Models and applications for educators, speech–language pathologists, psychologists, caregivers, and users.* San Diego, CA: Plural.

Electronic Sources

AAC Institute:
http://www.aacinstitute.org

AAC TechConnect:
http://www.aactechconnect.com

International Society for Augmentative and Alternative Communication:
http://www.isaac-online.org

Spectronics Inclusive Learning Technologies:
http://www.spectronicsinoz.com

"ATEval2GO" app by Smarty Ears

Form 10-1.

Augmentative and Alternative Communication Information and Needs Assessment

Name: _____ Age: _____ Date: _____

Examiner's Name: _____

Informants: Relationship to Client:

_____   _____

_____   _____

_____   _____

Instructions: For each modality ask the informant (1) whether the modality is used, and if it is to describe the client's current use of the modality, (2) to indicate the size of the client's vocabulary using the modality, and (3) to indicate how well the client is understood when using the modality. Use the spaces provided to record notes.

Modality	Description	Vocabulary Size	Intelligibility
Speech			
Vocalizations			
Sign language			

(continues)

Adapted from *Handbook of Augmentative and Alternative Communication* (pp. 157–159), by S. L. Giennen and D. C. DeCoste, 1997, Clifton Park, NY: Cengage Learning. Permission to reproduce for clinical use granted.

AUGMENTATIVE OR ALTERNATIVE COMMUNICATION

Form 10-1. continued

Modality	Description	Vocabulary Size	Intelligibility
Gesture/pointing			
Head nods			
Eye gaze			
Facial expressions			
AAC device			

(continues)

Form 10-1. continued

Modality	Description	Vocabulary Size	Intelligibility
Other			

Past AAC Experience

Instructions: Ask the informant the following questions. Record notes in the spaces provided.

Has this individual ever used a picture- or letter-based AAC device in the past? If yes, describe the system.

Name of device: _____ Length of time used: _____

Number of symbols: _____ Size of symbols: _____

Symbol system used: _____ Organization of symbols: _____

Access method: _____

What were the strengths and limitations of the AAC system described above?

Communication Environments

Instructions: Ask the informant to describe how the AAC will be used and with whom. Also determine barriers to using the AAC. Take notes in the spaces provided.

Environment	Description	Interaction Partner
Home		
School		

(continues)

Form 10-1. continued

Environment	Description	Interaction Partner
Work		
Community		
Other		

What barriers to AAC implementation exist in any of the environments listed above?

Mobility and Access

Instructions: Ask the informant to describe the client's mobility and access regarding use of an AAC system. Also determine specific mobility, seating, or positioning concerns.

Mobility	Description	Environment Used
Fully ambulatory		

(continues)

Form 10-1. continued

Mobility	Description	Environment Used
Ambulatory with assistance		
Manual wheelchair		
Power wheelchair		
Other		

Are there any mobility, seating, or positioning concerns that will affect the implementation of an AAC system? If yes, describe.

(continues)

Adapted from *Handbook of Augmentative and Alternative Communication* (pp. 157–159), by S. L. Giennen and D. C. DeCoste, 1997, Clifton Park, NY: Cengage Learning. Permission to reproduce for clinical use granted.

Form 10-1. continued

Functional Access	Description	Access Limitations
Left arm/hand		
Right arm/hand		
Head		
Left leg/foot		
Right leg/foot		
Eye gaze		

(continues)

Form 10-1. continued

Functional Access	Description	Access Limitations
Other		

Other Technologies

Instructions: Ask the informant what other technologies will need to be integrated with an AAC system. Record notes in the spaces provided.

Technology	Description	Environment Used
Wheelchair		
Computer		
Environmental controls		
Switch toys		

(continues)

AUGMENTATIVE OR ALTERNATIVE COMMUNICATION

Form 10-1. continued

Technology	Description	Environment Used
Other		

AAC Expectations

What goals could be achieved if the client had access to an AAC system?

Adapted from *Handbook of Augmentative and Alternative Communication* (pp. 157–159), by S. L. Giennen and D. C. DeCoste, 1997, Clifton Park, NY: Cengage Learning. Permission to reproduce for clinical use granted.

Form 10-2.

Visual Scanning and Tracking Checklist

Name: _____ Age: _____

Examiner's Name: _____

Date: _____

Instructions: Make the following observations. Mark a check (✔) if a statement describes the client. Record additional comments in the right-hand column.

Client is able to track from:

_____ Left to right _____

_____ Right to left _____

_____ Up and down _____

_____ Down and up _____

_____ Diagonally up and down, left to right _____

_____ Diagonally up and down, right to left _____

_____ Diagonally down and up, left to right _____

_____ Diagonally down and up, right to left _____

Client is able to:

_____ Read words (indicate size of print) _____

_____ Read phrases (indicate size of print) _____

_____ Recognize pictures or objects _____

_____ Recognize symbols _____

Client is able to:

_____ Visually focus on stimuli _____

_____ Scan stimuli for desired word/picture/symbol (circle one and indicate number of stimulus items in the field) _____

_____ Identify desired stimulus quickly/slowly (circle one and indicate seconds) _____

_____ Identify desired stimulus consistently _____

_____ Identify desired stimulus with cues (indicate type) _____

(continues)

Form 10-2. continued

Client demonstrates:

_____ Visual neglect (indicate areas) _____

_____ Nystagmus (oscillating movement of the eyeball) _____

_____ Strabismus (eyes turn in or out) _____

_____ Poor ability to move eyes together _____

_____ Difficulty seeing stimuli more than 12 inches away from face _____

Note any identifiable patterns of scanning, including where the client begins visually searching (e.g., at midline, top left, top right)

Chapter 11

ASSESSMENT OF STUTTERING AND CLUTTERING

Fluent speech flows in a rhythmic, smooth, and effortless manner. Disfluencies are disruptions of fluid speech. All speakers experience moments of disfluency. It is normal to occasionally repeat a sound or word, pause briefly mid-utterance, or interject extra syllables such as "uh" while speaking. It is not normal for disfluencies to handicap a speaker to the point of impairing communication or causing anxiety in the speaker or listener. When evaluating a client for a stuttering or cluttering disorder, the speech-language pathologist must consider many factors and discern whether the presenting problem is a disorder or a case of normal disfluency.

OVERVIEW OF ASSESSMENT

History of the Client

    Procedures

        Written Case History
        Information-Gathering Interview
        Information from Other Professionals

    Contributing Factors

        Medical or Neurological Factors
        Family History
        Sex, Motivation, and Levels of Concern

Assessment of Stuttering and Cluttering

    Procedures

        Screening
        Speech Sampling
        Stimulability

    Analysis

        Disfluency Indexes
        Associated Motor Behaviors
        Other Physiological Factors
        Rate of Speech
        Feelings, Attitudes, and Reactions to Speech

Orofacial Examination

Speech and Language Assessment

Hearing Assessment

Determining the Diagnosis

Providing Information (written report, interview, etc.)

DEFINING STUTTERING

Stuttering is perhaps the oldest known communicative disorder, and the most familiar among the lay population.[1] Most people are aware of celebrities or others who struggle with a stuttering disorder. Over the years, stuttering has been widely researched and many theories of etiology exist. Yet, despite these facts, the cause of stuttering remains somewhat of a mystery. We do know that:

- Stuttering can develop for no apparent reason.
- Stuttering is more common among boys than girls.
- Stuttering is more common among highly sensitive children.
- Some people are genetically predisposed to stutter.
- The onset of stuttering usually occurs before the age of 6.
- Most children experience a period of disfluent speech between the ages of 2 and 5; some outgrow it whereas others do not.
- Stuttering is variable. A person may be completely fluent in one situation and extremely disfluent in another.
- Some disfluency types are more indicative of a fluency disorder than others.
- Stuttering causes personal grief, fear, and frustration.

Disfluencies are often categorized by type. The disfluency types that are most typically associated with a stuttering disorder are part-word repetitions, monosyllabic whole-word repetitions, sound prolongations, silent pauses (blocks), and broken words. In contrast, the disfluency types that are more frequently associated with normal disfluency are interjections, revisions, multisyllabic whole-word repetitions, and phrase repetitions. The major disfluency types are as follows (from Hegde & Davis, 2005, p. 416):

Repetitions

Part-word repetitions	"What t-t-t-time is it?"
Whole-word repetitions	"*What-what-what* are you doing?"
Phrase repetitions	"*I want to-I want to-I want to* do it."

Prolongations

Sound/syllable prolongations	"*Lllllllet* me do it."
Silent prolongations	A struggling attempt to say a word when there is no sound.

----

1. This chapter focuses on developmental stuttering. Some researchers report two types of acquired stuttering: neurogenic stuttering (resulting from a neurological insult) and psychogenic stuttering (resulting from a psychologically traumatic event).

Interjections

Sound/syllable interjections	*"um . . . um* I had a problem this morning."
Whole-word interjections	"I had a *well* problem this morning."
Phrase interjections	"I had a *you know* problem this morning."

Silent Pauses

A silent duration within speech considered abnormal	"I was going to the [*pause*] store."

Broken Words

A silent pause within words	"It was won [*pause*] derful."

Incomplete Phrases

Grammatically incomplete utterances	*"I don't know how to* . . . Let us go, guys."

Revisions

Changed words, ideas	"I thought I will write a letter, *card.*"

SPEECH SAMPLING

The most important procedure for any evaluation of stuttering is a speech sample. Speech samples should be gathered from more than one session and, if possible, from more than one setting in order to obtain the most representative sample possible. Attempt to obtain samples that contain the fewest disfluencies, the most disfluencies, and the typical number of disfluencies present in the client's speech. Obtain samples from a variety of speaking situations, including oral reading, dialogue, and monologue. Also obtain samples when speaking to different audiences, including family members, friends, peers, and superiors. The collection of an adequate sample is critical because it is the primary basis on which most analyses and judgments about fluency are made.

Collect speech samples from:

- The clinic or testing site
- Outside the assessment area but still in proximity to it
- Home
- Classroom
- Playground
- Work environment
- Other places the client spends time and interacts with others

If it is not feasible to collect samples from different settings, ask the client or a parent to provide recorded samples for analysis. Because stuttering is variable, it is important to ask how typical the samples are. It could be quite embarrassing and damaging to one's credibility to make judgments and recommendations, only to learn later that the client's stuttering behaviors were uncharacteristic during the assessment.

Specific procedures and stimulus materials for collecting a speech sample were presented in Chapter 5. For the assessment of stuttering, the following materials from Chapter 5 may be particularly helpful:

- Pictures
- Narratives
- Reading Passages
- Syllable-by-Syllable Stimulus Phrases

After obtaining thorough and representative samples of the client's speech, the analysis phase of the assessment can begin. Specifically, determine:

- The total number of disfluencies
- Frequencies of different types of disfluencies
- Disfluency indexes
- The duration of individual instances of disfluency
- Speech rate
- Types and frequencies of accessory behaviors

DISFLUENCY INDEXES

A disfluency index refers to the percentage of disfluent speech present in a speech sample. Disfluency indexes should be determined in several different environments (the therapy room, outside, at home, at work, etc.), within different modes of speech (reading, spontaneous speech, etc.), and across more than one assessment session. The "Fluency Charting Grid," Form 11-1, and "Frequency Count for Disfluencies," Form 11-2, are methods for identifying and quantifying disfluencies. Use Form 11-1 to count the total number of disfluent and fluent productions and, for more sophisticated charting, to code each disfluency type. Form 11-2 can be used to tally occurrences of each type of disfluency. Form 11-2 may be preferable for charting short samples, or for more informal charting such as screenings.

Form 11-3, "Calculating the Disfluency Index," is helpful for assessing fluency. When determining a disfluency index, count each repetition of a sound, part of a word, whole word, or phrase only once. For example, *ba-ba-ba-ba-ball* is one disfluency, *I-want-I want-I want to go* is one disfluency, and *go-go-go-away* is also one disfluency.[2]

---

2. There are times when counting the number of repetitions per disfluency provides useful information. In the examples just provided, calculate the average number of repetitions per disfluency. But for calculating a disfluency index, do not count every repetition.

The Total Disfluency Index reflects *all* disfluencies produced by the client. For example, consider a 500-word sample with the following number of disfluencies:

75 repetitions
50 pauses
25 sound prolongations
____
150 total disfluencies

To calculate the Total Disfluency Index:

1. Count the total number of words in the speech sample (500 in this example).
2. Count the total number of disfluencies (150).
3. Divide the total disfluencies by the total words. In this example: $150 \div 500 = 0.30$.
4. Change to a percentage: $0.30 = 30\%$ Total Disfluency Index.

Separate indexes can also be determined for individual disfluency types. For example, to calculate a Total Repetitions Index (using the previous example data):

1. Count the total number of words in the speech sample (500 in this example).
2. Count the number of specified disfluencies (75 repetitions in this example).
3. Divide the total specified disfluency (repetitions) by the total words. In this example: $75 \div 500 = 0.15$.
4. Change to a percentage: $0.15 = 15\%$ Total Repetitions Index.

Indexes for any disfluency type can be calculated using the same method.

A third type of disfluency index reflects the percentage of each disfluency type based on the Total Disfluency Index. For this calculation, base the computation on the total number of disfluencies. Using the same example:

1. Count the total number of disfluencies in the speech sample (150 in this example).
2. Count the number of specified disfluencies (75 repetitions).
3. Divide the total specified disfluency (repetitions) by the total disfluencies. In this example: $75 \div 150 = 0.50$.
4. Change to a percentage: $0.50 = 50\%$ of all disfluencies present were repetitions.

Occasionally, a client will exhibit very few disfluencies, resulting in a normal disfluency index. However, some of the disfluencies exhibited will be long in duration and therefore indicate a possible fluency disorder. In these cases, time the duration of the disfluencies and determine a mean duration of disfluency. Time each disfluency with a stopwatch. Pauses or prolongations are most commonly measured, but the duration of repetitions can also be timed. For example, 10 disfluencies resulting in a total of 42 seconds yields an average duration of 4.2 seconds.

ACCESSORY BEHAVIORS

People who stutter often develop *accessory behaviors*, also called *secondary behaviors* in response to, or in anticipation of stuttering. These behaviors are reinforced and become habitual when the speaker has initial success in maneuvering out of or postponing disfluent speech. Accessory behaviors are learned responses to stuttering. They are present only during disfluent speech, and the speaker may or may not be aware of these behaviors. Although such behaviors are common, not all people who stutter exhibit them. These behaviors may include:

- Associated motor behaviors
- Physiologic responses
- Avoidance
- Expectancy

Associated motor behaviors are extraneous body movements. These visible displays of tension usually involve parts of the oralfacial mechanism and may include behaviors such as eye blinking, wrinkling the forehead, frowning, distorting the mouth, moving the head, and quivering the nostrils. Sometimes they include movements of body parts that are not normally associated with speech, such as movements of the arms, hands, legs, feet, or torso.

During the assessment, note all unusual movements the client exhibits. Form 11-4, "Assessment of Associated Motor Behaviors," is designed to help identify these extraneous movements. Note that the form lists the most common behaviors; it is not an exhaustive list of all the possible behaviors clients may exhibit. Once the behaviors are identified, chart their frequency in the same manner other disfluencies are charted.

A client may also exhibit abnormal physiological behaviors associated with stuttering. These may affect respiratory, phonatory, articulatory, and prosodic aspects of speech production. Form 11-5, "Assessment of Physiological Factors Associated with Stuttering," is provided to help identify several physiological factors that may be observed during an assessment. Clinicians need to carefully examine whether these factors are present during fluent and disfluent speech or only during disfluencies.

Avoidance is a learned response to unpleasant stimuli. Just as people learn to avoid touching a hot stove because it is painful to get burned, many people who stutter learn to avoid certain sounds, words, or speaking situations that are especially difficult for them. Stuttering clients occasionally circumlocute—or talk around a subject—to avoid disfluencies. Specifically, some stutterers tend to avoid difficult:

- Sounds
- Words
- Topics
- People (e.g., employer, teacher, strangers)
- Situations (e.g., ordering in a restaurant, talking on the telephone)
- Communicative events (e.g., public speaking, speaking with members of the opposite sex)

During the assessment, pay particular attention to avoidance behaviors. Ask probing questions during the interview and observe the client's speech during the speech sample.

Avoidance behaviors can be described as primary or secondary. Primary avoidances refer to the client's attempts to alter verbal output. Secondary avoidances are acts of reducing or ceasing verbal output. Examples of primary and secondary avoidances are provided next.

STUTTERING AND CLUTTERING

Primary Avoidances

- Starters: using words, sounds, gestures, or rituals to initiate speech.
- Postponements: silences (e.g., pretending to think), ritualistic acts (e.g., lip licking), or verbal stalling.
- Retrials: repeating a fluent utterance to "hurdle" a feared word or phrase.
- Circumlocutions: sound, word, or phrase substitutions.
- Antiexpectancies: altering the communicative text by speaking with an accent, imitating someone else's voice, overemphasizing articulation, speaking rhythmically, whispering, or singing.

Secondary Avoidances

- Reducing verbal output or not talking at all.
- Relying on others to communicate for them.

Expectancy, also known as *anticipation*, is the expectation of a disfluency before it occurs. Expectancies can occur for sounds, words, people, or specific situations. Some clients respond to expectancy by "pushing forward" into the disfluency. Others respond with avoidance behaviors. Obtain information about expectancy by observing and listening during speech tasks and interviews. Ask the client to report when he or she experiences expectancy.

SPEECH RATE

Specific procedures for assessing rate of speech are provided in Chapter 5. Assessing speech rate is an especially important element of the evaluation of stuttering. Evaluate:

- Overall rate including disfluencies
- Normal rate excluding disfluencies

These two measures often produce very different results. For example, a person who stutters may produce only a few words per minute when both fluent and disfluent segments are measured. But if only segments of fluent speech are analyzed, the same person may actually exhibit a fast rate of speech. A rapid speech rate, which can go undetected if only the overall rate is assessed, may be a major contributor to the fluency disorder.

ASSESSING FEELINGS AND ATTITUDES

Stuttering is a debilitating handicap that can cause feelings of great pain, anguish, and frustration. The person who stutters may be corrected, teased, ridiculed, mocked, chastised, avoided, isolated, pitied, or scorned because of the speech disorder. He or she is likely to experience negative feelings and attitudes as a result of the communication difficulty.

Erickson (1969) developed the *S-Scale*, a 39-item form used to assess stutterers' attitudes about various speaking situations. This scale was later modified into a 24-item scale by

Andrews and Cutler (1974) so that it could be readministered across time to assess progress. Researchers have reported conflicting results from studies of the *S-Scale* and its modified form. One criticism is that the items are not exclusive to stutterers and, therefore, they are not fully discriminative between people with normal and disordered fluency. However, people who stutter answer "true" to items on the scale more often than people who do not stutter.

Understanding a client's feelings and attitudes about his or her stuttering behavior may be helpful for making decisions about the client's care. Administering the modified S-Scale is useful for gathering this information. It is provided in Form 11-6, "The Modified S-Scale." For young children, the form can be adapted and completed by a parent by changing *I* to *my child*. The parent should answer from the child's point of view.

Because parents are likely to have fears, anxieties, and concerns of their own about a child's stuttering pattern, it is helpful to consider the attitudes and feelings of the parent as well as the child. A separate form, the "Parental Speech Chart," Form 11-8, can be completed to assess level of concern from the parent's point of view.

Bray, Kehle, Lawless, and Theodore (2003) used a form similar to the *Modified S-Scale* that is specifically for adolescent-age clients. Their "Adolescent Communication Questionnaire" is provided in Form 11-7.

CRITERIA FOR DIAGNOSING STUTTERING

Authorities do not agree on what constitutes a stuttering disorder versus normal nonfluent speech. This makes it difficult in some cases to diagnose. Clinicians must use professional judgment and experience to make an appropriate diagnosis. There are several factors to consider. A diagnosis of stuttering disorder is often made if one or more of these conditions exist:

- The client has a Total Disfluency Index of 10% or greater.
- The client's disfluency indexes for repetitions, prolongations, and intralexical pauses are 3% or greater.
- The duration of disfluencies is 1 second or longer.
- The most prevalent disfluency types are part-word repetitions, monosyllabic whole-word repetitions, sound prolongations, silent pauses, or broken words.
- Secondary accessory behaviors are present.
- The client's (or parent's) degree of concern is significant.

Making a diagnosis is sometimes more complicated when the client is a young child. Most clinicians agree that normally developing children experience a period of nonfluent speech. This typically occurs during the preschool years, between the ages of 2 and 5. Unfortunately there are no sure indicators that a child will naturally outgrow stuttering behavior. Professionals have varying opinions about diagnosing a fluency disorder and recommending therapy for children who stutter.

In general, a stuttering disorder requiring intervention is more likely if:

- The child is male.
- Stuttering has continued for 6 months or longer.

STUTTERING AND CLUTTERING

- Onset of stuttering occurred before the child's third birthday.
- The child demonstrates associated motor behaviors.
- Other speech or language disorders are present.
- The child or child's family have strong fears or concerns about stuttering.

When assessing a nonfluent child, it is also important to consider his or her language, articulation, and oral-motor skills. In some cases, an apparent "stuttering disorder" may actually be a secondary behavior of another communicative disorder.

Speech-language pathologists rely on experience, knowledge of stuttering, and professional judgment to make diagnoses and recommendations. Commercial assessment instruments are also available to assist in the assessment process. These include:

- *Behavior Assessment Battery (BAB) for School-Age Children Who Stutter* (Brutten & Vanryckeghem, 2007)
- *Stuttering Prediction Instrument for Young Children* (Riley, 1981)
- *Stuttering Severity Instrument (SSI-4)* (Riley, 2008)
- *Test of Childhood Stuttering (TOCS)* (Gillam, Logan, & Pearson, 2009)

STIMULABILITY

Stimulability of fluency refers to a client's responsiveness to techniques that improve fluency. Clinicians typically elicit fluent speech by using the same techniques that are used in treatment. Several of these techniques are described in Table 11-1.

Imitation and adequate instruction are key elements to successful stimulation. These techniques are used in combination with response-contingent management (specifically,

TABLE 11-1 Fluency Modification Techniques

TECHNIQUE	DESCRIPTION
Prolonged speech	The clinician seeks to prolong the client's duration of sounds, usually with a slow, well-controlled transition between sounds and syllables.
Gentle onset/airflow	The stutterer is directed to initiate vocalization with a stable egressive airflow and a gentle onset of phonation.
Reduced speech rate	The stutterer maintains a reduced rate of speech, usually beginning with single-word productions and advancing to longer, more complex utterances. Normal phrase boundaries and prosodic features are maintained.
Reduced articulatory effort	The client minimizes articulatory tension by bringing the specific articulatory patterns of ongoing speech into conscious attention.

Source: Adapted from "Diagnosis of fluency disorders," by J. M. Hutchinson, in *Diagnosis in Speech-Language Pathology* (p. 203), I.J. Meitus and B. Weisenberg (Eds.), Baltimore: University Park Press.

positive or negative reinforcement of desired responses and punishment of undesired responses). Stimulation usually begins at the single-word level and increases in incremental steps. The "Syllable-by-Syllable Stimulus Phrases" in Chapter 5 are especially useful for assessing stimulability of fluency in increasingly longer phrases.

CLUTTERING

Cluttering is a fluency disorder that often coexists with stuttering, but can also be present on its own. The characteristics of cluttering include:

- Rapid speech rate, which negatively affects other aspects of communication
- Excessive disfluencies (normal nonfluencies predominate)
- Coexisting disorders of language and/or articulation
- Monotone voice
- Indistinct "mumbling" speech; sound distortions and omissions are common.
- Errors present in connected speech are less pronounced or not present during single-word articulation tests or during more slowly produced speech segments.
- Telescoped errors—for example, *statistical* may become *stacal*, or *refrigerator* may become *reor*.
- Spoonerisms, in which sounds are transposed in a word, phrase, or sentence—for example, *hit the books* may be produced as *bit the hooks*, or *many people think so* may become *many thinkle peep so*.
- Lack of awareness of the speech disorder, at least initially. Clients who clutter are sometimes genuinely surprised when the disorder is diagnosed or when other people do not understand them.
- Short attention span, restlessness, and hyperactivity
- Poor handwriting
- Poor thought organization and expression
- Lack of rhythm or musical ability
- Difficulty in treatment. Establishing and maintaining a slower speech rate and generalizing treatment behaviors into everyday speech are often difficult

Table 11-2 describes differential characteristics of stuttering and cluttering.

Assessment

Because cluttering affects all four primary aspects of communication—articulation, language, voice, and fluency—its assessment must also include each of these areas. The procedures that usually provide the best information for diagnosing cluttering are articulation testing and spontaneous speech sampling. A thorough examination of language is also recommended.

STUTTERING AND CLUTTERING

TABLE 11-2   Differential Characteristics of Stuttering and Cluttering

STUTTERING	CLUTTERING
Client is aware of disfluencies.	Client is unaware of disfluencies.
Speech becomes less fluent when the client concentrates on being fluent.	Speech becomes more fluent when client concentrates on being fluent.
Spontaneous speech may be more fluent than oral reading or directed speech.	Spontaneous speech may be less fluent than oral reading or directed speech.
Speech is usually less fluent with strangers.	Speech is usually more fluent with strangers.
Brief verbalizations are often more difficult to control.	Brief verbalizations are often less difficult to control.
Structured retrials may not result in increased fluency.	Structured retrials may improve fluency.
More sound and syllable repetitions are present.	Fewer sound and syllable repetitions are present.
Fewer language problems (e.g., incomplete phrases, reduced linguistic complexity) are present.	More language problems are present.
Speech rate may be normal when disfluencies are omitted from speech rate calculation.	Speech rate may be produced at a very rapid, "machine gun" rate.
Fewer articulation errors are present.	Multiple articulation errors may be present.

The following procedures and stimulus materials may be helpful for completing an assessment of cluttering:

- "Reading Passages" (Chapter 5)
- "Speech and Language Sampling" (Chapter 5)
- "Evaluating Rate of Speech" (Chapter 5)
- "Determining Intelligibility" (Chapter 5)
- "Orofacial Examination Form" (Form 5-1)
- "Diadochokinetic Syllable Rates Worksheet" (Form 5-2)
- "Formal Tests" (Chapter 6)
- "Comparison of Sound Errors From an Articulation Test and Connected Speech" (Form 6-1)

The "Checklist of Cluttering Characteristics," Form 11-9, is designed to help compile and evaluate assessment findings. Normally, a cluttering client will not exhibit every associated characteristic. Consider the presenting behaviors in light of other assessment information to make an accurate diagnosis. Also be aware that some cases of apraxia or stuttering resemble cluttering, at least initially. It is important to be familiar with the differentiating characteristics of each disorder.

Stimulability

Once the cluttering behaviors are identified, it is important to see if the client can improve his or her speech. Two of the five techniques for eliciting improved fluency in Table 11-1 are also useful for cluttering, specifically *prolonged speech* and *reduced speech rate*. These are useful because excessive speech rate is a primary problem with a cluttering pattern. Another technique is borrowed from dysarthria therapy. Called *syllable-by-syllable attack*, it emphasizes that the client correctly produce every syllable in an utterance (see Darley, Aronson, & Brown, 1975; Rosenbek & LaPointe, 1985). To accomplish this, the client usually reduces his or her speech rate.

Even though the cluttering client usually exhibits errors of articulation, language, and voice, stimulation of all these deficits may not need to be the primary focus of stimulability assessment. In many cases, reducing the speech rate to a slower, more manageable speed reduces or eliminates the effects of these secondary characteristics. As with other disorders, stimulability should start at the most simple level and incrementally increase in complexity. The "Syllable-by-Syllable Stimulus Phrases" in Chapter 5 are especially useful for assessing stimulability across different syllable lengths.

CONCLUDING COMMENTS

The assessment of fluency disorders is an intriguing and challenging aspect of clinical work for speech-language pathologists. The behaviors exhibited vary considerably among individual clients, as do their reactions to these problems. The valid assessment of a fluency disorder is a prerequisite to effective clinical treatment. The clinician's understanding of the disorder, the patterns exhibited, and the client's (and caregiver's) reaction all enter into the diagnostic process. The absence of accurate knowledge and information precludes, or at least reduces, the chances of effectively diagnosing and treating the disorder.

SOURCES OF ADDITIONAL INFORMATION

Print Sources

Bloodstein, O., & Bernstein Rather, N. (2008). *A handbook on stuttering* (6th ed.). Clifton Park, NY: Cengage Learning.

Curlee, R. F. (2007). *Stuttering and related disorders of fluency* (3rd ed.). New York: Thieme.

Guitar, B. E. (2014). *Stuttering: An integrated approach to its nature and treatment* (4th ed.). Baltimore: Lippincott, Williams & Wilkins.

Ward, D. (2006). *Stuttering and cluttering*. London: Psychology Press.

Wingate, M. E. (2001). *Foundations of stuttering*. Burlington, MA: Elsevier.

Electronic Sources

American Speech-Language-Hearing Association:
http://www.asha.org

National Stuttering Association:
http://www.nsastutter.org

The Stuttering Foundation:
http://www.stutteringhelp.org

The Stuttering Homepage (Judith Kuster):
http://www.communicationdisorders.com (click "stuttering home page" in the quick index)

"Disfluency Index Counter" app by Smarty Ears

Form 11-1.

Fluency Charting Grid

Name: _____ Age: _____ Date: _____

Examiner's Name: _____

Instructions: Make an appropriate mark in each square for every word uttered using the suggested symbols (or make up your own) to indicate the type of disfluency present. The major categories of disfluencies are in bold print.

(•)	**No Disfluency**	**(I)**	**Interjection**
(R)	**Repetition**	(I-SS)	Sound/Syllable Interjection
(R-PW)	Part-Word Repetition	(I-Wd)	Whole-Word Interjection
(R-WW)	Whole-Word Repetition	(I-Ph)	Phrase Interjection
(R-P)	Phrase Repetition	**(SP)**	**Silent Pause**
(P)	**Prolongation**	**(BW)**	**Broken Word**
(P-Sd)	Sound Prolongation	**(Inc)**	**Incomplete Phrase**
(P-Si)	Silent Prolongation	**(Rev)**	**Revision**

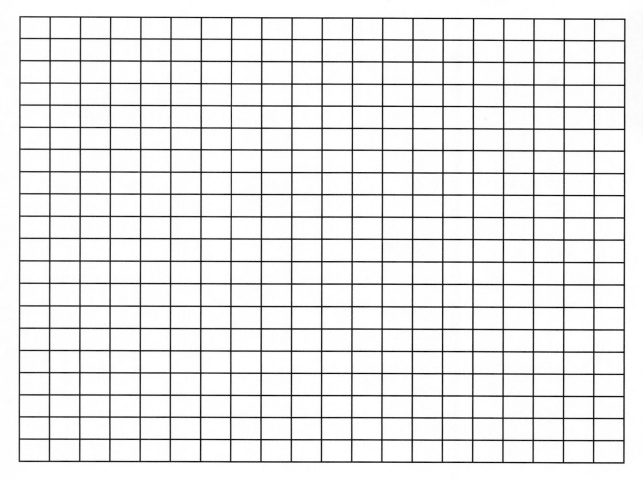

STUTTERING AND CLUTTERING

Form 11-2.

Frequency Count for Disfluencies

Name: _____ Age: _____ Date: _____

Examiner's Name: _____

Instructions: Make a check (✓) on the appropriate line each time the corresponding disfluency is produced.

Repetitions   **Totals**

   Part-Word _____ _____

   Whole-Word _____ _____

   Phrase _____ _____

Prolongations

   Sound _____ _____

   Silent _____ _____

Interjections

   Sound/Syllable _____ _____

   Whole-Word _____ _____

   Phrase _____ _____

Silent Pauses _____ _____

Broken Words _____ _____

Incomplete Phrases _____ _____

Revisions _____ _____

Form 11-3.

Calculating the Disfluency Index

Name: _____ Age: _____ Date: _____

Examiner's Name: _____

Instructions: Transfer findings from the "Fluency Charting Grid" (Form 11-1) to the appropriate blanks below to determine the Total Disfluency Index and/or the index for specific disfluency types. Calculate disfluency indexes for general or specific disfluency types. For example, *Repetitions* are general fluency types that consist of specific types: *Part-Word*, *Whole-Word*, and *Phrase Repetitions*. For calculation instructions, please refer back to the chapter.

Environment: _____

Sample Type: _____

Total Number of Words: _____

	Number of Disfluencies	Disfluency Index
Repetitions (R):	_____	_____
Part-Word (R-PW):	_____	_____
Whole-Word (R-WW):	_____	_____
Phrase (R-P):	_____	_____
Prolongations (P):	_____	_____
Sound (P-Sd):	_____	_____
Silent (P-Si):	_____	_____
Interjections (I):	_____	_____
Sound/Syllable (I-SS):	_____	_____
Whole-Word (I-Wd):	_____	_____
Phrase (I-Ph):	_____	_____
Silent Pauses (SP):	_____	_____
Broken Words (BW):	_____	_____
Incomplete Phrases (Inc):	_____	_____
Revisions (Rev):	_____	_____
TOTAL NUMBER OF DISFLUENCIES:	_____	_____

Comments:

STUTTERING AND CLUTTERING

Form 11-4.

Assessment of Associated Motor Behaviors

Name: _____ Age: _____ Date: _____

Examiner's Name: _____

Instructions: Check all associated motor behaviors the client exhibits. Use the right-hand column to describe behaviors or record frequency counts.

Eyes

_____ Blinking _____

_____ Shutting _____

_____ Upward movement _____

_____ Downward movement _____

_____ Vertical movement _____

_____ Other (specify) _____

Nose

_____ Flaring _____

_____ Dilation _____

_____ Wrinkling _____

_____ Other (specify) _____

Forehead

_____ Wrinkling/creasing _____

_____ Other (specify) _____

Head

_____ Shaking _____

_____ Upward movement _____

_____ Downward movement _____

_____ Lateral movement to right _____

_____ Lateral movement to left _____

_____ Other (specify) _____

(continues)

STUTTERING AND CLUTTERING

Form 11-4. continued

Lips

_____ Quivering _____

_____ Pursing _____

_____ Invert lower lip _____

_____ Other (specify) _____

Tongue

_____ Clicking _____

_____ Extraneous movement _____

_____ Other (specify) _____

Teeth

_____ Clenching _____

_____ Grinding _____

_____ Clicking _____

_____ Other (specify) _____

Jaw

_____ Clenching _____

_____ Opening _____

_____ Closing _____

_____ Other (specify) _____

Neck

_____ Tightening _____

_____ Twitching _____

_____ Upward movement _____

_____ Downward movement _____

_____ Lateral movement to the right _____

_____ Lateral movement to left _____

_____ Other (specify) _____

(continues)

Form 11-4. continued

Fingers

_____ Tapping _____

_____ Rubbing _____

_____ Clenching _____

_____ Excessive movement _____

_____ Clicking _____

_____ Other (specify) _____

Hands

_____ Fist clenching _____

_____ Wringing _____

_____ Splaying _____

_____ Other (specify) _____

Arms

_____ Excessive movement _____

_____ Banging against side _____

_____ Banging against leg _____

_____ Jerky movement _____

_____ Tensing _____

_____ Other (specify) _____

Legs

_____ Tensing _____

_____ Kicking _____

_____ Rapid movement _____

_____ Other (specify) _____

STUTTERING AND CLUTTERING

(continues)

Form 11-4. continued

Breathing

_____ Speaking on little air _____

_____ Unnecessary inhalation _____

_____ Jerky breathing _____

_____ Audible inhalation _____

_____ Audible exhalation _____

_____ Dysrhythmic _____

_____ Other (specify) _____

Others (describe):

Form 11-5.

Assessment of Physiological Factors Associated with Stuttering

Name: _____ Age: _____ Date: _____

Examiner's Name: _____

Instructions: Check all behaviors the client exhibits. Use the right-hand column to clarify or make additional comments.

Respiratory Factors

_____ Normal respiration at rest _____

_____ Normal respiration during speech _____

_____ Shallow breathing _____

_____ Audible inhalation _____

_____ Prolonged inhalation _____

_____ Audible exhalation (nonspeech) _____

_____ Gasping _____

_____ Arhythmical breathing _____

_____ Other (describe) _____

Phonatory Factors

_____ Normal phonatory functions _____

_____ Delays of phonatory onset _____

_____ Hard glottal attacks _____

_____ Pitch breaks _____

_____ Excessive pitch variations _____

_____ Too loud _____

_____ Too soft _____

_____ Alternating loudness _____

_____ Arhythmical breathing _____

_____ Other (describe) _____

(continues)

Source: Based on *Stuttering Treatment: A Comprehensive Clinical Guide* (p. 21), by G. B. Wells, 1987, Englewood Cliffs, NJ: Prentice Hall.

STUTTERING AND CLUTTERING

Form 11-5. continued

Articulatory Factors

_____ Normal articulatory contacts _____

_____ Easy articulatory contacts _____

_____ Hard articulatory contacts _____

_____ Normal articulation (place, manner) _____

_____ Other (describe) _____

Prosodic Factors

_____ Normal prosody _____

_____ Prolonged sound productions _____

_____ Excessive stressing _____

_____ Atypical stressing _____

_____ Other (describe) _____

Rate When Fluent

_____ Appropriate _____

_____ Excessively fast _____

_____ Excessively slow _____

Source: Based on *Stuttering Treatment: A Comprehensive Clinical Guide* (p. 21), by G. B. Wells, 1987, Englewood Cliffs, NJ: Prentice Hall.

Form 11-6.

The Modified S-Scale

Name: _____ Age: _____ Date: _____

Examiner's Name: _____

Instructions: Answer the following by circling "T" if the statement is generally true for you, or circle "F" if the statement is generally false for you. If the situation is unfamiliar or rare, judge it on an "If it was familiar ..." basis.*

T F   1.   I usually feel that I am making a favorable impression when I talk.

T F   2.   I find it easy to talk with almost anyone.

T F   3.   I find it very easy to look at my audience while talking in a group.

T F   4.   A person who is my teacher or my boss is hard to talk to.

T F   5.   Even the idea of giving a talk in public makes me afraid.

T F   6.   Some words are harder than others for me to say.

T F   7.   I forget all about myself shortly after I begin to give a speech.

T F   8.   I am a good mixer (in social settings).

T F   9.   People sometimes seem uncomfortable when I am talking to them.

T F   10.   I dislike introducing one person to another.

T F   11.   I often ask questions in group discussions.

T F   12.   I find it easy to keep control of my voice when speaking.

T F   13.   I do not mind speaking before a group.

T F   14.   I do not talk well enough to do the kind of work I'd really like to do.

T F   15.   My speaking voice is rather pleasant and easy to listen to.

T F   16.   I am sometimes embarrassed by the way I talk.

T F   17.   I face most speaking situations with complete confidence.

T F   18.   There are few people I can talk with easily.

T F   19.   I talk better than I write.

T F   20.   I often feel nervous while talking.

T F   21.   I often find it hard to talk when I meet new people.

T F   22.   I feel pretty confident about my speaking abilities.

T F   23.   I wish I could say things as clearly as others do.

T F   24.   Even though I knew the right answer, I have often failed to give it because I was afraid to speak out.

*Note that items 4, 5, 6, 9, 10, 14, 16, 18, 20, 23, and 24 are presumed to be true for people who stutter; the other items are presumed to be false.

STUTTERING AND CLUTTERING

Form 11-7.

Adolescent Communication Questionnaire

Name: _____ Age: _____

School: _____ Grade: _____

Date: _____

Instructions: We are interested in learning more about your speaking abilities and your confidence in various situations. Your responses are confidential.

On the left-hand side of the page, circle the number that would best represent your confidence in the situation described. Assume that 1 means "No way, I would be too uptight to speak" and 5 means "No problem, I would be very confident speaking."

1	2	3	4	5	1. Talking with a parent about a movie.
1	2	3	4	5	2. Talking to a brother or sister at the dinner table.
1	2	3	4	5	3. Talking with three friends during lunch at school.
1	2	3	4	5	4. Talking with a large group of friends during lunch at school.
1	2	3	4	5	5. Answering the telephone.
1	2	3	4	5	6. Talking with the teacher during class.
1	2	3	4	5	7. Talking with the principal.
1	2	3	4	5	8. Asking a friend to come to your house after school.
1	2	3	4	5	9. Arguing with a brother or sister.
1	2	3	4	5	10. Asking a parent if you can spend the night at a friend's house.
1	2	3	4	5	11. Telling a new friend about your family.
1	2	3	4	5	12. Telling your teacher your birth date.
1	2	3	4	5	13. Calling your friend on the telephone.
1	2	3	4	5	14. Asking your parent if you can go to bed later than usual.
1	2	3	4	5	15. Talking to a family member on the telephone.
1	2	3	4	5	16. Explaining how to play a game to your friends.

(continues)

Form 11-7. continued

1	2	3	4	5	17. Asking a librarian for help in finding a book.
1	2	3	4	5	18. Talking with a friend alone.
1	2	3	4	5	19. Asking a sales clerk how much an item costs.
1	2	3	4	5	20. Telling a police officer your home address.
1	2	3	4	5	21. Calling a store to find out what time it opens.
1	2	3	4	5	22. Talking to a teacher alone after class.
1	2	3	4	5	23. Reading aloud to a whole class.
1	2	3	4	5	24. Reading aloud to five classmates.
1	2	3	4	5	25. Reading aloud to your family.
1	2	3	4	5	26. Speaking to your pet.
1	2	3	4	5	27. Raising your hand to ask the teacher a question.
1	2	3	4	5	28. Answering a question in class.
1	2	3	4	5	29. Asking a question in class.
1	2	3	4	5	30. Ordering food at a restaurant.
1	2	3	4	5	31. Telling a joke.
1	2	3	4	5	32. Giving a book report in front of the class.
1	2	3	4	5	33. Taking a speaking part in a school play.
1	2	3	4	5	34. Reading aloud just to your teacher.
1	2	3	4	5	35. Talking with a large group of your friends.
1	2	3	4	5	36. Talking aloud to yourself with no one else there.
1	2	3	4	5	37. Talking with the school secretary.
1	2	3	4	5	38. Reading a book aloud with no one else in the room.
1	2	3	4	5	39. Talking to your teacher on the telephone.

Form 11-8.

Parental Speech Chart

Name: _____ Age: _____

Informant's Name: _____ Date: _____

Instructions: Indicate each disfluency present and factors surrounding the disfluency. This is a general worksheet; it does not need to be absolutely precise. Do the best you can, and write down any questions or thoughts you have, so you can mention them to the speech-language pathologist.

Date/Time	Type of difficulty (repeating sounds or words, prolongations, etc.)	Tension or struggle?	Reaction to disfluency? Aware of difficulty?	Topic of conversation	Whom was the child talking to? What did the other person do?	Did you notice anything that preceded the disfluency?

(continues)

STUTTERING AND CLUTTERING

Form 11-8. continued

Date/Time	Type of difficulty (repeating sounds or words, prolongations, etc.)	Tension or struggle?	Reaction to disfluency? Aware of difficulty?	Topic of conversation	Whom was the child talking to? What did the other person do?	Did you notice anything that preceded the disfluency?

Form 11–9.

Checklist of Cluttering Characteristics

Name:_____ Age:_____ Date:_____

Examiner's Name: _____

Instructions: Check each characteristic your client exhibits. Include additional comments on the right-hand side.

_____ Indistinct speech _____

_____ Minimal pitch variation _____

_____ Minimal stress variation _____

_____ Monotone voice _____

_____ More errors on longer units _____

_____ Rapid rate _____

_____ Sound distortions _____

_____ Spoonerisms _____

     _____ Within words _____

     _____ Within phrases/sentences _____

_____ Telescoping _____

     _____ Sounds _____

     _____ Words _____

     _____ Parts of phrases _____

_____ Speech improves when concentrating on fluency _____

_____ Speech improves when speech rate is reduced _____

_____ Speech improves during shorter intervals _____

_____ Structured retrials improve fluency _____

_____ Relatively few sound or syllable repetitions _____

_____ Presence of language problems _____

_____ Improved speech is somewhat difficult to stimulate _____

_____ Improved speech does not tend to generalize _____

_____ Client not very aware of speech problem _____

_____ Client not very concerned about speech problem _____

STUTTERING AND CLUTTERING

Chapter 12

ASSESSMENT OF VOICE AND RESONANCE

- **Overview of Assessment**

- **Anatomy for Voice and Resonance**

- **Categories of Voice Disorders**

- **The Multidisciplinary Team**

- **Screening**

- **Client History and Present Concerns**

- **Perceptual and Instrumental Examination of Voice**

  Evaluation of Pitch

  Evaluation of Vocal Intensity

  Evaluation of Vocal Quality

  Assessing Respiratory Support for Speech

  Maximum Phonation Time

  S/Z Ratio

- **Assessment Hardware and Software**

- **Assessment of Resonance**

- **Two Special Populations: Alaryngeal Clients and Clients with Cleft Lip and/or Palate**

- **Assessment of Alaryngeal Clients**

  Alaryngeal Communication Options

- **Assessment of Clients with Cleft Lip and/or Palate**

- **Concluding Comments**

- **Sources of Additional Information**

- **Chapter 12 Forms**

415

Vocal production occurs via vibration of the vocal folds as air is pushed up by the respiratory system and passes through the glottis. The umbrella term for a voice disorder is *dysphonia* (faulty phonation), or, in some situations, *aphonia* (no phonation). Features of the voice are *pitch*, *quality*, and *loudness*. Resonance is affected by conditions of the vocal tract. Features of resonance are *nasal resonance* and *oral resonance*. Disorders of voice and resonance are distinct, yet they are often addressed together in professional literature. Assessment procedures for both conditions are presented in this chapter because of the overlapping nature of portions of the assessment process. The chapter concludes with assessment procedures for two special populations that are associated with a voice or resonance disorder: alaryngeal clients and clients with cleft lip and/or palate.

Voice and resonance evaluation and management is a specialized science within our profession. A clinician should not enter into an evaluation without proper experience or supervision. This chapter is provided as a resource and aid; however, it is not possible to provide depth of information, or necessary training on specified equipment, in a text of this nature.

OVERVIEW OF ASSESSMENT

History of the Client
  Procedures
      Written Case History
      Information-Getting Interview
      Information from Other Professionals
  Contributing Factors
      Environmental and Behavioral Factors
      Medical and Neurological Factors
      Psychological Factors
      Motivation and Concern
Assessment of Voice
  Procedures
      Screening
      Auditory-Perceptual Judgments
      Aerodynamic Measures
      Acoustic Measures
      Imaging
      Stimulability
Assessment of Resonance
  Procedures
      Screening
      Auditory-Perceptual Judgments
      Velopharyngeal Function
      Acoustic Measures
      Stimulability

Orofacial Examination
Hearing Considerations
Determining the Diagnosis
Providing Information (written report, interview, etc.)

ANATOMY FOR VOICE AND RESONANCE

Healthy voice production requires normal and synchronized participation of the respiratory system (lungs, diaphragm, ribs, and abdominal and chest muscles), the vibratory system (larynx, vocal folds, and glottis), and the resonating system (pharyngeal, oral, and nasal cavities). See Figure 12-1 for a pictorial representation of the voice mechanism. Figure 12-2 shows normal vocal folds open and closed. Figure 12-3 shows some of the most common vocal fold pathologies.

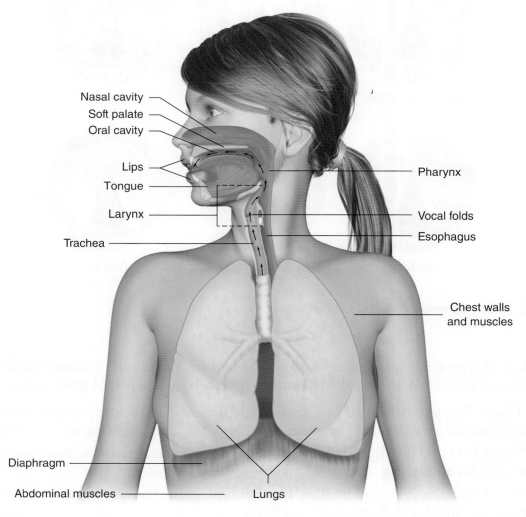

FIGURE 12-1. Anatomy of the Vocal Mechanism

VOICE AND RESONANCE

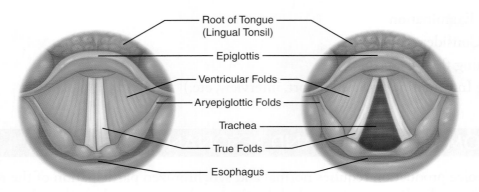

FIGURE 12-2.   The Vocal Folds

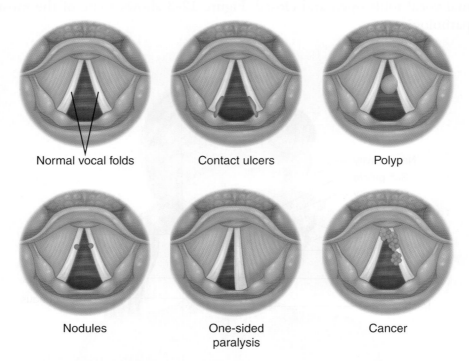

FIGURE 12-3.   Common Vocal Fold Pathologies

Medical apps that explore anatomy for voice and resonance can be downloaded for use on tablets. A few that are especially relevant to speech-language pathologists include:

- "Upper Respiratory Virtual Lab" by Georgia Regents University: provides three-dimensional simulation of the upper respiratory tract, highlighting laryngeal anatomy.
- "Vocal Folds ID" by Blue Tree Publishing, Inc.: offers images and animations of the vocal folds and larynx.
- "Vocal Pathology: Polyps" by Blue Tree Publishing, Inc.: offers images and animations of normal and disordered vocal folds.

CATEGORIES OF VOICE DISORDERS

There are four primary categories of voice disorders, grouped according to etiology:

1. *Functional disorders*: nonorganic disorders that result from vocal misuse or abuse. The most common conditions are vocal nodules, contact ulcers, and granuloma.

2. *Neurogenic disorders*: organic disorders that result from illness, disease, or damage to the nervous system. Conditions may include partial or complete vocal fold paralysis, spasmodic dysphonia, and voice associated with Parkinson's disease and amyotrophic lateral sclerosis (ALS).

3. *Psychogenic disorders*: disorders that result from psychological and emotional conflict such as extreme stress or anxiety. Resultant voice disorders may include tense voice, aphonia, and mutational falsetto.

4. *Alaryngeal communication*: voice production without a larynx, usually because of a tracheostomy or because the larynx has been partially or completely removed. Communication options include artificial larynx, electrolarynx, and pseudoglottis.

It is important to realize that, in some situations, these categories may seem to overlap. For example, a speaker with a neurogenic disorder may misuse his or her voice in an effort to compensate for poor respiratory support, and thus develop a secondary functional voice disorder. Or a speaker may be distraught following a laryngectomy, adding an emotional component (know that the resultant voice disorder would not be considered a psychogenic disorder). Also, some conditions can occur in more than one category depending on etiology. For example, aphonia could be caused by a functional disorder, psychogenic disorder, or alaryngeal communication.

THE MULTIDISCIPLINARY TEAM

Voice and resonance disorders are typically managed by a team. At minimum, the team consists of a laryngologist, the speech-language pathologist, and the client. Other members of the team may include a primary care physician, neurologist, allergist, gastroenterologist, pulmonologist, orthodontist, radiologist, plastic surgeon, psychologist, psychiatrist, nurse, audiologist, social worker, teacher, music or drama specialist, voice coach, family members, or others. Including the client as an integral member of the team is imperative. Without the client's cooperation and participation during the diagnostic and decision-making period, progress with treatment will not be possible.

The role of the speech-language pathologist is primarily to describe and characterize the features of the voice, determine if the features differ from the norm, and, if a disorder is present, explore intervention approaches that will improve the client's voice. The speech-language pathologist will also make recommendations and referrals as appropriate. Many speech-language pathologists who specialize in disorders of voice physically share office space with laryngologists, providing an ideal environment for professional collaboration.

VOICE AND RESONANCE

SCREENING

A screen for voice and resonance disorders can be accomplished with a few quick and easy tasks. For example, ask the client to:

- Imitate words and phrases of varying lengths
- Count to 20
- Recite the alphabet
- Read a short passage
- Talk conversationally for a couple of minutes
- Prolong the following vowels for 5 seconds each: /ɑ/, /ʌ/, /i/, /u/, /æ/.
- Produce sustained /s/ and /z/ for calculation on an s/z ratio (described later in this chapter)

During the screen, listen carefully to the client's resonance, tone, pitch, and loudness. Any perceived deviation from normal suggests that further evaluative measures should be pursued.

CLIENT HISTORY AND PRESENT CONCERNS

Thoroughly gathering historical information and evaluating a client's current perceptions and concerns is an important aspect of a complete evaluation. Obtain copies of all relevant professional reports. In some situations, these reports will already be available. In other situations, the speech-language pathologist may need to make referrals for additional evaluation. In either case, a treatment program should not be initiated until all appropriate medical evaluations have been completed, as therapy may prove detrimental in some situations.

In addition to the standard case history queries, these issues or questions should be considered:

- How is the client's voice impacting his or her daily life?
- Has there been previous medical or surgical treatment for a laryngeal pathology?
- Has there been previous treatment for a voice or resonance disorder?
- Are there craniofacial anomalies?
- Has there been laryngeal trauma?
- Does the client have a neurological condition?
- Does the client have a hearing loss?
- Has the client experienced a hormonal disturbance?
- What ethnocultural variables might influence the client's voice and resonance?

It is particularly helpful to understand how a client perceives his or her own voice. Form 12-1, "The Voice Handicap Index (VHI)," was designed by a team of professionals to quantify the psychosocial consequences of voice disorders. It consists of three subscales: the functional prompts evaluate the impact of a person's voice on daily activities, the emotional prompts evaluate the client's affective response to his or her voice, and the physical prompts evaluate the client's own perceptions of vocal quality. Page 1 of Form 12-1 is the

TABLE 12-1   Self-Perceived Voice Severity per the Voice Handicap Index

SCALE	MILD	MODERATE	SEVERE
Functional	10–11	12–17	18+
Physical	16–18	19–22	23+
Emotional	8–12	13–19	20+
Total	34–43	44–60	61+

Source: Adapted from "The Voice Handicap Index (VHI): Development and validation," by Barbara H Jacobson, Alex Johnson, Cynthia Grywalski, Alice Silbergleit, Gary Jacobson, Michael S. Benninger, 1997, *American Journal of Speech-Language Pathology*, 6(3), pp. 66–70.

questionnaire portion of the VHI and is to be given to the client to complete. Page 2 is for clinical use for calculating results. The data in Table 12-1 can be used to interpret findings.

Forms 12-2 and 12-3 offer checklists that are helpful for identifying behaviors that may be contributing to a voice disorder. Form 12-2, "Vocally Abusive Behaviors Checklist—Adult," is most appropriate for adults and Form 12-3, "Vocally Abusive Behaviors Checklist—Children and Youth," is for younger clients.

PERCEPTUAL AND INSTRUMENTAL EXAMINATION OF VOICE

The perceptual component of an evaluation is the somewhat subjective "human" piece of the assessment. What does the voice sound like, and does it draw attention to itself in a negative way? On the other hand, instrumental examination provides the objective data that validate and quantify perceptual judgments. Instruments provide acoustic, aerodynamic, and/or imaging-based analysis. Both perceptual and instrumental assessment measures are important aspects of a complete evaluation.

For both perceptual and instrumental examination it is important to collect multiple representative samples of the client's speech. Specific procedures for collecting a speech sample were described in Chapter 5. The "Conversation Starters for Eliciting a Speech-Language Sample," "Pictures," "Narratives," and "Reading Passages" are possible resource materials. The clinician can also ask the client to perform serial tasks, such as count to 20, name the days of the week, name the months of the year, or recite the alphabet. Listen to and observe the client, and note the following:

- Pitch
- Intensity
- Vocal quality
- Vocal habits (including abusive behaviors)
- Resonance
- Respiratory support
- Posture, tension, and behaviors

VOICE AND RESONANCE

Use a high-quality audio-recording device, or, better, a video device so that behaviors can be heard and viewed. Ask the client to provide samples from other environments, such as the workplace, school, entertainment venues, and home. Do not delete files, as they are helpful for location comparisons and to assess changes over time.

Evaluation of Pitch

Pitch, or frequency, is expressed in cycles per second, or Hertz (Hz) and is a measure of the speed of vocal fold vibration. Frequency is influenced by vocal fold mass, length, and tension. During an assessment, determine a client's fundamental frequency, range, and best pitch.

The *fundamental frequency* (F_0), also called *habitual pitch*, is the average pitch that a client uses during speaking and reading. Table 12-2 presents normal fundamental frequencies for males and females of various ages, and includes the approximated equivalent note value on a piano or pitch pipe.

Several methods exist for determining a client's fundamental frequency. The most objective way is to use an assessment instrument or computer software program. If such a device is not available, analyze recorded samples of the client's speech. Use a musical instrument

TABLE 12-2 Normal Fundamental Frequencies

AGE (YRS)	AVERAGE HZ	NOTE	RANGE HZ	NOTES
infant	500	B_4		
1–2	400	G_4	340–470	E_4–$A\#_4$
3	300	D_4	255–360	C_4–$F\#_4$
4–8	275	$C\#_4$	210–340	$G\#_3$–F_4
9–12	243	B_3	195–290	G_3–D_4
13	210	$G\#_3$	140–280	$C\#_3$–$C\#_4$
14–18 female	223	A_3	175–270	F_3–$C\#_4$
20–29 female	233	$A\#_3$	190–275	$F\#_3$–$C\#_4$
30–40 female	197	G_3	171–222	F_3–A_3
40–50 female	188	$F\#_3$	168–208	E_3–$G\#_3$
50–60 female	209	$G\#_3$	176–241	F_3–B_3
60–70 female	189	$F\#_3$	143–235	$C\#_3$–$A\#_3$
80–90 female	210	$G\#_3$	170–249	E_3–B_3
14–18 male	160	E_3	105–215	$G\#_2$–A_3
20–29 male	119	$A\#_2$		
30–40 male	112	A_2		
40–50 male	107	$G\#_2$		
50–60 male	118	$A\#_2$		
60–70 male	112	A_2		
80–90 male	146	D_3		

Note: Blank cells indicate data unavailable.

(e.g., piano or pitch pipe) to match the client's pitch at several different moments in the sample. An average can be approximated from those pitches. A quick way to estimate a client's habitual pitch for screening purposes is to ask a yes-no question and have the client reply with "mmm-hhmm" (yes) or "hhmm-mmm" (no). The pitch the client uses for the "mmm" syllable is often the client's habitual pitch.

Also determine the client's *pitch range*. Ask the client to phonate "ah" at a comfortable pitch and glissando up to the highest note possible. Identify the pitch at the top of the range. Repeat twice. To determine bottom of the range, ask the client to glissando down to the lowest note possible. The highest and lowest pitches elicited determine vocal range.

For most speakers, habitual pitch is also their *best pitch*. In some cases, however, a person may habitually speak at a frequency that is not ideal and may be abusive to vocal structures. During an assessment, explore pitches at which the client's voice is least effortful and most natural sounding. As a general guideline, best pitch for a male speaker is approximately 25% above the lowest pitch in his range, and best pitch for a female is approximately 18% above the lowest pitch in her range.

Jitter, also called *pitch perturbation*, is a measure of the minuscule variations in fundamental frequency from cycle to cycle. Jitter is determined using sensitive instrumentation. Jitter values in normal voices range from 0.2% to 1%. Higher measurements indicate interference with vocal fold vibration.

Evaluation of Vocal Intensity

Vocal intensity, or loudness, is measured in decibels (dB). Vocal intensity is a reflection of the amplitude of vocal fold vibrations. The greater the amplitude, the greater the perceived loudness. Vocal intensity is controlled by the amount of airflow coming up from the lungs and the amount of resistance by the vocal folds to the airflow. Table 12-3 presents normal conversational intensity and range data.

Consider if the client's habitual loudness is appropriate for the setting, and whether there is normal or abnormal variation in loudness levels used. Also assess the client's ability to vary vocal intensity during informal tasks. Ask him or her to whisper, speak softly, speak loudly, and shout. To assess range, ask the client to count upward from one, starting with a soft voice and increasing vocal intensity with each number.

Shimmer, also called *amplitude perturbation*, is a measure of the miniscule variations in amplitude from cycle to cycle. Shimmer values below 0.5 dB are normal in the human voice. Like jitter, shimmer is measured using sensitive instrumentation.

TABLE 12-3   Normal Vocal Intensity—Averages and Ranges

Whisper	10 dB
Quiet voice	35–40 dB
Normal conversational voice	60–80 dB
Loud voice	80 dB
Shouting	90 dB
Minimum intensity	50 dB
Maximum intensity	100 dB

Evaluation of Vocal Quality

Vocal qualities are the general characteristics of a person's voice. Until recently, there was not a standardized process for perceptual assessment of vocal quality. In 2002, the American Speech-Hearing-Language Association (ASHA) formed a team of professionals to remedy the void. As a result, the *Consensus Auditory-Perceptual Evaluation of Voice (CAPE-V)* was developed. It is reprinted in this text as Form 12-4.

The six standard attributes of vocal quality, as defined by the CAPE-V, are:

- Overall severity: a global and integrated impression of voice deviance
- Roughness: a perceived irregularity in the voicing source
- Breathiness: audible air escape in the voice
- Strain: a perception of excessive vocal effort; hyperfunction
- Pitch: the perceptual correlate of fundamental frequency (Does the speaker's voice sound too high or too low considering his or her gender, age, and culture?)
- Loudness: the perceptual correlate of intensity (Does the speaker's voice sound too soft or too loud considering his or her age, gender, and culture?)

Additional attributes may include:

- Diplophonia: simultaneous production of two different pitches
- Fry: a rhythmic creaking or popping quality that occurs below the lowest note of a speaker's pitch range. It is normal at the end of phrases and sentences on occasion, but problematic if habitual.
- Falsetto: the use of a pre-pubescent voice in adulthood
- Asthenia: a weak, thin voice
- Aphonia: absence of voice
- Pitch instability: involuntary pitch changes
- Tremor: a rhythmic fluctuation of vocal loudness and/or pitch
- Wet/gurgling voice: a wet quality to the voice

Normal vocal quality is in the ears of the listener. There is huge variation in what is considered normal. In general, vocal quality is abnormal if it draws negative attention to itself and/or has a negative impact on the speaker's daily life. Many qualities, such as mild roughness, are sometimes validated by society, but they can lead to significant functional vocal pathologies.

Assessing Respiratory Support for Speech

Good respiratory support is critical for normal vocal production. Some clients with voice disorders demonstrate poor breathing habits. During the assessment, observe the client's respiratory behavior following instruction to "take a deep breath" and during connected speech. Note the following:

- Tension in upper chest, shoulders, face and/or neck
- Shallow inhalation

- Noisy inhalation
- Mouth breathing
- Running out of air
- Weak voice
- Fatigue

Maximum Phonation Time

Maximum phonation time (MPT) is a measure of glottic efficiency. The sequence of administration is as follows:

1. Ask the client to take a deep breath and exhale "ah" (or other vowel) at a comfortable pitch and loudness, sustaining as long as possible. Time the production using a stopwatch or other instrument.
2. Repeat for two more trials.
3. Record the longest phonation as MPT.

MPT may vary significantly among speakers with normally functioning vocal folds. Typical adult males can sustain vowel sounds for 25 to 35 seconds and adult females can sustain vowel sounds for 15 to 25 seconds. In general, glottic insufficiency is a concern for speakers who are able to sustain vowel sounds for fewer than 10 seconds.

S/Z Ratio

The **s/z ratio** is another widely used test for measuring respiratory and phonatory efficiency. Because /s/ and /z/ are produced the same way, except for voicing, a speaker with normal phonatory function will sustain both sounds for approximately the same amount of time. Sequence of administration is as follows:

1. Ask the client to take a deep breath and sustain /s/ for as long as possible. Time the production using a stopwatch or other instrument. Repeat twice.
2. Ask the client to take a deep breath and sustain /z/ for as long as possible. Time the production using a stopwatch or other instrument. Repeat twice.
3. Divide the longest /s/ by the longest /z/.

Interpret findings according to the following guidelines:

- A 1.0 ratio with normal duration for both phonemes (approximately 10 seconds for children and 20 to 25 seconds for adults) indicates normal respiratory and vocal function.
- A ratio above 1.0 with normal duration of /s/ and reduced duration of /z/ indicates vocal fold pathology. The higher the ratio is above 1.0, the greater the likelihood that a laryngeal pathology exists.
- A 1.0 ratio with reduced duration for both sounds indicates respiratory inefficiency.

ASSESSMENT HARDWARE AND SOFTWARE

Objective analysis of voice and resonance is possible with the use of specialized hardware or software. These tools often provide the objective counterpart to perceptual assessment. They range from simple apps to sophisticated and comprehensive assessment systems. Instruments that assess acoustic properties quantify aspects of voice such as fundamental frequency, range, intensity, quality, tremor, jitter, shimmer, maximum phonation time, and vocal efficiency. Instruments that analyze aerodynamic properties measure aspects of respiration that affect voice and speech production such as phonatory flow rates and volumes, subglottic pressure, resistance, vital capacity, s/z ratio, and maximum phonation time. Imaging techniques allow direct viewing of the larynx and vocal folds.

Some of the most commonly used hardware and software tools for assessment of resonance and voice include the following:

- Aerophone II: an instrument that measures aerodynamic properties of speech including sound pressure levels, airflow, and air pressure.
- Computerized Speech Lab (CSL; KayPENTAX): a complete hardware and software system for acoustic analysis of multiple aspects of voice, speech, and fluency.
- Digital endoscope: a fiberoptic tube fitted with a light and camera that can be directed into the oral cavity for visual viewing of the larynx. A stroboscope is a type of endoscope that emits a pulsing light, as opposed to constant light, allowing for a motionless or slow motion effect when viewing the vocal folds.
- Electroglottograph: a noninvasive instrument that measures vocal fold contact during voice production and aids in assessment of abductory function of the vocal folds.
- Fundamental Frequency Indicator: a computerized instrument that measures multiple aspects of pitch, including habitual pitch, best pitch, and pitch range.
- Multi-Dimensional Voice Program (MDVP: KayPENTAX): a powerful software tool that analyzes multiple aspects of vocal quality and their interactive effects on one another.
- Nasometer (KayPENTAX): an instrument that quantifies nasality by measuring acoustic energy in the mouth and nose during speech.
- Phonatory Function Analyzer: a computerized instrument that measures aerodynamic and acoustic properties of speech including airflow rate, volume of expired air, vocal frequency, and pitch.
- "Pitch Analyzer" (by Ting Wang): a simple app that identifies pitch frequency, amplitude, and equivalent note name and location on a music staff and keyboard.
- Pratt (Boersma & Weenink, 2014): a software program that analyzes multiple acoustic aspects of speech and voice. It can be downloaded free from the Internet at http://www.praat.org.
- Visi-Pitch (KayPENTAX): a hardware/software system that measures several aspects of voice and speech, including fundamental frequency, pitch range and intonation, intensity, glottal attack, and stress patterns.
- "Voice Test" (by Danube Team): a simple app that provides basic measures of fundamental frequency, shimmer, and jitter.

Form 12-5, "Assessment of Voice Worksheet," is helpful for recording and summarizing findings from a voice assessment.

ASSESSMENT OF RESONANCE

Resonance disorders result from faulty sound vibration in the oral, nasal, and/or pharyngeal cavities. They should not be confused with voice disorders, which result from faulty laryngeal function, although both influence perceptions of a speaker's voice. Normal resonance occurs when air for speech is directed through the oral cavity, by closure of the velopharyngeal port, during production of all vowels and oral consonants, and directed through the nasal cavity during production of nasal consonants, specifically /m/, /n/, and /ŋ/.

The most common disorders of resonance are:

- Disorders due to incomplete closure of the velopharyngeal port:
  - *Hypernasality*: occurs when there is too much sound vibration in the nasal cavity during vowels and voiced oral consonants.
  - *Nasal emissions*: occurs when air escapes through the nose during speech.
  - *Phoneme-specific velopharyngeal dysfunction*: occurs when there is audible nasal emission on only certain sounds (usually /s/ and /z/). It results from velopharyngeal mislearning, not dysfunction, and is not a structural issue.

- Disorders due to an obstruction:
  - *Hyponasality*: occurs when there is too little sound vibration in the nasal cavity during nasal consonants. Phoneme /m/ sounds like /b/, /n/ sounds like /d/, and /ŋ/ sounds like /g/.
  - *Cul-de-sac resonance*: occurs when airflow in the oral cavity is obstructed, often by enlarged tonsils, resulting in a muffled voice quality.

A quick assessment of resonance can be accomplished by making a nasal listening tube from a bendy straw or piece of tubing. The clinician places one end of the tube in his or her ear and the other end at the client's nostril. The client is then asked to speak conversationally or perform a targeted speech task. Assess findings according to the following guidelines:

- If the clinician hears sound through the tube during production of vowels or plosives, hypernasality is indicated.

- If minimal or no sound is heard through the tube during production of nasal sounds, hyponasality or cul-de-sac resonance is indicated.

This assessment technique allows the clinician to test each naris separately to obtain more discriminative information.

To assess velopharyngeal function specifically, gently pinch the client's nose closed and ask him or her to repeat some of the nonnasal sentences containing pressure consonants presented in Table 12-4. The pressure consonants require a great amount of intraoral air pressure to produce. Hypernasality is identified if excessive nasal pressure is felt or if nasopharyngeal snorting occurs.

Assimilation nasality occurs when nonnasal sounds that precede or follow nasal consonants are also nasalized. To evaluate, instruct the client to repeat the following words and phrases with nasal sounds. Listen carefully for the presence of assimilation nasality. Pay particular attention to the client's speech rate in relation to the severity of the assimilation nasality. Is the assimilation nasality more noticeable at a faster speech rate? Is it eliminated at a slower speech rate?

TABLE 12-4 The Pressure Consonants

These words and phrases can be used to detect nasal emissions and hypernasality.

/p/	paper	pepper	top
	Pass the pepper.	papa's puppy	up top
	Please put the supper up.		
/b/	Bob	baby	bib
	baby's tub	baby's bib	the bear cub
	Baby's bib is by the tub.		
/k/	cake	hockey	kick
	Kathy's cake	kid's breakfast	broke his truck
	Katie's breakfast was cake.		
/g/	gave	forgot	hug
	Give it here.	Go get the sugar.	bib hog
	Gary gave sugar to the dog.		
/t/	two	guitar	hat
	tabletop	top hotel	hit the light
	Terry took the top hat.		
/d/	day	today	good
	Dave did it.	Ted cried.	good bread
	Dick was louder with David.		
/f/	fall	laughter	off
	feed father	before relief	half a loaf
	Fred carefully fed his calf.		
/v/	view	review	five
	very evil	every cover	have to drive
	Vicki loves to drive.		
/s/	sit	icy	House
	Suzie said so.	It's icy.	It's rice.
	Sarah spilled the sausage by the box.		
/z/	zero	busy	his
	Zack is lazy.	Easy does it.	those eyes
	Zack was too busy to choose.		
/ʃ/	ship	ashes	wish
	ship-shape	wishy-washy	fresh radish
	She washed a bushel of fish.		
/ʒ/	visual	usual	prestige
	beige corsage	visual pleasure	usual prestige
	a casual corsage		
/tʃ/	chalk	teacher	batch
	child's chair	richest butcher	each pitch
	Chip reached for the teacher's watch.		
/θ/	thought	birthday	bath
	thirsty father	third birthday	through both
	Thought I'd get a toothbrush for both.		
/ð/	they	father	bathe
	their father	the leather	They bathe.
	Their other brother likes to bathe.		

Words and Phrases with Multiple Nasal Sounds

man	man on the moon
many	home on the range
my mommy	Mickey and Minnie Mouse
my imagination	Manny's mommy made me mad on Monday.

Compensatory articulatory productions, usually pharyngeal or glottal sounds, may occur if there is velopharyngeal dysfunction. These productions may linger even after the structural defect has been repaired, requiring articulation treatment. Some of the more common compensatory patterns are noted in the following list. Phonetic symbols used during transcription are provided in parentheses.

- *Glottal stops* (/ʔ/): The vocal folds are used in an effort to produce plosive consonants. This strategy is frequently detected in cleft palate speech.
- *Pharyngeal stops* (/ʡ/, unvoiced; /ʕ/ voiced): Produced by lingual contact with the posterior pharyngeal wall.
- *Mid-dorsum palatal stops* (/ɟ/, unvoiced; /ɟ/ voiced): The mid-dorsum of the tongue makes contact with the mid-palate.
- *Pharyngeal fricatives* (/ʜ/, unvoiced; /ʕ/ voiced): Produced by narrowing the pharyngeal airway through linguapharyngeal constriction. These are attempted substitutes for sibilant fricatives.
- *Velar fricatives* (/χ/, unvoiced; /ɣ/ voiced): Fricatives are produced in the approximate place where /k/ and /g/ are normally produced.
- *Nasal fricatives* (/m̃/, /ñ/, /ŋ̃/): Excessive nasal emission is used as a substitute for consonants. These are also referred to as "nasal snorts," "nasal rustles," or "nasal friction."
- *Posterior nasal fricatives* (/fŋ/): Produced when the velum or uvula approximates the posterior pharyngeal wall of the nasopharynx. The back of the tongue may elevate in an attempt to assist in velopharyngeal closure.
- *Nasal grimaces*: A narrowing of the nostrils produced in an attempt to control nasal emission and inefficient use of the air source.

To assess hyponasality, instruct the client to repeat the sentences containing nasal sounds listed previously. Listen carefully for appropriateness of resonance. Then have him or her repeat the sentences while you gently pinch the client's nose closed. If unoccluded and occluded productions sound the same, hyponasality is present.

The procedures described in this section for assessing velopharyngeal dysfunction may not be adequate for identifying mild or borderline instances. Instruments and/or software programs that measure aerodynamic factors or allow direct viewing of the velopharyngeal mechanism may be required, such as a nasometer, the MDVP (described earlier), or a nasopharyngoscope. These tools require prior training and expertise before using.

Clients diagnosed with hypernasality or generalized nasal emission should be referred to a craniofacial medical doctor for further assessment. These are structural defects requiring surgical management. Hyponasality or cul-de-sac resonance typically results from obstruction in the vocal tract, and should be assessed by a laryngologist. Speech intervention is appropriate when a client demonstrates phoneme-specific nasality, nasal emission due to faulty articulation, or a compensatory articulation disorder that persists following surgical management of velopharyngeal dysfunction.

TWO SPECIAL POPULATIONS: ALARYNGEAL CLIENTS AND CLIENTS WITH CLEFT LIP AND/OR PALATE

Assessment of Alaryngeal Clients

Laryngectomy is the surgical removal of all or part of the larynx. Most commonly, laryngectomy is performed to remove cancerous tumors, or, in the case of traumatic injury, to remove a larynx that is severely damaged and not repairable. Obvious and immediate changes occur to the physiology of the speech mechanism as a result of a laryngectomy. Figure 12-4 shows the anatomical changes. The major respiratory and vocal changes are summarized in Table 12-5.

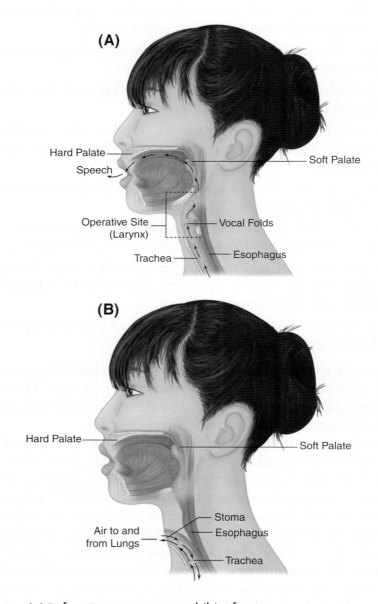

FIGURE 12-4. Larynx (a) Before Laryngectomy and (b) After Laryngectomy

Source: Adapted from InHealth Technologies.

TABLE 12-5 Pre- and Postoperative Changes in Respiratory Structures and Behaviors

PREOPERATIVE	POSTOPERATIVE
The patient could inhale air into the lungs through the nose or the mouth or both.	The patient can take air into the lungs only through the stoma in the neck.
The patient could exhale air from the lungs through the nose or the mouth or both.	The patient can exhale lung air only through the stoma in the neck.
The air inhaled through the nose was warmed, moistened, and filtered en route to the lungs.	The air taken into the stoma passes rapidly into the lungs without the benefit of passing through upper respiratory tract passages.
The respiratory tract was continuous from the lungs through the bronchi, trachea, and larynx to the pharynx, mouth, and nose.	The tracheal stump is sutured to, and terminates at, the stoma. No communication exists between the mouth, nose, pharynx and the trachea, bronchi, and lungs.
	Pulmonary air is exhaled directly through the stoma.

Source: Adapted from *Manual of Voice Treatment: Pediatrics Through Geriatrics* (p. 436), by M. L. Andrews, 2006, Clifton Park, NY: Cengage Learning.

Because the vocal mechanism is completely or partially gone, oral communication is profoundly impaired. A primary responsibility of the speech-language pathologist is to help the client establish an adequate postoperative means of communication as soon as possible. Assessment involves preoperative and postoperative consultations. Prior to the preoperative visit, consult the client's physician and review all relevant medical records to learn as much information as possible about the surgery. Form 12-6, "Alaryngeal Assessment," may be used to collect this information.

The preoperative consultation with the client provides an opportunity to describe the effects of surgery on communication and discuss post-surgery communication options. Other objectives are given in the following list. During this initial visit, be sensitive to just how much information the client is prepared to receive. Some of the information may need to be repeated or deferred until the postoperative consultation.

- Determine what the client already knows.
- Be positive about post-surgery outcomes.
- Instruct the client to be patient with him- or herself as a new mode of communication is learned.
- Correct misunderstandings, reinforce correct information, and provide new information.
- Provide information about support groups.
- Encourage family involvement.
- If the client is amenable, have a rehabilitated alaryngeal speaker visit the client and family.

- Discuss communication options.
- Provide printed information about laryngectomy, postoperative care, and alaryngeal communication options.
- Informally assess cognition and speech and language skills.
- Informally observe or assess writing skills.

The postoperative visit provides opportunity to review information provided preoperatively and focuses on more detailed discussion and demonstration of alaryngeal communication options. Encourage the client to try a variety of options that are suitable considering his or her needs and situation. The selection of one option does not preclude the use of another.

Alaryngeal Communication Options

There are three primary alaryngeal communication options:

- An *artificial larynx* is an electronic or mechanical instrument that provides a sound source as speech is shaped by the articulators. Some devices are held against the neck, whereas others have a tube that is placed in the oral cavity. In many cases, an artificial larynx is a first means of alaryngeal communication following surgery.
- *Esophageal speech* relies on a client's remaining anatomical structures to produce an internal source of sound. The speaker takes air in through the mouth, traps it in the throat, and then releases it back through the mouth, articulating normally. Esophageal speech is difficult to master.
- A *tracheoesophageal puncture (TEP)* is a surgical procedure whereby a surgeon makes a small hole in the common wall shared by the trachea and esophagus and fits it with a one-way shunt valve. The speaker inhales air into the lungs through the stoma, and then covers the stoma to direct the air through the valve and into the esophagus, which vibrates and creates a sound source for speech. This is one of the more common alaryngeal communication options.

All three alaryngeal communication options have advantages and disadvantages. These are summarized in Table 12-6.

In some cases, one option is used initially and another is used later. For example, an artificial larynx is often selected as an immediate form of communication while a client awaits healing of the region for later use of TEP.

ASSESSMENT OF CLIENTS WITH CLEFT LIP AND/OR PALATE

Orofacial clefts are malformations that occur early in the gestational period when the tissues in the mouth or lip area, or both, do not fuse together properly. Clefts vary in size, extent, and severity, and therefore have varying impact on normal speech development. Figure 12-5 shows normal structures, unilateral and bilateral cleft lip, cleft palate, and unilateral and bilateral cleft lip and palate.

Surgical closure of a cleft before single-word development begins (at approximately age 1) often precludes the development of cleft-related speech problems. This is not always the case, however. A primary characteristic of cleft palate speech is faulty resonance.

TABLE 12-6   Advantages and Disadvantages of the Three Primary Alaryngeal Communication Options

	ARTIFICIAL LARYNX
Advantages:	Easy to use
	Speech is generally intelligible
	Suitable for use immediately after surgery in most cases
	Can be an interim source of communication
Disadvantages:	Mechanical, "robot-like" vocal quality
	Draws attention to the speaker
	Requires good articulation skills
	Requires the use of one hand
	ESOPHAGEAL SPEECH
Advantages:	Does not require reliance upon a mechanical device
	Both hands are free while speaking
	Vocal productions are the client's "own voice"
	More natural sounding than electromechanical devices
Disadvantages:	Difficult to learn (approximately one-third of laryngectomees are unable to learn esophageal speech)
	Client may need to learn to habitually speak in shorter phrases
	Vocal intensity is sometimes insufficient
	Client may have a hoarse voice quality
	Potential articulatory errors, excessive stoma noise, "klunking," and facial grimacing need to be overcome during the learning process
	TRACHEOESOPHAGEAL SPEECH
Advantages:	Most natural voice quality of all alaryngeal communication options
	Greater pitch and intensity range than esophageal speech
	Easier and faster to learn than esophageal speech
	Clients can effectively produce sentences of normal length
Disadvantages:	Requires additional surgery
	Maintenance of the prosthesis is required
	Manual occlusion of the stoma is required if a tracheostoma valve is not used
	Some risk of aspiration of the prosthesis

VOICE AND RESONANCE

Children with clefts are also at increased risk for voice and articulation disorders due to their efforts to compensate for structural abnormalities. Many of the worksheets and guidelines provided in this chapter for assessment of voice and resonance are appropriate for assessing clients with clefts. Additionally, worksheets and guidelines in other chapters are also useful for basic assessment protocols.

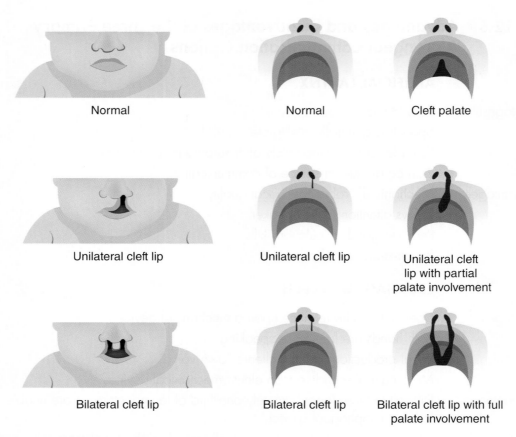

FIGURE 12-5 Clefts of the Lip and Palate

Language disorders are not necessarily associated with clefts, as many children in this population develop language normally. However, children with clefts often have language disorders due to cleft-related hearing loss, negative social and emotional factors, or cognitive delay, especially if the cleft coexists with other conditions.

An orofacial examination is an important component of a complete evaluation of a client with a cleft. In addition to the traditional elements of an orofacial examination, these factors should be considered when assessing a client with a cleft lip and/or palate:

- Type of cleft
- Stage and adequacy of repair
- Presence of other facial abnormalities such as fistulas or labial pits
- Presence of a submucosal cleft. This is often indicated by a bifid uvula, reduced or asymmetrical palatal movement, translucency or thinning of musculature at the velum midline, or a palpable notch on the posterior edge of the hard palate.
- Perceived length of the velum
- Perceived depth of the nasopharynx
- Shape of the alveolar ridge (e.g., notched, cleft, wide, collapsed)

Articulation considerations specific to clients with clefts include:

- Possible hypernasality during production of pressure consonants
- Increased hypernasality during vowel production
- Possible nasal emission, especially during production of sibilants /s/ and /z/
- Possible presence of less common phonological processes
- Worsened nasality during connected speech, as opposed to individual word productions

Form 12-7, "Checklist for the Assessment of Clients with Clefts," is provided to help summarize information gathered during the speech-language evaluation. Other assessment instruments that are helpful for evaluating clients with clefts include:

- *Great Ormand Street Speech Assessment*: *A Screening Assessment of Cleft Palate Speech* (Sell, Harding, & Grunwell, 1994)
- Several assessment protocols in *Communicative Disorders Related to Cleft Lip and Palate* (5th ed.) (Bzoch, 2004)

Feeding concerns may be a primary focus of care for infants with clefts. More information about pediatric feeding and swallowing is presented in Chapter 15.

CONCLUDING COMMENTS

The evaluation of voice and resonance is multifaceted. Respiratory, vibratory, and resonatory systems all influence perceptions of voice. A thorough case history, physical examination, perceptual evaluation, and instrumental analysis are all important aspects of a complete assessment. The speech-language pathologist typically works with a team of professionals to provide appropriate services to clients. Alaryngeal clients and clients with cleft lip and/or palate often present with voice and/or resonance disorders.

SOURCES OF ADDITIONAL INFORMATION

Print Sources

Boone, D. R., McFarlane, S. C., Von Berg, S. L., & Zraick, R. I. (2013). *The voice and voice therapy* (9th ed.). Upper Saddle River, NJ: Pearson.

Bzoch, K. R. (Ed.). (2004). *Communicative disorders related to cleft lip and palate* (5th ed.). Austin, TX: Pro-ed.

Kummer, A. W. (2014). *Cleft palate & craniofacial anomalies: Effects on speech and resonance* (3rd ed.). Clifton Park, NY: Cengage Learning.

Peterson-Falzone, S., Hardin-Jones, M. A., & Karnell, M. P. (2009). *Cleft palate speech* (4th ed.). St. Louis, MO: Mosby.

VOICE AND RESONANCE

Verdolini, K., Rosen, C. A., & Branski, R. C. (Eds.). (2006). *Classification manual for voice disorders—I.* Mahwah, NJ: Lawrence Erlbaum Associates.

Electronic Sources

Johns Hopkins Voice Center:
http://www.gbmc.org/voice

The Voice Foundation:
http://voicefoundation.org/

International Association of Laryngectomees:
http://www.theial.com/ial/

Laryngectomy Life:
http://www.laryngectomylife.com

Cleft Palate Foundation:
http://www.cleftline.org

Form 12-1.

Voice Handicap Index (VHI)

Name: _____ Date: _____

Examiner: _____

Instructions: These are statements that many people have used to describe their voices and the effects of their voices on their lives. For each statement, circle the response that indicates how frequently you have the same experience.

		0 = Never	1 = Almost Never	2 = Some-times	3 = Almost Always	4 = Always
F1.	My voice makes it difficult for people to hear me.	0	1	2	3	4
P2.	I run out of air when I talk.	0	1	2	3	4
F3.	People have difficulty understanding me in a noisy room.	0	1	2	3	4
P4.	The sound of my voice varies throughout the day.	0	1	2	3	4
F5.	My family has difficulty hearing me when I call them throughout the house.	0	1	2	3	4
F6.	I use the phone less often than I would like.	0	1	2	3	4
E7.	I'm tense when talking with others because of my voice.	0	1	2	3	4
F8.	I tend to avoid groups of people because of my voice.	0	1	2	3	4
E9.	People seem irritated with my voice.	0	1	2	3	4
P10.	People ask, "What's wrong with your voice?"	0	1	2	3	4
F11.	I speak with friends, neighbors, or relatives less often because of my voice.	0	1	2	3	4
F12.	People ask me to repeat myself when speaking face to face.	0	1	2	3	4
P13.	My voice sounds creaky and dry.	0	1	2	3	4
P14.	I feel as though I have to strain to produce voice.	0	1	2	3	4
E15.	I feel other people don't understand my voice problem.	0	1	2	3	4
F16.	My voice difficulties restrict my personal and social life.	0	1	2	3	4
P17.	The clarity of my voice is unpredictable.	0	1	2	3	4

(continues)

Source: From *The Voice Handicap Index (VHI): Development and Validation* (1997), by B. H. Jacobson, A. Johnson, C. Grywalski, A. Silbergleit, G. Jacobson, and M. S. Benninger, *American Journal of Speech–Language Pathology*, Vol 6(3), 66-70. Reprinted with permission.

VOICE AND RESONANCE

Form 12-1. continued

	0 = Never	1 = Almost Never	2 = Some-times	3 = Almost Always	4 = Always
P18. I try to change my voice to sound different.	0	1	2	3	4
F19. I feel left out of conversations because of my voice.	0	1	2	3	4
P20. I use a great deal of effort to speak.	0	1	2	3	4
P21. My voice is worse in the evening.	0	1	2	3	4
F22. My voice problem causes me to lose income.	0	1	2	3	4
E23. My voice problem upsets me.	0	1	2	3	4
E24. I am less outgoing because of my voice problem.	0	1	2	3	4
E25. My voice makes me feel handicapped.	0	1	2	3	4
P26. My voice "gives out" on me in the middle of speaking.	0	1	2	3	4
P27. I feel annoyed when people ask me to repeat myself.	0	1	2	3	4
E28. I feel embarrassed when people ask me to repeat myself.	0	1	2	3	4
E29. My voice makes me feel incompetent.	0	1	2	3	4
E30. I'm ashamed of my voice problem.	0	1	2	3	4

Note. The letter preceding each item corresponds to the subscale (E = emotional subscale, F = functional subscale, P = physical subscale).

(continues)

Source: From *The Voice Handicap Index (VHI): Development and Validation* (1997), by B. H. Jacobson, A. Johnson, C. Grywalski, A. Silbergleit, G. Jacobson, and M. S. Benninger, *American Journal of Speech–Language Pathology*, Vol 6(3), 66-70. Reprinted with permission.

Form 12-1. continued

Voice Handicap Index Summary

Instructions: Record score for each question below. Calculate totals for each subscale.

	F	P	E
1.	_____		
2.		_____	
3.	_____		
4.		_____	
5.	_____		
6.	_____		
7.			_____
8.	_____		
9.			_____
10.		_____	
11.	_____		
12.	_____		
13.		_____	
14.		_____	
15.			_____
16.	_____		
17.		_____	
18.		_____	
19.	_____		
20.		_____	
21.		_____	
22.	_____		
23.			_____
24.			_____
25.			_____
26.		_____	
27.		_____	
28.			_____
29.			_____
30.			_____

Totals: F _____ + P _____ + E _____ = _____

Source: From *The Voice Handicap Index (VHI): Development and Validation* (1997), by B. H. Jacobson, A. Johnson, C. Grywalski, A. Silbergleit, G. Jacobson, and M. S. Benninger, *American Journal of Speech–Language Pathology*, Vol 6(3), 66-70. Reprinted with permission.

VOICE AND RESONANCE

Form 12-2.

Vocally Abusive Behaviors Checklist—Adult

Name: _____ Date: _____

Instructions: These are behaviors that are potentially harmful to your vocal system. Rate each behavior according to the following scale. Use the Comments column on the right-hand side to add any additional information.

0 = Never

1 = Rarely

2 = Occasionally

3 = Often

4 = Always

Rating   Comments

_____ Alcohol consumption _____

_____ Allergies _____

_____ Arguing with peers, spouse, others _____

_____ Athletic activities involving yelling _____

_____ Breathing through the mouth _____

_____ Caffeine consumption (coffee, chocolate, etc.) _____

_____ Calling others from a distance _____

_____ Coughing or sneezing loudly _____

_____ Dehydration _____

_____ Drug use (prescription and nonprescription) _____

_____ Environmental pollutants exposure _____

_____ Grunting during exercise or lifting _____

_____ Laughing hard _____

_____ Nightclub social talking _____

_____ Pitch too high or low _____

_____ Poor posture _____

_____ Post-nasal drip _____

_____ Religious chanting _____

_____ Singing frequently (amateur or professional) _____

_____ Smoking _____

(continues)

Form 12-2. continued

Rating Comments

_____ Speaking for prolonged periods _____

_____ Speaking in noisy environments (specify) _____

_____ Speaking in smoky environments _____

_____ Speaking while in the car _____

_____ Speaking while tense _____

_____ Speech presentations _____

_____ Teaching or instructing _____

_____ Telephone used frequently _____

_____ Theater participation _____

_____ Throat clearing _____

_____ Upper respiratory infections _____

_____ Vocalizing with hard attacks _____

_____ Whispering for prolonged periods _____

_____ Other _____

Form 12-3.

Vocally Abusive Behaviors Checklist—Children and Youth

Name: _____ Date: _____

Instructions: These are behaviors that are potentially harmful to your vocal system. Rate each behavior according to the following scale. Use the Comments column on the right-hand side to add any additional information.

0 = Never

1 = Rarely

2 = Occasionally

3 = Often

4 = Always

Rating   Comments

_____ Allergies _____

_____ Arcade talking _____

_____ Arguing with peers, siblings, others _____

_____ Athletic activities involving yelling _____

_____ Breathing through the mouth _____

_____ Caffeine consumption (soda, chocolate, etc.) _____

_____ Calling others from a distance _____

_____ Cheerleading or pep squad participation _____

_____ Coughing or sneezing loudly _____

_____ Debate team participation _____

_____ Dehydration _____

_____ Drug use (prescription and nonprescription) _____

_____ Environmental pollutants exposure _____

_____ Grunting during exercise or lifting _____

_____ Laughing hard _____

_____ Pitch too high or low _____

_____ Poor posture _____

_____ Post-nasal drip _____

_____ Religious chanting _____

_____ Singing frequently (amateur or professional) _____

(continues)

VOICE AND RESONANCE

Form 12-3. continued

Rating   Comments

_____ Speaking for prolonged periods _____

_____ Speaking in noisy environments (specify) _____

_____ Speaking while in the car _____

_____ Speaking while tense _____

_____ Sports participation _____

_____ Theater participation _____

_____ Throat clearing _____

_____ Upper respiratory infections _____

_____ Vocalizing animal or motor noises _____

_____ Vocalizing with hard attacks _____

_____ Whispering for prolonged periods _____

_____ Yelling or screaming _____

_____ Other _____

Form 12-4.

Consensus Auditory-Perceptual Evaluation of Voice (CAPE-V)[1]

Name: _____ Age: _____ Date: _____

Examiner: _____

The following parameters of voice quality will be rated upon completion of the following tasks:

1. Sustained vowels, /a/ and /i/ for 3–5 seconds of duration each.
2. Sentence production:

   a. The blue spot is on the key again.   d. We eat eggs every Easter.
   b. How hard did he hit him?   e. My mama makes lemon muffins.
   c. We were away a year ago.   f. Peter will keep at the peak.

3. Spontaneous speech in response to: "Tell me about your voice problem." or "Tell me how your voice is functioning."

> **Legend:** C = Consistent I = Intermittent
> MI = Mildly Deviant
> MO = Moderately Devaint
> SE = Severely Deviant

						SCORE
Overall Severity	_____			C	I	___/100
	MI	MO	SE			
Roughness	_____			C	I	___/100
	MI	MO	SE			
Breathiness	_____			C	I	___/100
	MI	MO	SE			
Strain	_____					
	MI	MO	SE			
Pitch	(Indicate the nature of the abnormality: _____			C	I	___/100
	MI	MO	SE			
Loudness	(Indicate the nature of the abnormality: _____			C	I	___/100
	MI	MO	SE			
_____	_____			C	I	___/100
	MI	MO	SE			
_____	_____			C	I	___/100
	MI	MO	SE			

COMMENTS ABOUT RESONANCE: NORMAL   OTHER (Provide description): _____

ADDITIONAL FEATURES (for example, diplophonia, fry, falsetto, asthenia, aphonia, pitch instability, tremor, wet/gurgly, or other relevant terms):

[1] Source: From "*Consensus Auditory-Perceptual Evaluation of Voice: Development of a standardized clinical protocol*" by Gail B. Kempster, Bruce R. Gerratt, Katherine Verdolini Abbott, Julie Barkmeier-Kraemer, and Robert E. Hillman, 2009, *American Journal of Speech-Language Pathology, 18*, pp. 124–132.

VOICE AND RESONANCE

Form 12-5.

Assessment of Voice Worksheet

Name: _____ Date: _____

Occupation _____

Examiner's Name: _____ Date: _____

Summarize salient findings from case history and client interview:

Summarize impact of voice on daily activities:

Summarize salient findings from oral-motor assessment:

Record general observations (e.g., tension, neurological signs, posture, emotion):

Record general phonatory behaviors (frequent throat clearing or coughing, signs of allergy or cold, hard glottal attacks, etc.):

VOICE AND RESONANCE

Form 12-5. continued

Loudness

During conversational speech: too soft   too loud   normal

Variations in loudness? yes/no _____

Ask client to vary loudness to determine range and control. Record observations:

    Whisper:

    Speak softly:

    Speak loudly:

    Increase loudness while counting from 1–20:

    Stability:

Additional and/or supplemental objective measures (including shimmer, dB levels, range, etc.):

Pitch

During conversational speech: monotone   too high   too low   normal

Variations in frequency? yes/no _____

Fundamental frequency:

Best pitch:

Ask client to vary pitch to determine range and control. Record observations:

    Top of range:

    Bottom of range:

    Smoothness:

    Stability:

Additional and/or supplemental objective measures (including jitter, fundamental frequency, range, etc.):

Quality

During conversational speech:

    Breathy:

    Harsh:

    Hoarse:

    Rough:

    Strained:

    Asthenia:

    Aphonia:

    Tremor:

    Fry:

    Other:

Form 12-5. continued

S/Z ratio:

Maximum phonation time (MPT):

Additional and/or supplemental objective measures (including spectrum analysis, etc.):

Respiratory Support

Observe during conversational speech:

>Tension in upper chest, shoulders, face, neck:

>Inhalation (shallow or noisy):

>Mouth breathing:

>Asthenia:

>Fatigue:

>Running out of air:

>Speaking on inhalation:

S/Z ratio:

Maximum phonation time (MPT):

Additional and/or supplemental objective measures (including vital capacity, resistance, flow rates/volumes, subglottic pressure):

Stimulability for Improved Voice

Easy onset:

Postural shift:

Loudness shift (increase or decrease):

Pitch shift (increase or decrease):

Laryngeal manipulation:

Other:

FORM 12-6.

Alaryngeal Assessment

Name: _____ Age: _____ Date: _____

Occupation: _____

Employer: _____

Examiner's Name: _____

Medical History

Surgery type and extent: _____

_____

_____

Date of surgery: _____

Surgeon: _____

History of present problems: _____

_____

Previous treatment of problem: _____

_____

Previous speech therapy: _____

_____

Radiation treatment: _____

_____

Other health factors: _____

_____

Medications: _____

Previous surgeries: _____

_____

Current Status

Living situation: _____

Family/friends support: _____

Cognitive status: _____

Emotional status: _____

VOICE AND RESONANCE

Form 12-6. continued

Communication strategies: _____

_____

Hearing: _____

Vision: _____

Dental: _____

Chewing: _____

Swallowing: _____

_____

Taste: _____

Smell: _____

Tongue: if resectioned, how much? _____

    Range of motion: _____

    Reconstruction or prosthesis: _____

Possible Communication Scenarios

Artificial larynx: _____

Tracheoesophageal speech: _____

Esophageal speech: _____

Additional Notes and Recommendations:

FORM 12-7.

Checklist for the Assessment of Clients with Clefts

Name:_____ Age: _____ Date:_____

Primary Care Physician: _____

Type of Cleft: _____

Date of Surgery: _____

Other Conditions and Medical History: _____

_____

_____

Examiner's Name: _____

Orofacial Examination

Instructions: Administer a standard orofacial examination (you may wish to use Form 5-1, "Orofacial Examination Form"). Additionally, make observations about the following orofacial features. Check and circle each item noted. Include descriptive comments in the right-hand margin.

_____ Type of cleft: lip/palate/lip and palate (describe) _____

_____ Adequacy of cleft repair: good/fair/poor _____

_____ Other facial abnormalities: absent/present (describe) _____

_____ Submucosal cleft: absent/present _____

_____ Labial pits in lower lip: absent/present _____

_____ Labiodental fistulas: absent/present _____

_____ Alveolar fistulas: absent/present _____

_____ Palatal fistulas: absent/present _____

_____ Velar fistulas: absent/present _____

_____ Perceived length of velum: normal/short/long _____

_____ Perceived depth of nasopharynx: normal/shallow/deep _____

_____ Shape of the alveolar ridge: notched/cleft/wide/collapsed _____

_____ Notes from standard orofacial examination _____

_____

_____

Form 12-7. continued

Assessment of Voice

Instructions: Evaluate the client's voice, paying particular attention to possible cleft-related problems. Check deficits that are present and indicate severity. Record additional notes in the right-hand margin. (You may also use Form 12-5, "Assessment of Voice Worksheet," for a more detailed analysis.)

    1 = Mild

    2 = Moderate

    3 = Severe

_____ Pitch variation is reduced _____

_____ Vocal intensity is reduced _____

_____ Vocal quality is hoarse/harsh/breathy (circle) _____

_____ Vocal quality is strangled _____

_____ Client produces glottal stops in place of plosives and fricatives _____

_____ Client attempts to mask hypernasality and nasal emission _____

_____ Client strains voice to achieve adequate pitch change and loudness _____

_____ Client strains voice in attempt to increase speech intelligibility _____

Assessment of Resonance and Velopharyngeal Integrity

Instructions: Evaluate the client's voice, listening for the following qualities of resonance. Check each characteristic the client exhibits and indicate severity. Record additional notes in the right-hand margin.

    1 = Mild

    2 = Moderate

    3 = Severe

_____ Hypernasality _____

_____ Nasal emission _____

_____ Cul-de-sac resonance _____

_____ Hyponasality _____

Form 12-7. continued

Instructions: Ask the client to produce the pressure consonants /p/, /b/, /k/, /g/, /t/, /d/, /f/, /v/, /s/, /z/, /ʃ/, /ʒ/, /tʃ/, /θ/, and /ð/ in words and phrases, and listen for hypernasality and nasal emissions. Check the appropriate observations below.

_____ Velopharyngeal function is adequate (no nasal emissions or hypernasality)

_____ Velopharyngeal function is inadequate (nasal emissions or hypernasality present)

_____ Further testing using objective instrumentation is necessary

_____ Nasal emissions and hypernasality are consistent

_____ Nasal emissions and hypernasality are inconsistent

Assessment of Articulation and Phonology

Instructions: Listen to the client's articulatory accuracy. Pay particular attention to the client's production of stop-plosives, fricatives, and affricates, which are most likely to be negatively affected by a cleft. Indicate severity and make additional comments in the right-hand margin.

    1 = Mild

    2 = Moderate

    3 = Severe

_____ Stop-plosive errors _____

_____ Fricative errors _____

_____ Affricate errors _____

_____ Glide errors _____

_____ Liquid errors _____

_____ Nasal errors _____

_____ Vowel errors _____

_____ Error patterns are consistent _____

_____ Error patterns are inconsistent _____

_____ Further assessment is recommended _____

VOICE AND RESONANCE

Form 12-7. continued

Instructions: Check the following compensatory strategies the client uses during speech production and indicate severity. Make additional comments in the right-hand margin.

1 = Mild

2 = Moderate

3 = Severe

_____ Glottal stops _____

_____ Pharyngeal stops _____

_____ Mid-dorsum palatal stops _____

_____ Pharyngeal fricatives _____

_____ Velar fricatives _____

_____ Nasal fricatives _____

_____ Posterior nasal fricatives _____

_____ Nasal grimaces _____

Summary

Instructions: Check areas that require further assessment. Make additional comments in the right-hand margin.

_____ Articulation—cleft-related _____

_____ Articulation—non-cleft-related _____

_____ Cognition _____

_____ Hearing _____

_____ Language _____

_____ Velopharyngeal integrity _____

_____ Voice _____

Chapter 13

ASSESSMENT OF NEUROCOGNITIVE DISORDERS

This chapter focuses on the assessment of neurocognitive speech and language disorders that have a major impact on communication—specifically, aphasia, right hemisphere syndrome, traumatic brain injury, and dementia. These conditions are most commonly associated with adults, although they can affect any age group. The qualifying marker for classification as a neurocognitive disorder is a decline, either suddenly or over time, in cognitive function.

OVERVIEW OF ASSESSMENT

History of the Client

    Procedures

        Written Case History

        Information-Getting Interview

        Information from Other Professionals

    Contributing Factors

        Medical Diagnosis

        Pharmacological Factors

        Age

        Intelligence, Motivation, and Levels of Concern

Assessment of Aphasia

    Procedures

        Screening

        Speech and Language Sampling

        Formal Testing

        Cognitive Skills Evaluation

    Analysis

        Expressive/Receptive Abilities

        Types of Errors

        Intelligibility

Assessment of Right Hemisphere Syndrome

    Procedures

        Screening

        Speech and Language Sampling

        Formal Testing

        Cognitive Skills Evaluation

    Analysis

        Cognitive-Linguistic Abilities

        Types of Errors

        Visual-Perceptual Abilities

Assessment of Clients with Traumatic Brain Injury

    Procedures

        Screening

Speech and Language Sampling
Formal Testing
Cognitive Skills Evaluation
Analysis
Expressive/Receptive Abilities
Types of Errors
Intelligibility
Assessment of Clients with Dementia (Major Neurocognitive Disorder)
Procedures
Screening
Behavioral Observations
Formal Testing
Analysis
Expressive-Receptive Abilities
Severity of Impairment
Functional Potential
Orofacial Examination
Hearing Assessment
Determining the Diagnosis
Providing Information (written report, interview, etc.)

ASSESSMENT OF APHASIA

Aphasia is defined as a loss of language function due to an injury to the brain in an area associated with the comprehension and production of language. Aphasia is most often caused by a stroke or cerebral vascular accident (CVA). Other etiologies include accident, tumor, infection, toxicity, and metabolic and nutritional disorders that affect brain function. Aphasia can have multiple ramifications. Every client will be different depending on a variety of factors, including the site of the injury, the severity of the injury, and the uniqueness of the individual. The fact that clients may vary so dramatically from one another makes it challenging to clearly define aphasia in terms of a set of behaviors and deficits.

Experts have different opinions about how aphasia ought to be classified or indeed whether classifications should exist at all. These differences of opinion are due to the fact that the brain functions to integrate all aspects of language, and an injury to a particular site typically affects all language modalities to one degree or another. Therefore, clear-cut symptoms following a brain injury simply do not exist. On the other hand, classification systems do help us clarify broad categories of language deficiencies based on the site of the injury even though there is a degree of variation from one client to another.

Table 13-1 summarizes several types of aphasia according to one of the most commonly used classification systems. The aphasia types are differentiated according to fluent and nonfluent characteristics. Keep in mind when using this type of classification system that aphasia is not always so easily simplified. In practice, a clinician will typically not find "textbook

TABLE 13-1   Types and Characteristics of Aphasia

TYPE	CHARACTERISTICS
Nonfluent Aphasias	
Broca's aphasia	Agrammatism
	Effortful speech
	Short, telegraphic phrases
	Presence of apraxia
	Marked naming problems
	Slow speech rate, lacking intonation
	Poor reading and writing ability
	Relatively good auditory comprehension
Transcortical motor aphasia	Intact repetition
	Lack of spontaneous speech
	Naming problems
	Short, telegraphic sentences
	Good articulation
	Agrammatism
	Paraphasias
Isolation aphasia	Marked naming difficulty
	Severely impaired comprehension
	Mild to moderately impaired repetition skills
Global aphasia	All language functions severely affected
	Severe deficits in comprehension and production
	Naming problems
	Difficulty with gestural skills
	Impaired reading and writing
Fluent Aphasias	
Wernicke's aphasia	Fluent but meaningless speech
	Severe auditory comprehension deficit
	Jargon, paraphasias, and neologisms
	Good articulation and intonation
	Naming difficulties
	Poor reading comprehension
	Writing deficits
Conduction aphasia	Marked difficulty repeating words and phrases
	Only minor comprehension problems
	Good articulation and prosody
	Naming problems
	Recognition of errors with attempts to self-correct

TYPE	CHARACTERISTICS
Transcortical sensory aphasia	Intact repetition
	Poor auditory comprehension
	Naming difficulties
	Paraphasias
Anomic aphasia	Marked naming problems
	Near-normal language
	Good comprehension
	Good repetition skills
	Relatively good auditory comprehension
	Good articulation
	Good grammatical structures

Source: Adapted from *PocketGuide to Assessment in Speech-Language Pathology* (3rd ed.), by M. N. Hegde, 2007, Clifton Park, NY: Cengage Learning.

cases" of the different types of aphasia. In reality, aphasia is manifest differently in every client, and the lines separating one type from another are not clearly defined.

Although there is variation from one aphasic client to the next, there are certain behaviors and deficits of communication that are characteristic of aphasia. These include:

- Impaired auditory comprehension
- Impaired verbal expression
- Presence of paraphasias
- Perseveration
- Agrammatism, or grammatical errors
- Nonfluent speech or nonmeaningful fluent speech
- Impaired prosodic features of speech
- Difficulty repeating words, phrases, and sentences
- Problems with naming and word finding (anomia)
- Impaired reading ability (alexia or dyslexia)
- Impaired writing ability (agraphia or dysgraphia; possibly confounded by loss of use of the dominant right hand due to hemiparesis)
- In bilingual clients, unequal impairment between the two languages
- Pragmatic deficits
- Difficulty using or understanding gestures

When completing an evaluation of aphasia, identify strengths and deficiencies within all these areas in order to make the most complete and realistic diagnosis and treatment plan for

NEUROCOGNITIVE DISORDERS

the client. Several formal tests are available for the assessment of aphasia. Some of the most commonly used published tests include:

- *Aphasia Diagnostic Profiles (ADP)* (Helm-Estabrooks, 1992)
- *Boston Assessment of Severe Aphasia (BASA)* (Helm-Estabrooks, Ramsberger, Morgan, & Nicholas, 1989)
- *Boston Diagnostic Aphasia Examination (BDAE-3)* (Goodglass, Kaplan, & Barresi, 2000)
- *Comprehensive Aphasia Test (CAT)* (Swiburn, Porter, & Howard, 2004)
- *Examining for Aphasia: Assessment of Aphasia and Related Impairments (EFA-4)* (La Pointe & Eisenson, 2008)
- *Quick Assessment for Aphasia* (Tanner & Culbertson, 1999)
- *Reading Comprehension Battery for Aphasia (RCBA-2)* (La Pointe & Horner, 1998)
- *Western Aphasia Battery Revised (WAB-R)* (Kertesz, 2006)

Tasks for identifying skills and deficits of aphasic clients are found in Form 13-1 "Evaluation of Aphasia." These evaluation procedures are based on principles and tasks common to many examinations of aphasia. The materials in Form 13-1 allow the clinician to assess a variety of receptive and expressive skills by using simple tasks that vary in difficulty. In the "Comments" sections, make specific notes about the client's behaviors, such as delayed responses (include length of time), self-corrections, numbers and types of cues provided by the therapist, perseverations, visual neglect, response accuracy (e.g., incorrect response but correct response class), and so forth. Gain as much relevant information as possible for a complete assessment.

Although failure to respond correctly to some items may be the result of aphasia, incorrect responses may also be the result of other disorders (e.g., language deficiencies secondary to severe hearing impairment, visual impairment, mental impairment, poor academic skills, schizophrenia). Know the client's medical history! Aphasia results from a neurological insult. The symptoms have a sudden onset (at the time of neurological insult), not a gradual onset as in the case of other disorders that have similar symptoms. To accurately assess aphasia, obtain as much information as possible about the nature of the disorder, including events surrounding its onset, communicative abilities prior to its onset, and results of any related neurological assessments (e.g., magnetic resonance imaging [MRI], computerized tomographic [CT] scan).

The test items are not score-based or criterion-based. Rather, the tasks are designed to identify strengths and weaknesses. When administering the items, include tasks from each section. Administer entire sections or sample from within each section. The tasks are arranged in an easy to difficult sequence; sample some of the more difficult tasks before assuming a client does or does not have a deficit in that given area.

ASSESSMENT OF RIGHT HEMISPHERE SYNDROME

Traditionally, the left hemisphere of the brain is known as the hemisphere of language function. However, both cerebral hemispheres perform specific tasks that complement and are integrated with tasks that are specific to the opposite hemisphere. Simply stated, both hemispheres are vitally important for normal and functional communication. The left hemisphere is primarily responsible for basic language functions, such as phonology, syntax, and simple-level semantics. The right hemisphere is primarily responsible for complex linguistic processing and the nonverbal, emotional aspects of communication.

Injury to the right hemisphere of the brain results in a unique set of deficits that can significantly affect a person's ability to communicate and function appropriately in his or her environment. As with other neurologically based disorders, outcomes from right hemisphere damage can vary significantly from one client to another. However, there are specific impairments that are characteristic of right hemisphere damage. These are summarized from Brookshire (2003) and Tompkins (1995) and fall into four categories:

Perceptual and Attentional Deficits

- Neglect of the left visual field
- Difficulty with facial recognition (prosopagnosia)
- Difficulty with constructional tasks
- Impulsivity, distractibility, and poor attention to tasks
- Excessive attention to irrelevant information
- Denial of deficits (anosognosia)

Affective Deficits

- Difficulty expressing emotions
- Difficulty recognizing emotions of others
- Depression
- Apparent lack of motivation

Communicative Deficits

- Difficulty with word retrieval
- Impaired auditory comprehension
- Reading and writing deficits
- Impaired prosodic features of speech
- Difficulty with pragmatics
- Dysarthria

Cognitive Deficits

- Disorientation
- Impaired attention
- Difficulty with memory
- Poor integration of information
- Difficulty with logic, reasoning, planning, and problem solving
- Impaired comprehension of inferred meanings
- Difficulty understanding humor

NEUROCOGNITIVE DISORDERS

Many of the characteristics of right hemisphere syndrome are similar to those of aphasia, resulting from left hemisphere damage. To assist in the differential diagnosis of these two disorders, see Table 13-2.

The "Cognitive–Linguistic Evaluation," Form 13-2, is an informal assessment designed to identify specific problem areas that may be present in a client with a right cerebral hemisphere injury. There are also a variety of other assessment materials included in this book that may be helpful. These include:

- "Evaluation of Aphasia," Form 13-1. Selected subsections may be used to assess memory, logic, reasoning, problem solving, auditory processing, thought organization, reading, and writing.
- "Assessment of Pragmatic Skills," Form 7-8. This worksheet may be useful for assessing a variety of pragmatic responses.
- "Assessment of Clients with Traumatic Brain Injury," Form 13-3. Selected questions in this behavioral profile may be helpful for gathering specific information from family members or other caregivers.

TABLE 13-2 Differential Characteristics of Right Hemisphere Syndrome and Aphasia

APHASIA	RIGHT HEMISPHERE SYNDROME
Significant or dominant problems in naming, fluency, auditory comprehension, reading and writing	Only mild problems in naming, fluency, auditory comprehension, reading, and writing
No left-sided neglect	Left-sided neglect
No denial of illness	Denial of illness
Speech is generally relevant	Speech is often irrelevant, excessive, rambling
Generally normal affect	Often lack of affect
Intact recognition of familiar faces	Possible impaired recognition of familiar faces
Simplification of drawings	Rotation and left-sided neglect
No significant prosodic defect	Significant prosidic defect
Appropriate humor	Inappropriate humor
May retell the essence of a story	May retell only nonessential, isolated details (no integration)
May understand implied meanings	Understands only literal meanings
Pragmatic impairments less striking	Pragmatic impairments more striking (eye contact, topic maintenance, etc.)
Although limited in language skills, communication is often good	Although possessing good language skills, communication is very poor
Pure linguistic deficits are dominant	Pure linguistic deficits are not dominant

Source: *PocketGuide to Assessment in Speech-Language Pathology* (3rd ed., pp. 39–40), by M. N. Hegde, 2008, Clifton Park, NY: Cengage Learning.

- "Reading Passages" (Chapter 5). These may be useful for assessing reading ability and visual function.
- "Narratives" (Chapter 5). These may be useful for assessing memory and thought organization.

Several commercially available sources for assessment are listed here. Keep in mind that many of them were not developed for evaluating right hemisphere syndrome specifically. However, administered in their entirety or in selected subsections, they can be adapted for such use.

- *Boston Diagnostic Aphasia Examination* (Goodglass, Kaplan, & Barresi, 2000)
- *Communicative Abilities of Daily Living (CADL-2)* (Holland, Frattali, & Fromm, 1999)
- *Discourse Comprehension Test* (2nd ed.) (Brookshire & Nicholas, 1997)
- *Mini Inventory of Right Brain Injury (MIRBI-2)* (Pimental & Knight, 2000)
- *Revised Token Test (RTT)* (McNeil & Prescott, 1978)
- *Ross Information Processing Assessment (RIPA-2)* (Ross-Swain, 1996)
- *Ross Information Processing Assessment—Geriatric (RIPA-G)* (Ross-Swain & Fogle, 1996)
- *Ross Information Processing Assessment—Primary (RIPA-P)* (Ross-Swain, 1999)

ASSESSMENT OF CLIENTS WITH TRAUMATIC BRAIN INJURY

A traumatic brain injury (TBI) is the result of an acute assault on the brain. There are two subcategories of TBIs: penetrating injuries and closed-head injuries. Penetrating injuries occur when an object, such as a bullet or a knife, penetrates the skull and rips through the soft brain tissue, damaging nerve fibers and nerve cells. The neurological damage is focal (localized) and the resulting behaviors vary, depending on the severity and location of the injury. Closed-head injuries are incurred from the collision of the head with an object or surface that does not penetrate the skull. Even though the skull remains intact, the brain can be severely damaged. The damage is diffuse (nonlocalized), and the resulting behaviors vary depending on the severity and location(s) of the injury.

Considering the varying nature of a TBI, one can understand why there is no such thing as a typical brain injury. Also, a brain injury can occur at any age. These factors pose a unique challenge to the clinician attempting to assess the communicative skills of a client who has suffered a head injury. A uniform set of symptoms characteristic of all TBIs does not exist. However, some commonly seen consequences of brain injury include:

- Inconsistency
- Attention deficits
- Impaired memory
- Impaired language
- Disorientation to time and place
- Poor organization
- Impaired reasoning
- Reduced ability to write or draw
- Anomia

NEUROCOGNITIVE DISORDERS

- Restlessness
- Irritability
- Distractibility
- High frustration and anxiety
- Aggressive behavior
- Inconsistent responses
- Disorders of smell and taste
- Poor judgment
- Poor control of emotions
- Denial of disability
- Poor self-care

These behaviors vary depending upon the type of injury, the severity, the cerebral systems involved, the presence of additional neuromedical variables (e.g., extended coma, cerebral hemorrhage), the client's age, and the pre-trauma status.

A person who has suffered a TBI normally experiences a period of unconsciousness at the time of injury. It may last for only a few seconds, or for many days or months. The Glasgow Coma Scale (GCS) is a frequently used scoring system for assessing levels of conciousness following TBI. It is based on objective measures of eye opening (E), verbal response (V), and motor response (M). The score is expressed as individual categories and as a summation of the three categories (e.g., E3 + V3 + M4 = GCS10). Total scores range from 3 (comatose) to 15 (grossly neurologically intact). The GCS and interpretive information is presented in Table 13-3.

Another frequently used rating system is The Rancho Levels of Cognitive Functioning. It is helpful for identifying cognitive status in clients with recent-onset, severe head injuries. There are eight levels, each identified with a Roman numeral. The Rancho Levels of Cognitive Functioning with specific cognitive characteristics are presented in Table 13-4.

TABLE 13-3　Glasgow Coma Scale

Eye Opening (E)		Motor Response (M)	
Spontaneous	4	Normal	6
To verbal command	3	Localizes pain	5
To pain	2	Withdraws from pain (flexion)	4
No response	1	Decorticate (flexion) rigidity	3
		Decerebrate (extension) rigidity	2
Verbal Response (V)		No response	1
Normal conversation	5		
Disoriented conversation	4	Interpretation of total score:	
Words, but not coherent	3	Mild injury = 13–15 points	
Incomprehensible sounds	2	Moderate injury = 9–12 points	
No response	1	Severe injury (comatose) = 3–8 points	

TABLE 13-4 The Rancho Levels of Cognitive Functioning

LEVEL OF COGNITIVE FUNCTIONING:	CHARACTERISTIC BEHAVIORS:
Level I *No response*	Unresponsive to any stimuli Appears to be in a deep sleep
Level II *Generalized response*	Limited, inconsistent, and nonpurposeful responses Often responds to pain only May open eyes, but does not focus on anything in particular
Level III *Localized response*	Purposeful responses May follow simple commands May focus on presented object May turn heard toward loud noises
Level IV *Confused, agitated*	Heightened state of activity, confusion, and disorientation Aggressive behavior Unable to do self-care Unaware of present events Agitation appears related to internal confusion
Level V *Confused, inappropriate, but not agitated*	Non-agitated Appears alert, but confused Responds to simple commands Distractible Does not concentrate on tasks Occasional agitated responses to external stimuli Does not learn new information May experience frustration as elements of memory return
Level VI *Confused, appropriate*	Serious memory problems Some awareness of self and others Can relearn old skills, such as activities of daily living Difficulty learning new skills
Level VII *Automatic, appropriate*	Appears appropriately oriented Performs all self-care activities Minimal or absent confusion Shallow recall for recent events and discussions Increased awareness of self and interaction in the environment Lacks insight into condition Decreased judgment and problem solving Lacks realistic planning for future
Level VIII *Purposeful, appropriate*	Alert and oriented Recalls and integrates past events Learns new activities and can continue without supervision Independent in home and living skills Capable of driving Some defects in stress tolerance, judgment, and abstract reasoning persist May function at reduced levels in society

The assessment of clients with TBI will vary depending upon many factors, including the client's age, severity of the injury, and current level of consciousness. Before meeting with the client, obtain a thorough case history. Research the type and severity of the head injury, the date of onset, and the cerebral areas affected. Obtain evaluation dates and results from other assessments (e.g., CT scans, MRIs). Review GCS ratings and Rancho Levels, noting changes across time. It is important to continually review the client's medical chart during the assessment process and treatment because of the significant changes that often occur following a brain injury.

The direct assessment will typically include the following considerations:

- Visuospatial, visuomotor, and visuoconstructional abilities
- General motor functioning
- General emotional functioning
- Chewing and swallowing abilities
- Pragmatic behaviors
- Speech
- Expressive and receptive language abilities
- Cognitive and intellectual abilities, including memory, processing, reasoning judgment, and problem-solving
- Execution of activities of daily living

Several formal speech and language assessment instruments that are appropriate for assessing the communicative effects of TBI include:

- *Boston Diagnostic Aphasia Examination* (3rd ed.) (Goodglass, Kaplan, & Barresi, 2000)
- *Brief Test of Head Injury* (Helm-Estabrooks & Hotz, 1991)
- *The Cognitive Assessment of Minnesota* (Rustad et al., 1993)
- *Cognitive Linguistic Quick Test (CLQT)* (Helm-Estabrooks, 2001)
- *Communication Activities of Daily Living (CADL-2)* (Holland, Frattali, & Fromm, 1999)
- *Ross Information Processing Assessment* (2nd ed.) *(RIPA-2)* (Ross-Swain, 1996)
- *Ross Information Processing Assessment—Primary (RIPA-P)* (Ross-Swain, 1999)
- *Scales of Cognitive Ability for Traumatic Brain Injury* (Adamovich & Henderson, 1992)
- *Western Aphasia Battery—Revised (WAB-R)* (Kertesz, 2006)

Form 13-3, "Assessment of Clients with Traumatic Brain Injury," is a worksheet for informally evaluating clients with a TBI. Ask a family member, nurse, or other caregiver to serve as the informant. Ideally, the form is to be completed over an extended period of time (1 to 2 days) by someone who spends a significant amount of time with the client. Some less impaired clients may be able to answer the questions themselves.

Other resources included in this manual may also be helpful for assessing clients with TBI. For example:

- Form 13-2, "Cognitive–Linguistic Evaluation," is appropriate for assessing memory, orientation, auditory processing and comprehension, problem solving, reasoning, thought organization, visual processing, and graphic expression.

- Selected subsections of Form 13-1, "Evaluation of Aphasia," are appropriate for assessing memory, logic, reasoning, semantic concepts, problem solving, and language skills.
- Form 7-8, "Assessment of Pragmatic Skills", is appropriate for assessing a variety of pragmatic behaviors.
- "Reading Passages" and "Narratives" in Chapter 5 are appropriate for assessing memory and language organization.

Because these materials are not designed specifically for assessing the effects of TBI, be creative in selecting and administering stimulus items. Keep in mind the behaviors to be assessed, and adapt the assessment materials as needed.

ASSESSMENT OF CLIENTS WITH DEMENTIA (MAJOR NEUROCOGNITIVE DISORDER)

Major neurocognitive disorder, more commonly known as dementia, is characterized by progressive deterioration of memory, orientation, intellectual ability, and behavioral appropriateness. It generally progresses from a very mild to a very severe cognitive impairment over the course of months or even years. This section on the assessment of dementia focuses on irreversible dementias, but there are forms of dementia that are reversible. For example, certain medications can cause symptoms of dementia. Depression can manifest in dementia-like behaviors. Also, certain medical conditions such as tumors or infections may result in dementia. These reversible forms of dementia are generally treated by other health care professionals, yet it is still important for the speech-language pathologist to be knowledgeable about nonreversible dementias and conditions related to reversible dementia.

The most common form of progressive, irreversible dementia is Alzheimer's disease. Other dementias include multi-infarct dementia (MID), Pick's disease, Parkinson's disease (PD), Huntington's disease (HD), Wilson's disease, supranuclear palsy, Creutzfeldt-Jakob disease, and Korsakoff's syndrome. Most dementias follow a general pattern of progression. We have divided this pattern into three stages, although there may be variability from one client to another and from one dementia type to another. The following stages are primarily related to dementia of the Alzheimer's type; however, several other forms of dementia have similar patterns of progression.

Stage 1: Early Dementia

- Slow, insidious onset
- Some memory loss
- Word-finding problems
- Poor attention span
- Disorientation
- Reasoning and judgment problems
- Difficulty with abstract concepts
- Empty speech at times
- Intact automatic speech

- Intact articulation and phonological skills
- Intact syntactic skills
- Mechanics of writing and reading intact, although meaning may be obscured
- Possible anxiety, depression, agitation, and apathy
- Attitude of indifference toward deficits

Stage 2: Intermediate Dementia

- Increasing memory loss (The client may forget the names of loved ones, although usually remembers his or her own name.)
- Increasing word-finding deficits
- Decreasing orientation
- Empty speech
- Poor topic maintenance
- Intact automatic speech
- Intact articulation and phonological skills
- Intact syntactic skills
- Mechanics of writing and reading still intact, although meaning is more obscured
- Wandering
- Unable to take care of own needs
- Inability to perform complex tasks
- Perseveratory behaviors such as chewing or lip smacking
- Withdrawal from challenging situations
- Personality and emotional changes such as delusional behaviors, obsessive behaviors, anxiety, agitation, and previously nonexistent violent behaviors

Stage 3: Advanced Dementia

- Severely impaired memory
- Profound intellectual deterioration
- Severely impaired verbal abilities, speech is meaningless or absent.
- Unable to participate in social interaction
- Physical debilitation
- Aimless wandering
- Restlessness and agitation
- Possible violent outbursts
- The client requires assistance for all activities of daily living.

During the speech-language evaluation, the case history questions are especially important for determining the etiology and prognosis of a client's dementia. As many of the client's primary caregivers and family members as possible need to be consulted to offer details related to the onset and progression of the client's condition. In addition to traditional case history questions, the clinician may also want to ask:

- What behaviors were first noticed and when?
- How have the behaviors changed over time?
- Was the onset sudden or gradual?
- What other events were occurring in the client's life at the time of onset?
- What is the client's psychiatric history?
- What problems is the client having taking care of his or her daily needs?
- How has the client attempted to compensate for his or her deficits?
- How do you and others currently communicate with the client?

One frequently used dementia assessment tool is the *Mini-Mental State Examination (MMSE)* (Folstein, Folstein, & McHugh, 1975/2001). It is often used as an initial test for a possible diagnosis of dementia. The examination is quick to administer, only taking about 10 minutes, and the outcome can provide direction for further assessment. The examination measures memory, orientation, and cognitive abilities. Other commercially available assessment tools include:

- *Alzheimer's Quick Test (AQT) Assessment of Temporal-Parietal Function* (Wiig, Nielsen, Minthon, & Warkentin, 2002)
- *Cognitive-Linguistic Quick Test* (Helm-Estabrooks, 2001)

Each can be used as a screening tool for identification of neurologic dysfunction.

If the outcome of a dementia screening test indicates a need for further evaluation, there are several commercially available assessment tools for dementia. Take care to select testing materials that are appropriate for the client's level of cognition and awareness because assessment tools vary widely in their focus, length, and application. Some evaluative tools to consider include:

- *Arizona Battery for Communication Disorders of Dementia (ABCD)* (Bayles & Tomoeda, 1993)
- *Communication Activities of Daily Living (CADL-2)* (Holland, Fratalli, & Fromm, 1999)
- *Dementia Rating Scale (DRS-2)* (Mattis, Jurica, & Leitten, 2001)
- *Functional Linguistic Communication Inventory* (Bayles & Tomoeda, 1995)
- *Ross Information Processing Assessment—Geriatric (RIPA-G)* (Ross-Swain & Fogle, 1996)
- *Severe Impairment Battery* (Saxton, McGonigle, Swihart, & Boller, 1993). This test is appropriate for a client who scores less than eight on the MMSE.

There are also assessment materials in this book that can be adapted for evaluating a client with a dementia disorder. For example, subsections of the "Cognitive–Linguistic Evaluation" (Form 13-2) are appropriate for assessing orientation, memory, auditory processing and comprehension, thought organization, and pragmatics. The "Evaluation of Aphasia," Form 13-1, is useful for assessing memory, semantic concepts, and language skills. The "Assessment of Pragmatic Skills," Form 7-8, can be adapted for the assessment of a variety of pragmatic skills. The "Reading Passages" (Chapter 5) can be adapted for the assessment of reading comprehension and memory of written material. The "Pictures" (Chapter 5) can be used to evaluate thought organization, confrontational naming, and language skills. Finally, the "Narratives" (Chapter 5) can be used to assess auditory comprehension and memory.

CONCLUDING COMMENTS

The basic principles and methods for the assessment of four neurologically based disorders have been addressed in the preceding sections. Each disorder presents a different pattern of symptoms and communicative behaviors. Even though each neurologically based disorder is a distinct clinical entity, many clients are affected by several disorders simultaneously. This requires the clinician to carefully evaluate a variety of communicative skills and abilities. The clinician must determine a hierarchy of clinical importance for each disorder diagnosed. It is important to view the "whole picture" and prioritize immediate and less-immediate needs for making appropriate diagnostic and treatment decisions.

SOURCES OF ADDITIONAL INFORMATION

Print Sources

Bayles, K. A., & Tomoeda, C. K. (2013). *MCI and Alzheimer's dementia: Clinical essentials for assessment and treatment of cognitive-communication disorders.* San Diego, CA: Plural.

Brookshire, R. H. (2007). *Introduction to neurogenic communication disorders* (7th ed.). St. Louis, MO: Mosby.

Hegde, M. N. (2006). *Coursebook on aphasia and other neurogenic language disorders* (3rd ed.). Clifton Park, NY: Cengage Learning.

Helm-Estabrooks, N., & Albert M. L. (2013). *Manual of aphasia and aphasia therapy* (3rd ed.). Austin, TX: Pro-ed.

Hux, K. (2010). *Assisting survivors of traumatic brain injury: The role of speech–language pathologists* (2nd ed.). Austin, TX: Pro-ed.

Manasco, M. H. (2014). *Introduction to neurogenic communication disorders.* Burlington, MA: Jones and Bartlett Learning.

Electronic Sources

American Speech-Language-Hearing Association:
http://www.asha.org

National Aphasia Association:
http://www.aphasia.org

Alzheimer's Association:
http://www.alz.org

Dementia.com:
http://www.dementia.com

Brain Injury Association of America:
http://www.biausa.org

Brain Trauma Foundation:
http://www.braintrauma.org

Form 13-1.

Evaluation of Aphasia

Name: _____ Age: _____ Date: _____

Primary Care Physician: _____

Medical Diagnosis: _____

Date of Incident: _____

Condition Prior to Incident: _____

Date of CT Scan/MRI: _____ Findings: _____

Relevant Medical History: _____

_____

_____

Medications: _____

Examiner's Name: _____

Instructions: Administer selected sections or all sections as appropriate for the client. Specific instructions are provided under each subheading.

Conversational Speech

Use pictures or converse with the client to stimulate speech, noting specific difficulties the client exhibits.

Agrammatism _____

Anomia _____

Circumlocution _____

Disfluency _____

Effortful speech _____

Jargon _____

Paraphasia _____

Perseveration _____

Telegraphic speech _____

Other _____

(continues)

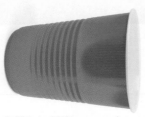

© NikolayN/Shutterstock.com

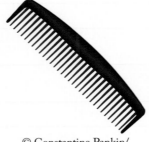

© didora/Shutterstock.com

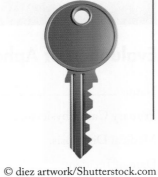

© diez artwork/Shutterstock.com

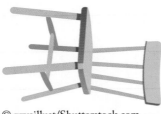

© zzveillust/Shutterstock.com

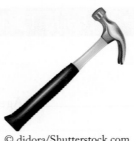

© Constantine Pankin/
Shutterstock.com

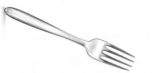

© Oleksii Natykach/Shutterstock.com

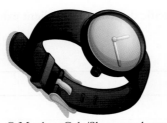

© Matthew Cole/Shutterstock.com

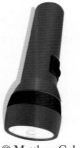

© Matthew Cole/
Shutterstock.com

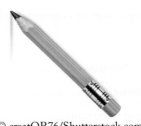

© creatOR76/Shutterstock.com

(continues)

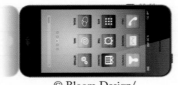

© Bloom Design/
Shutterstock.com

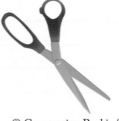

© Constantine Pankin/
Shutterstock.com

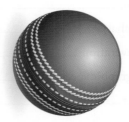

© Christos Georghiou/
Shutterstock.com

Form 13-1. continued

Recognition of Common Nouns

Name each picture on the left-hand page one at a time and have the client point to the picture requested. If the client is unable to point, observe eye gaze. Record responses in the first colum of the checklist on the right-hand side.

Naming Common Nouns

Use the same pictures and ask the client to name each item. Record responses on the checklist in the middle column of the right-hand side.

Recognition of Common Functions

Use the same pictures and ask the client to identify the correct item for the following questions. Record responses in the third column of the checklist on the right-hand side.

What do you eat with?

What do you use to see at night?

What do you use to write something?

What do you use to talk to someone who is not in the room with you?

What do you use to hit a nail?

What do you use to cut paper?

What do you use to unlock the door?

What do you sit on?

What do you use on your hair?

What do you drink out of?

What do you use to play a game with?

What do you use to tell time?

Checklist for Common Nouns and Functions

	Recognition of Word	Naming Word	Recognition of Functions
fork			
key			
ball			
flashlight			
chair			
hammer			
scissors			
watch			
pencil			
comb			
cup			
telephone			

(continues)

NEUROCOGNITIVE DISORDERS

Form 13-1. continued

Yes-No Questions

Ask the following questions to evaluate appropriateness of yes and no responses. Score a plus (+) or minus (−) for correct or incorrect responses.

_____ Are you sitting on a chair? _____

_____ Are we in Paris, France? _____

_____ Is a book an animal? _____

_____ Is a dog an animal? _____

_____ Are you wearing a swimsuit? _____

_____ Am I an adult? _____

_____ Do you butter toast with a comb? _____

_____ Do frogs swim? _____

_____ Do cars fly? _____

_____ Do trains carry people? _____

Following Commands

Ask the client to carry out each of the following commands. Make sure your client waits until you have finished the entire command before responding.

One-Part Command

_____ Touch your nose. _____

_____ Raise your hand. _____

_____ Look at the door. _____

Two-Part Command

_____ Touch your head, then your mouth. _____

_____ Clap your hands, then touch your knees. _____

_____ Nod your head twice, then close your eyes. _____

_____ Touch your chair, then clap twice. _____

(continues)

Form 13-1. continued

Three-Part Command

_____ Nod your head, clap your hands, then make a fist. _____

_____ Look at the door, look at me, then close your eyes. _____

_____ Touch your chin, then your nose, then raise your hand. _____

Repeating Phrases

Read each phrase and ask the client to repeat it. Syllabic complexity of each phrase increases as you read down the list (the number of syllables for each phrase is indicated in parentheses). Note the syllable length at which the client exhibits difficulty.

_____ (1) Cap _____

_____ (1) Boat _____

_____ (2) Laughing _____

_____ (2) Not now _____

_____ (3) Piano _____

_____ (3) Forty-two _____

_____ (4) Geography _____

_____ (4) It's time to go. _____

_____ (5) Magnifying glass _____

_____ (5) The car was dirty. _____

_____ (6) Personal computer _____

_____ (6) Put everything away. _____

_____ (7) Revolutionary War _____

_____ (7) She is not very happy. _____

_____ (8) Mechanical engineering _____

_____ (8) The letter arrived yesterday. _____

_____ (9) Recreational motorcycle _____

_____ (9) Put it in the microwave oven. _____

(continues)

NEUROCOGNITIVE DISORDERS

Form 13-1. continued

Logic Questions

Ask the following questions to evaluate logic and problem-solving skills. Suggested answers are provided, but other responses may also be appropriate.

_____ Why do you store ice in the freezer? (so it won't melt) _____

_____

_____ Why do you brush your teeth? (so you don't get cavities, to clean them, etc.) _____

_____

_____ Why don't people swim outdoors in the winter? (it's too cold) _____

_____

_____ Why don't people eat house plants? (they aren't edible, they are for decoration, etc.) _____

_____

_____ What would you do if your car ran out of gas? (call someone for help, walk to a gas station, etc.) ___

_____

_____ What would you do if you couldn't find a friend's phone number? (look it up in a phone book, ask someone else, call information, etc.) _____

_____

_____ How could you learn about current news if you didn't have a newspaper? (listen to the radio, watch television, etc.) _____

_____

_____ How could you get downtown if you didn't have a car? (take a bus, walk, etc.) _____

_____

Sequencing

Ask the client to describe the steps necessary to complete the following tasks. Make a note of difficulties with thought organization or sequencing.

_____ Make a sandwich _____

_____ Wash a car _____

(continues)

Form 13-1. continued

———— Prepare a frozen dinner ———————————————————————

———— Change a light bulb ———————————————————————————

———— Write and send a letter ———————————————————————

Definition of Terms

Ask the client to define each of the terms below. Note behaviors such as paraphasias and circumlocutions.

———— Car ———

———— Tree ——

———— Window ——

———— Bathe ——

———— Shopping ————————————————————————————————————

———— Cloudy ——

———— Solo ——

———— Tricky ——

———— Northern ——————————————————————————————————————

———— Controversial —————————————————————————————————

———— Fleeting ——————————————————————————————————————

———— Content ——

———— Opinion —————————————————————————————————————

(continues)

NEUROCOGNITIVE DISORDERS

Form 13-1. continued

6	3	8
11	29	49
173	207	151
297	2,046	7,921
one	six	four
nine	seven	three
thirteen	twenty-two	seventeen
thirty-three	forty-one	ninety-one

one hundred and twenty-seven

two hundred and twelve

two thousand and forty-four

(continues)

Form 13-1. continued

Number Recognition

Ask the client to identify each number on the left-hand page. Circle correct responses and mark a slash (/) through incorrect responses.

8	3	6
49	29	11
151	207	173
7,921	2,046	297

Numeric Word Recognition

Ask the client to read each number on the left-hand page. Circle correct responses and mark a slash (/) through incorrect responses.

four	six	one
three	seven	nine
seventeen	twenty-two	thirteen
ninety-one	forty-one	thirty-three

one hundred and twenty-seven

two hundred and twelve

two thousand and forty-four

(continues)

NEUROCOGNITIVE DISORDERS

baby

radio

ordinary

sometimes

Put it away.

Open the door.

They don't want any.

peanut butter and honey

What happened to the flowers?

Send it to your friend before Thursday.

(continues)

Form 13-1. continued

Reading Words and Sentences Orally

Ask the client to read each word or sentence on the left-hand side of the page. Make a note of specific difficulties.

baby _____

radio _____

ordinary _____

sometimes _____

Put it away. _____

Open the door. _____

They don't want any. _____

peanut butter and honey _____

What happened to the flowers? _____

Send it to your friend before Thursday. _____

Writing Words and Sentences

Give the client a blank sheet of unlined paper and a pencil or pen. Ask him or her to write the following words and sentences. Observe ease of writing and make a note of paraphasic or spelling errors, incomplete sentences, and overall legibility.

car _____

tree _____

summer _____

I saw her. _____

We ate dinner. _____

They went outside. _____

The television set was broken. _____

He is saving his money *for* a rainy day. _____

It's too bad they can't come tomorrow. _____

I would rather have chicken than spaghetti. _____

(continues)

NEUROCOGNITIVE DISORDERS

Form 13-1. continued

```
  1        7        5        3        8       11
 +7       +2       +3       -2       -5       -2
____     ____     ____     ____     ____     ____


  9       13       12       17       16       56
 +3       +4       +7       -7      -12       -9
____     ____     ____     ____     ____     ____


 77       17      107       72       82      171
+58       +4      +92      -13      -14      -83
____     ____     ____     ____     ____     ____
```

(continues)

Form 13-1. continued

Mathematic Calculations (Addition and Subtraction)

Ask the client to calculate the problems on the left-hand page. Circle correct responses and make a slash (/) through incorrect responses.

Subtraction

$$\begin{array}{r} 8 \\ -5 \\ \hline 3 \end{array} \qquad \begin{array}{r} 3 \\ -2 \\ \hline 1 \end{array}$$

$$\begin{array}{r} 16 \\ -12 \\ \hline 4 \end{array} \qquad \begin{array}{r} 17 \\ -7 \\ \hline 10 \end{array}$$

$$\begin{array}{r} 82 \\ -14 \\ \hline 68 \end{array} \qquad \begin{array}{r} 72 \\ -13 \\ \hline 59 \end{array}$$

$$\begin{array}{r} 11 \\ -2 \\ \hline 9 \end{array}$$

$$\begin{array}{r} 56 \\ -9 \\ \hline 47 \end{array}$$

$$\begin{array}{r} 171 \\ -83 \\ \hline 88 \end{array}$$

Addition

$$\begin{array}{r} 1 \\ +7 \\ \hline 8 \end{array} \qquad \begin{array}{r} 7 \\ +2 \\ \hline 9 \end{array} \qquad \begin{array}{r} 5 \\ +3 \\ \hline 8 \end{array}$$

$$\begin{array}{r} 9 \\ +3 \\ \hline 12 \end{array} \qquad \begin{array}{r} 13 \\ +4 \\ \hline 17 \end{array} \qquad \begin{array}{r} 12 \\ +7 \\ \hline 19 \end{array}$$

$$\begin{array}{r} 77 \\ +58 \\ \hline 135 \end{array} \qquad \begin{array}{r} 17 \\ +4 \\ \hline 21 \end{array} \qquad \begin{array}{r} 107 \\ +92 \\ \hline 199 \end{array}$$

(continues)

NEUROCOGNITIVE DISORDERS

Form 13-1, continued

$$
\begin{array}{r}
3 \\
\times 2 \\
\hline
\end{array}
\qquad
\begin{array}{r}
7 \\
\times 1 \\
\hline
\end{array}
\qquad
\begin{array}{r}
3 \\
\times 3 \\
\hline
\end{array}
\qquad
3\overline{)9}
\qquad
2\overline{)4}
\qquad
7\overline{)42}
$$

$$
\begin{array}{r}
4 \\
\times 3 \\
\hline
\end{array}
\qquad
\begin{array}{r}
5 \\
\times 5 \\
\hline
\end{array}
\qquad
\begin{array}{r}
9 \\
\times 3 \\
\hline
\end{array}
\qquad
9\overline{)27}
\qquad
7\overline{)56}
\qquad
9\overline{)81}
$$

$$
\begin{array}{r}
13 \\
\times 14 \\
\hline
\end{array}
\qquad
\begin{array}{r}
23 \\
\times 17 \\
\hline
\end{array}
\qquad
\begin{array}{r}
19 \\
+26 \\
\hline
\end{array}
\qquad
12\overline{)36}
\qquad
6\overline{)126}
\qquad
9\overline{)144}
$$

(continues)

Form 13-1. continued

Mathematic Calculations (Multiplication and Division)

Ask the client to calculate the problems on the left-hand page. Circle correct responses and make a slash (/) through incorrect responses.

Division

$$7\overline{)42} \quad \overset{6}{}$$

$$2\overline{)4} \quad \overset{2}{}$$

$$3\overline{)9} \quad \overset{3}{}$$

$$9\overline{)81} \quad \overset{9}{}$$

$$7\overline{)56} \quad \overset{8}{}$$

$$9\overline{)27} \quad \overset{3}{}$$

$$9\overline{)144} \quad \overset{16}{}$$

$$6\overline{)126} \quad \overset{21}{}$$

$$12\overline{)36} \quad \overset{3}{}$$

Multiplication

$$\begin{array}{r} 3 \\ \times 2 \\ \hline 6 \end{array} \qquad \begin{array}{r} 7 \\ \times 1 \\ \hline 7 \end{array} \qquad \begin{array}{r} 3 \\ \times 3 \\ \hline 9 \end{array}$$

$$\begin{array}{r} 4 \\ \times 3 \\ \hline 12 \end{array} \qquad \begin{array}{r} 5 \\ \times 5 \\ \hline 25 \end{array} \qquad \begin{array}{r} 9 \\ \times 3 \\ \hline 27 \end{array}$$

$$\begin{array}{r} 13 \\ \times 14 \\ \hline 52 \\ +130 \\ \hline 182 \end{array} \qquad \begin{array}{r} 23 \\ \times 17 \\ \hline 161 \\ +230 \\ \hline 391 \end{array} \qquad \begin{array}{r} 19 \\ \times 26 \\ \hline 114 \\ +380 \\ \hline 494 \end{array}$$

NEUROCOGNITIVE DISORDERS

Form13-2.

Cognitive–Linguistic Evaluation

Name: _____ Age: _____ Date: _____

Primary Care Physician: _____

Medical Diagnosis: _____

Date of Incident: _____

Condition Prior to Incident: _____

Date of CT Scan/MRI: _____ Findings: _____

Relevant Medical History: _____

_____

_____

Medications: _____

Examiner's Name: _____

Instructions: Administer selected sections or all sections as appropriate for the client. Specific instructions are provided under each subheading. Make additional observations in the right-hand column. The client will need a pen or pencil to complete the writing portion of the evaluation.

Orientation and Awareness

Ask the client the following questions. Score a plus (+) or minus (−) for correct or incorrect responses.

_____ What day is it? _____

_____ What month is it? _____

_____ What year is it? _____

_____ What season is it? _____

_____ Approximately what time do you think it is? _____

_____ What state are we in? _____

_____ What city are we in? _____

_____ What county are we in? _____

_____ Where do you live? _____

_____ What is the name of this building? _____

_____ Why are you in the hospital? _____

_____ How long have you been here? _____

(continues)

Form 13-2. continued

Orientation and Awareness (continued)

_____ When did you have your accident? _____

_____ What kind of problems do you have because of your accident? _____

_____ What is my name? _____

_____ What is my profession? _____

_____ Who is your doctor? _____

_____ About how much time has passed since we started talking together today? _____

Memory

Immediate Memory. Ask the client to repeat the following sequences or sentences. Score a plus (+) or minus (−) for correct or incorrect responses.

_____ 0, 7, 4, 2 _____

_____ 8, 6, 0, 1, 3 _____

_____ 2, 9, 1, 4, 6, 5 _____

_____ Car, duck, ring, shoe _____

_____ Rain, desk, ladder, horse, cake _____

_____ The keys were found under the table. _____

_____ He always reads the newspaper before he has breakfast. _____

_____ After their victory, the baseball team had pizza and watched a movie. _____

Ask the client to retell this story:

_____ Helen had a birthday party at the petting zoo. Ten of her friends came.

_____ All the children laughed when a goat was found eating the cake and ice cream.

Recent Memory. Ask the client the following questions. Score a plus (+) or minus (−) for correct or incorrect responses.

_____ What did you have for breakfast? _____

_____ What did you do after dinner last night? _____

_____ What did you do after breakfast this morning? _____

_____ What else have you done today? _____

(continues)

Form 13-2. continued

Recent Memory (continued)

_____   Have you had any visitors today or yesterday? _____

_____   What other therapies do you receive? _____

_____   Who is your doctor? _____

_____   How long have you been a resident here? _____

Long-Term Memory. Ask the client the following questions. Score a plus (+) or minus (−) for correct or incorrect responses.

_____   Where were you born? _____

_____   When is your birthday? _____

_____   What is your husband's/wife's name? _____

_____   How many children do you have? _____

_____   How many grandchildren do you have? _____

_____   Where did you used to work? _____

_____   How much school did you complete? _____

_____   Where did you grow up? _____

_____   How many brothers and sisters do you have? _____

Auditory Processing and Comprehension

Ask the client the following questions. Score a plus (+) or minus (−) for correct or incorrect responses.

_____   Is your last name Williams? _____

_____   Is my name Jim? _____

_____   Are you wearing glasses? _____

_____   Do you live on the moon? _____

_____   Have you had dinner yet? _____

_____   Do cows eat grass? _____

_____   Do fish swim? _____

_____   Do four quarters equal one dollar? _____

_____   Are there 48 hours in a day? _____

_____   Is Alaska part of the United States? _____

(continues)

NEUROCOGNITIVE
DISORDERS

Form 13-2. continued

Problem Solving

Ask the client the following questions. Score a plus (+) or minus (−) for correct or incorrect responses.

_____ What would you do if you locked your keys in your house? _____

_____ What would you do if your mail did not get delivered? _____

_____ What would you do if you could not find your doctor's phone number? _____

_____ What would you do if your TV stopped working? _____

_____ What would you do if you forgot to put the milk away when you got home from the grocery store?

Logic, Reasoning, Inference

Ask the client what is wrong with these sentences. Score a plus (+) or minus (−) for correct or incorrect responses.

_____ He put salt and pepper in his coffee. _____

_____ Six plus one is eight. _____

_____ I put my socks on over my shoes. _____

_____ Hang up when the phone rings. _____

_____ The dog had four kittens. _____

Ask the client what these expressions mean. Score a plus (+) or minus (−) for correct or incorrect responses.

_____ Haste makes waste. _____

_____ An apple a day keeps the doctor away. _____

_____ When it rains it pours. _____

_____ He's a chip off the old block. _____

_____ Beauty is only skin deep. _____

Ask the client the following questions. Score a plus (+) or minus (−) for correct or incorrect responses.

_____ What is worn on your feet, knit, and used to keep you warm? _____

_____ What has a bushy tail, climbs trees, and stores nuts? _____

_____ What is thin and lightweight, used to wipe tears, and used during a cold? _____

(continues)

Form 13-2. continued

Logic, Reasoning, Inference (continued)

_____ How are a sweater, pants, and a blouse alike? _____

_____ How are orange juice, soda, and milk alike? _____

Thought Organization

Ask the client to answer the following questions or tasks. Score a plus (+) or minus (−) for correct or incorrect responses.

_____ What does the word "affectionate" mean? _____

_____ What does the word "deliver" mean? _____

_____ What are the steps you follow to wash your hair? _____

_____ What are the steps you follow to make your bed? _____

_____ How would you plan a meal for two dinner guests? _____

Calculation

Ask the client to answer the following questions. Score a plus (+) or minus (−) for correct or incorrect responses.

_____ If you went to the mall and spent $8.00 in one store and $7.50 in another store, how much did you spend? _____

_____ If tomatoes cost $1.50 per pound and you bought 2 pounds, how much did you spend on tomatoes? _____

_____ If you went to the store with $3.00 and returned home with $1.75, how much did you spend? _____

_____ If toothbrushes cost $3.00 each and you have $10.00, how many toothbrushes can you buy? _____

_____ If you have a doctor's appointment at 10:30 and it takes you 30 minutes to get there, what time should you leave? _____

(continues)

Form 13-2. continued

Reading and Visual Processing

Ask the client to read the six words in each row and cross out the one that does not belong. Score a plus (+) or minus (−) for correct or incorrect responses.

____ Cow   Apple   Carrot   Cheese   Banana   Oatmeal

____ Desk   Chair   Blue   Bed   Couch   Table

Ask the client to read the following sentences and do what they say. Score a plus (+) or minus (−) for correct or incorrect responses.

____ Look at the ceiling. _____

____ Point to the door, then blink your eyes. _____

____ Sing Happy Birthday. _____

Ask the client to read the following paragraph out loud and answer the questions about it. Score a plus (+) or minus (−) for correct or incorrect responses.

Mark and Rick are brothers. They both entered a tennis tournament, hoping to win the $1,000 grand prize. Mark won his first two matches, but was eliminated after losing the third match. Rick made it all the way to the semi-finals. He lost, but was awarded a can of tennis balls as a consolation prize.

____ Are Mark and Rick cousins? _____

____ What sport did they play? _____

____ What was the grand prize? _____

____ Did one of them win the grand prize? _____

____ Which one did the best in the tournament? _____

(continues)

Form 13-2. continued

Show the client these two clocks and ask what time the clocks say. Score a plus (+) or minus (−) for correct or incorrect responses.

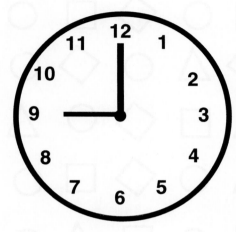
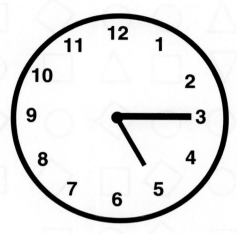

Now ask the client to copy the clocks below. Note accuracy of construction.

(continues)

NEUROCOGNITIVE DISORDERS

Form 13-2. continued

Ask the client to put an x through all the circles on this page. Note the client's attention to the left half of the page.

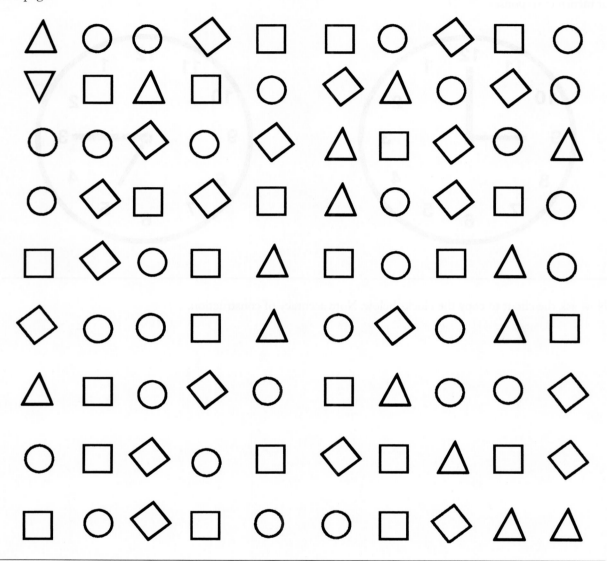

(continues)

Form 13-2. continued

Write your name.

Write today's date.

Write a short description of what you have done today in speech therapy.

(continues)

Form 13-2. continued

Writing

Ask the client to complete the writing tasks presented on the previous page. Observe accuracy of response, completeness and organization of response, legibility, and observance of left visual field. Make comments in the right margin.

Write your name. _____

Write today's date. _____

Write a short description of what you have done today in speech therapy. _____

_____

Pragmatics and Affect

Check all behaviors observed during your assessment.

_____ Inappropriate physical proximity _____

_____ Inappropriate physical contacts _____

_____ Left visual field neglect _____

_____ Poor eye contact _____

_____ Lack of facial expression _____

_____ Gestures (inappropriate, absent) _____

_____ Lack of prosodic features of speech (intensity, pitch, rhythm) _____

_____ Poor topic maintenance _____

_____ Lack of appropriate turn taking _____

_____ Perseveration _____

_____ Presupposition (too much, too little) _____

_____ Inappropriately verbose _____

_____ Lack of initiation _____

_____ Easily distracted _____

_____ Frequent interruptions _____

_____ Impulsive _____

_____ Poor organization _____

_____ Incompleteness _____

Form13-3.

Assessment of Clients with Traumatic Brain Injury

Name: _____ Age: _____ Date: _____

Primary Care Physician: _____

Medical Diagnosis: _____

Date of Incident: _____

Condition Prior to Incident: _____

Date of CT Scan/MRI: _____ Findings: _____

Relevant Medical History: _____

_____

_____

Medications: _____

Examiner's Name: _____

Informant's Name: _____

Instructions: Observe the client over an extended period of time and then answer each question.

Is the client aware of personal orientation (e.g., time, place)?

Does the client attend to stimuli?

How long can the client attend to a task (in seconds or minutes)?

(continues)

Form 13-3. continued

What distracts the client the most (e.g., someone entering the room, noise from a TV or radio, too much visual stimulation, etc.)?

Is the client able to shift attention from one activity to another?

Is the client able to attend to more than one activity at a time (e.g., converse while preparing a meal)?

Does the client attend to certain activities better than others?

    What are the most difficult activities?

    What are the easiest activities?

Is the client able to follow immediate directions?

Is the client able to follow complex directions?

(continues)

Form 13-3. continued

Is the client able to remember things that happened earlier that day?

Is the client able to remember things that happened earlier that month or year?

Is the client able to recall events that happened many years ago?

Is the client able to remember future activities (e.g., take the garbage out this afternoon, or take the roast out of the oven in 1 hour)?

Is the client able to shift from one activity to another without difficulty?

Is the client able to follow a conversation that shifts from one topic to another?

Is the client able to change the topic appropriately during a conversation?

(continues)

NEUROCOGNITIVE DISORDERS

Form 13-3. continued

What strategies does the client use to complete tasks?

Is the client aware of the strategies used?

How does the client respond to the question, "How did you do that?"

How does the client respond to problem-solving situations?

What are some things the client is able to problem-solve?

What are some things the client is unable to problem-solve?

How does the client respond to stressful situations?

What kinds of everyday tasks does the client have difficulties with?

What are some things that the client needs to do on a daily basis?

Is the client having difficulty with any of these things? If yes, identify.

(continues)

Form 13-3. continued

Is the client able to convey thoughts in writing?

Is the client able to use good judgment during everyday tasks?

Does the client seem to have good safety awareness?

What is the client's behavior like at home (passive, aggressive, compulsive, etc.)?

Please add additional comments about the client's behaviors and abilities.

ASSESSMENT OF MOTOR SPEECH DISORDERS

Motor speech disorders result from neurological damage that affects the muscles used for speech or the motor programming for speech. The most common motor speech disorders are dysarthria and apraxia. This chapter highlights the differences between these two communicative disorders and summarizes procedures for assessment.

OVERVIEW OF ASSESSMENT

History of Client

    Procedures

        Written Case History

        Information-Getting Interview

        Information from Other Professionals

    Contributing Factors

        Medical Diagnosis

        Pharmacological Factors

        Age

        Intelligence, Motivation, Levels of Concern

Assessment of Dysarthia and Apraxia

    Procedures

        Screening

        Speech Sampling

        Motor Speech Assessment

        Formal Testing

        Stimulability

    Analysis

        Types of Errors

        Consistency of Errors

        Intelligibility

        Rate of Speech

        Prosody

        Respiratory Support

Orofacial Examination

Hearing Assessment

Determining the Diagnosis

Providing Information (written report, interview, etc.)

THE CRANIAL NERVES AND THE BRAIN

The 12 cranial nerves perform the critical task of sending sensory and motor information to all the muscles of the body. It is helpful to have an understanding of these nerves and their functions when assessing neurological impairments. This information is summarized in Table 14-1. The cranial nerves that are directly related to speech, language, swallowing, or hearing are indicated with an asterisk in the table.

It is may also be helpful to have a visual image of the brain for personal review or when providing information to clients and their caregivers. Such an image is provided in Figure 14-1.

TABLE 14-1   The Cranial Nerves–Types and Functions

NERVE	TYPE	FUNCTION	
I	Olfactory	Sensory	Smell
II	Optic	Sensory	Vision
III	Oculomotor	Motor	Movement of eyeball, pupil, upper eyelid
IV	Trochlear	Motor	Movement of superior oblique eye muscle
V*	Trigeminal	Mixed	Tactile facial sensation, movement of muscles for chewing
VI	Abducens	Motor	Open the eyes
VII*	Facial	Mixed	Taste, movement of facial muscles
VIII*	Acoustic	Sensory	Hearing and equilibrium
IX*	Glossopharyngeal	Mixed	Taste, gag, elevation of palate and larynx for swallow
X*	Vagus	Mixed	Taste, elevation of palate, movement of pharynx and larynx
XI*	Accessory	Motor	Turn head, shrug shoulders, movement of palate, pharynx, and larynx
XII*	Hypoglossal	Motor	Movement of tongue

*Indicates nerves that are most directly related to speech, language, swallowing, or hearing.

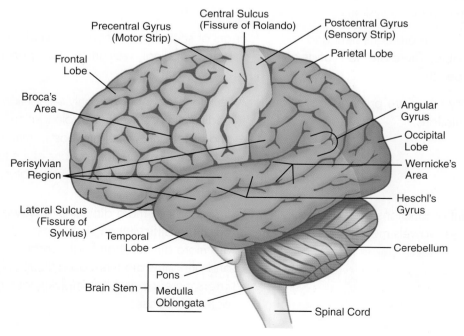

FIGURE 14-1.   The Brain

The areas that may have the greatest negative impact on speech and language when damaged are Broca's area and Wernicke's area, although damage to any cerebral area has the potential to impact functional communication.

DIFFERENTIAL CHARACTERISTICS OF DYSARTHRIA AND APRAXIA

Dysarthria and apraxia are both motor speech disorders that affect verbal expression. These disorders are sometimes confused with each other, especially by beginning clinicians. However, their symptoms are actually quite different. It is important to understand the differences between the two disorders to make an appropriate diagnosis. The general differences between dysarthria and apraxia are outlined in Table 14-2.

TABLE 14-2 Differential Characteristics of Dysarthria and Apraxia

DYSARTHRIA	APRAXIA
All processes of speech are affected (including respiration, phonation, resonance, articulation, and prosody).	The speech process for articulation is primarily affected. Prosody may also be abnormal.
There is a change in muscle tone secondary to neurologic involvement that results in difficulty with voluntary and involuntary motor tasks (such as swallowing, chewing, and licking).	There is a change in motor programming for speech secondary to neurologic involvement, but muscle tone is not affected. Involuntary motor tasks typically are not affected.
Speech errors result from a disruption in muscular control of the central and peripheral nervous systems.	Speech errors result from a disruption of the message from the motor cortex to the oral musculature.
Errors of speech are consistent and predictable. There are no islands of clear speech.	Errors of speech are inconsistent and unpredictable. Islands of clear, well-articulated speech exist.
Articulatory errors are primarily distortions and omissions.	Articulatory errors are primarily substitutions, repetitions, additions, transpositions, prolongations, omissions, and distortions (which are least common). Most errors are close approximations of the targeted phoneme. Errors are often perseveratory or anticipatory.
Consonant productions are consistently imprecise; vowels may be neutralized.	Consonants are more difficult than vowels; blends are more difficult than singletons; initial consonants are more difficult than final consonants; fricatives and affricates are the most difficult consonants. Errors increase as the complexity of the motor pattern increases.

DYSARTHRIA	APRAXIA
The speech rate may be slow and labored; strain, tension, and poor breath support may be apparent.	A prosodic disorder may occur as a result of compensatory behaviors (stopping, restarting, and difficulty initiating phonation and correct articulatory postures).
Speech intelligibility is often reduced as the speaking rate increases.	Speech intelligibility sometimes increases as the speaking rate increases.
Increases in word/phrase complexity result in poorer articulatory performance.	Increases in word/phrase complexity result in poorer articulatory performance.

ASSESSMENT OF DYSARTHRIA

Dysarthria is a motor speech disorder that results from muscular impairment. Muscular weakness, slowness, or incoordination can affect all the basic processes of speech—respiration, phonation, resonance, articulation, and prosody. Articulation errors are the most common feature of dysarthria, followed by impairments of voice, resonance, and fluency. Dysarthria is sometimes confused with apraxia of speech, also a motor speech disorder associated with expressive speech impairment, but the two disorders are quite different. A primary differentiating characteristic is that dysarthria is associated with muscular impairment; apraxia of speech is not.

There are six types of dysarthria, each characterized by a different etiology and different speech behaviors. During a diagnostic evaluation, it is easy to confuse the dysarthrias, because many of their characteristics overlap and more than one type may be present. Drs. Arnold Aronson and Frederick Darley of the Mayo Clinic pioneered research into the differential characteristics of the dysarthrias. Their work has led to a standard classification system for identifying the different dysarthrias in clinical practice. A summary of their work and a listing of potential etiologies for each dysarthria are presented in Table 14-3.

To complete an assessment of dysarthria, complete an orofacial examination and obtain a good speech sample at structured levels (according to syllabic length) and in continuous speech. These samples will be the basis for identifying the primary speech characteristics the client exhibits. Suggestions for obtaining a speech sample are found in other sections of this book. The "Reading Passages" and "Syllable-by-Syllable Stimulus Phrases" in Chapter 5 may be helpful for obtaining a sample. Three frequently used tests for evaluating dysarthric speech are:

- *Assessment of Intelligibility of Dysarthric Speech* (Yorkston, Beukelman, & Traynor, 1984)
- *Frenchay Dysarthria Assessment (2nd. ed.) (EDA-2)* (Enderby & Palmer, 2008)
- *Quick Assessment for Dysarthria* (Tanner & Culbertson, 1999)

Form 14-1, "Identifying Dysarthria," is another useful tool for analyzing a client's speech and identifying the type of dysarthria present.

MOTOR SPEECH DISORDERS

TABLE 14-3 Differentiating the Six Dysarthrias

TYPE	SITE OF LESION	POSSIBLE CAUSES	PRIMARY SPEECH CHARACTERISTICS
Flaccid	Lower motor neuron	Viral infection	Hypernasality
		Tumor	Imprecise consonants
		Cerebrovascular accident (CVA)	Breathiness
			Monopitch
		Congenital conditions	Nasal emission
		Disease	
		Palsies	
		Trauma	
Spastic	Upper motor neuron	CVA	Imprecise consonants
		Tumor	Monopitch
		Infection	Reduced stress
		Trauma	Harsh voice quality
		Congenital condition	Monoloudness
			Low pitch
			Slow rate
			Hypernasality
			Strained-strangled voice
			Short phrases
Mixed (flaccid and spastic)	Upper and lower motor neuron	Amyotrophic lateral sclerosis	Imprecise consonants
			Hypernasality
		Trauma	Harsh voice quality
		CVA	Slow rate
			Monopitch
			Short phrases
			Distorted vowels
			Low pitch
			Monoloudness
			Excess and equal stress
			Prolonged intervals
Ataxic	Cerebellar system	CVA	Imprecise consonants
		Tumor	Excess and equal stress
		Trauma	Irregular articulatory breakdowns
		Congenital condition	
		Infection	Distorted vowels
		Toxic effects	Harsh voice
			Loudness control problems
			Variable nasality

TYPE	SITE OF LESION	POSSIBLE CAUSES	PRIMARY SPEECH CHARACTERISTICS
Hypokinetic	Extrapyramidal system	Parkinsonism Drug-induced	Monopitch Reduced stress Monoloudness Imprecise consonants Inappropriate silences Short rushes of speech Harsh voice Breathy voice
Hyperkinetic	Extrapyramidal system	Chorea Infection Gilles de la Tourette's syndrome Ballism Athetosis CVA Tumor Dystonia Drug-induced Dyskinesia	Imprecise consonants Distorted vowels Harsh voice quality Irregular articulatory breakdowns Strained-strangled voice Monopitch Monoloudness

Source: "Neuropathologies of Speech and Language: An Introduction to Patient Management," (2nd ed., pp. 76–77) by R.T. Wertz, in *Clinical Management of Neurogenic Communication Disorders*, D.F. Johns (Ed.), 1985, Boston: Little Brown and Co.

ASSESSMENT OF APRAXIA

Apraxia is a motor disorder resulting from neurological damage. It is characterized by an inability to execute volitional (purposeful) movements despite having normal muscle tone and coordination. In other words, the muscles are capable of normal functioning, but faulty programming from the brain prevents the completion of precise, purposeful movements.

There are three types of apraxia: limb, oral, and verbal. Limb apraxia is associated with volitional movements of the arms and legs. The client may be unable to wave good-bye or make a fist on command, even though the muscular strength and range of motion necessary to complete the tasks are present and the client is able to automatically perform the tasks. The client with oral apraxia may be unable to protrude the tongue or smack the lips volitionally. Oral apraxia is sometimes confused with the third type, verbal apraxia, as they both involve orofacial muscles, but they are not the same. Verbal apraxia is a disorder of motor programming for the production of speech. The client with verbal apraxia has difficulty positioning and sequencing muscles involved in the volitional production of phonemes. Clients may exhibit one, two, or all three types of apraxia. Verbal apraxia is the most common type and limb apraxia is the least common type. Form 14-2, "Checklists for Limb, Oral, and Verbal Apraxia," is provided to help identify the type(s) of apraxia a client exhibits.

This section on the assessment of apraxia focuses on the assessment of *apraxia of speech (AOS)* in adults or as a result of neurological insult. Childhood apraxia of speech, which presents itself as a developmental concern, is presented in Chapter 6. AOS may also be referred to as *acquired apraxia*, *verbal apraxia*, or *dyspraxia*. AOS is characterized by difficulty sequencing sounds in connected speech. It can be caused by a stroke, traumatic brain injury, dementia, a brain tumor, or a progressive neurological disorder. Shipley, Recor, and Nakamura (1990) list 25 characteristics of AOS, including specific diagnostic features. Summarized excerpts from their work are as follows:[1]

- The number of misarticulations increases as the complexity of the speech task increases.
- Misarticulations occur on both consonants and vowels. Articulation errors occur more frequently on consonant clusters than on singletons. Vowels are misarticulated less frequently than consonants.
- Sounds in the initial position are affected more often than sounds in the medial or final positions.
- The frequency of specific sound errors is related, at least in part, to the frequency of occurrence in speech. More errors are noted with less frequently occurring sounds.
- Sound substitutions, omissions, distortions, and additions are all observed. The most frequent misarticulations are substitutions and omissions.
- Articulation errors and struggle behaviors increase as the length and complexity of the target word, phrase, or sentence increases.
- Speech production is variable. It is common for a person with AOS to produce a sound, syllable, word, or phrase correctly on one occasion and then incorrectly on another. It is also common to observe several different misarticulations for the same target sound.
- Struggling behaviors (such as groping to position the articulators correctly) are observed in many patients with AOS.
- Automatic speech activities (such as counting to 10 or naming the days of the week) tend to be easier and more error-free than volitional speech. Reactive speech (such as "thank you" or "I'm fine") is also easier for clients with apraxia to produce.
- Metathetic errors (errors of sound or syllable transposition) are common. For example, the client may say *snapknack* for *knapsack* or *guspetti* for *spaghetti*.
- "Syllable collapses" may occur. Syllable collapses are not commonly reported in the literature, but can be common. The client reduces or disrupts the number of syllables in motorically complex words or phrases. For example, a client might say *glost gers* for

---

1. Adapted from *Sourcebook of Apraxia Remediation Activities* (pp. 2–5), by K. G. Shipley, D. B. Recor, and S. M. Nakamura, 1990, Oceanside, CA: Academic Communication Associates. Copyright 1990 by Academic Communication Associates. Adapted with permission.

Los Angeles Dodgers or *be neers* for *Tampa Bay Buccaneers.* In both examples, the number of syllables is collapsed and the remaining syllables are inaccurately produced.

- Receptive language abilities are often, but not always, superior to expressive abilities. However, the language skills are separate from the apraxia.

- People with apraxia of speech are usually aware of their incorrect articulatory productions. Therefore, they may be able to identify many of their own correct and incorrect productions without feedback from the clinician.

- AOS can occur in isolation or in combination with other communicative disorders such as dysarthria, delayed speech or language development, aphasia, and hearing loss.

- Oral apraxia and limb apraxia may or may not be present with verbal apraxia. Often, an individual with oral apraxia will also have verbal apraxia.

- Severity varies from client to client. Some clients cannot volitionally produce a target vowel such as /a/. Others have speech that is fine until they attempt to produce motorically challenging phrases such as *statistical analysis* or *theoretical implications.*

The "Identifying Apraxia" worksheet (Form 14-3) may help confirm or rule out AOS. Use this worksheet in conjunction with the "Checklists for Limb, Oral, and Verbal Apraxia" for a more thorough evaluation. Evaluate the client's speech during automatic speech, spontaneous speech, and oral reading. To obtain a sample of automatic speech, ask the client to count to 50, name the days of the week, name the months of the year, or perform a similar task. To obtain the spontaneous speech sample, ask the client to describe pictures, describe the plot of a movie, or talk about hobbies or other interests. To obtain the oral reading sample, have the client read a section from a book, a popular magazine, or one or more of the reading passages from Chapter 5 of this manual.

Be sure to compare the errors found in different speech contexts. Clients with apraxia of speech usually exhibit multiple errors in spontaneous speech and oral reading, whereas fewer or no errors are exhibited during automatic speech. If the client exhibits an excessive number of errors during automatic speech, dysarthria may be present.

Published tests for the diagnosis of apraxia of speech include:

- *Apraxia Battery for Adults (ABA-2)* (Dabul, 2000)
- *Quick Assessment for Apraxia of Speech* (Tanner & Culbertson, 1999)

CONCLUDING COMMENTS

Dysarthria and apraxia are motor speech disorders caused by neurological damage. Dysarthria is characterized by muscular weakness, and apraxia is characterized by poor programming of the speech muscles. These motor speech disorders often coexist with other neurocognitive disorders, voice or resonance disorders, and/or dysphagia.

SOURCES OF ADDITIONAL INFORMATION

Print Sources

Duffy, J. R. (2013). *Motor speech disorders: Substrates, differential diagnosis, and management* (3rd ed.). St. Louis, MO: Mosby.

Freed, D. B. (2012). *Motor speech disorders: Diagnosis and treatment* (2nd ed.). Clifton Park, NY: Cengage Learning.

Yorkston, K. M., Beukelman, D. R., & Stand, E. A. (2010). *Management of motor speech disorders in children and adults* (3rd ed.). Austin, TX: Pro-ed.

Electronic Sources

American Speech-Language-Hearing Association:
http://www.asha.org

Form 14-1.

Identifying Dysarthria

Name: _____ Age: _____ Date: _____

Examiner's Name: _____

Instructions: Identify the speech characteristics noted during the speech sample.

Flaccid Dysarthria (lower motor neuron involvement)

_____ Hypernasality

_____ Imprecise consonants

_____ Breathiness

_____ Monopitch

_____ Nasal emission

Spastic Dysarthria (upper motor neuron involvement)

_____ Imprecise consonants

_____ Monopitch

_____ Reduced stress

_____ Harsh voice quality

_____ Monoloudness

_____ Low pitch

_____ Slow rate

_____ Hypernasality

_____ Strained-strangled voice quality

_____ Short phrases

Mixed Dysarthria (upper and lower motor neuron involvement)

_____ Imprecise consonants

_____ Hypernasality

_____ Harsh voice quality

_____ Slow rate

_____ Monopitch

_____ Short phrases

(continues)

Adapted from "The Dysarthrias: Diagnosis, Description, and Treatment," by J. C. Rosenbeck and L. L. LaPointe in *Clinical Management of Neurogenic Communication Disorders,* 2nd ed. (p. 100), by D. F. Johns (ed.), 1985, Boston: Little, Brown and Co.

MOTOR SPEECH DISORDERS

Form 14-1. continued

Mixed Dysarthria (continued)

_____ Distorted vowels

_____ Low pitch

_____ Monoloudness

_____ Excess and equal stress

_____ Prolonged intervals

Ataxic Dysarthria (cerebellar involvement)

_____ Imprecise consonants

_____ Excess and equal stress

_____ Irregular articulatory breakdowns

_____ Distorted vowels

_____ Harsh voice

_____ Loudness control problems

_____ Variable nasality

Hypokinetic Dysarthria (parkinsonism)

_____ Monopitch

_____ Reduced stress

_____ Monoloudness

_____ Imprecise consonants

_____ Inappropriate silences

_____ Short rushes of speech

_____ Harsh voice

_____ Breathy voice

Hyperkinetic Dysarthria (dystonia and choreathetosis)

_____ Imprecise consonants

_____ Distorted vowels

_____ Harsh voice quality

_____ Irregular articulatory breakdowns

_____ Strained-strangled voice quality

_____ Monopitch

_____ Monoloudness

Adapted from "The Dysarthrias: Diagnosis, Description, and Treatment," by J. C. Rosenbeck and L. L. LaPointe in *Clinical Management of Neurogenic Communication Disorders,* 2nd ed. (p. 100), by D. F. Johns (ed.), 1985, Boston: Little, Brown and Co.

Form 14-2.

Checklists for Limb, Oral, and Verbal Apraxia

Name: _____ Age: _____ Date: _____

Examiner's Name: _____

Instructions: Select several items from each section and ask the client to complete the task or repeat the utterance. Many items are provided to offer a wide range of tasks; you do not need to complete each item. Score each presented item as correct (+ or ✓) or incorrect (− or 0). Transcribe errors phonetically on the right-hand side. Also note accompanying behaviors such as delays with initiation, struggling, groping, or facial grimacing. The diagnosis of apraxia is made by evaluating the nature and accuracy of movement, as well as the type and severity of error patterns present.

Limb Apraxia

_____ Wave hello or goodbye _____

_____ Make a fist _____

_____ Make the "thumbs up" sign _____

_____ Make the "okay" sign _____

_____ Pretend you're zipping your coat _____

_____ Pretend you're combing your hair _____

_____ Pretend you're petting a dog _____

_____ Pretend you're turning a doorknob _____

_____ Pretend you're hitting a baseball (or golf ball) _____

_____ Pretend you're tieing a shoe _____

_____ Pretend you're using scissors to cut a piece of paper _____

_____ Pretend you're knocking on a door _____

_____ Pretend you're writing _____

_____ Pretend you're going to make a fire _____

_____ Pretend you're going to make coffee _____

_____ Pretend you're going to drive a car out of a driveway _____

Oral Apraxia

_____ Smile _____

_____ Open your mouth _____

_____ Blow _____

_____ Whistle _____

(continues)

Form 14-2. continued

Oral Apraxia (continued)

_____ Puff out your cheeks _____

_____ Show me your teeth _____

_____ Chatter your teeth as if you are cold _____

_____ Pucker your lips _____

_____ Bite your lower lip _____

_____ Smack your lips _____

_____ Lick your lips _____

_____ Stick out your tongue _____

_____ Touch your nose with the tip of your tongue _____

_____ Move your tongue in and out _____

_____ Wiggle your tongue from side to side _____

_____ Click your tongue _____

_____ Clear your throat _____

_____ Cough _____

_____ Alternately pucker and smile _____

Verbal Apraxia

Ask client to repeat after you

_____ love—loving—lovingly _____

_____ jab—jabber—jabbering _____

_____ zip—zipper—zippering _____

_____ soft—soften—softening _____

_____ hope—hopeful—hopefully _____

_____ hard—harden—hardening _____

_____ thick—thicken—thickening _____

_____ please—pleasing—pleasingly _____

_____ sit—city—citizen—citizenship _____

_____ cat—catnip—catapult—catastrophe _____

_____ strength—strengthen—strengthening _____

_____ door—doorknob—doorkeeper—dormitory _____

(continues)

Form 14-2. continued

Verbal Apraxia (continued)

_____ Tornado _____

_____ Radiator _____

_____ Artillery _____

_____ Linoleum _____

_____ Inevitable _____

_____ Delegation _____

_____ Probability _____

_____ Cauliflower _____

_____ Declaration _____

_____ Refrigeration _____

_____ Unequivocally _____

_____ Thermometer _____

_____ Parliamentarian _____

_____ Catastrophically _____

_____ Disenfranchised _____

_____ Statistical analysis _____

_____ Alternative opinion _____

_____ Regulatory authority _____

_____ Ruthlessly malicious _____

_____ Barometric pressure _____

_____ Indescribably delicious _____

_____ Mississippi River _____

_____ Tallahassee, Florida _____

_____ Kalamazoo, Michigan _____

_____ Boston, Massachusetts _____

_____ Sacramento, California _____

_____ Madison Square Garden _____

_____ Minneapolis, Minnesota _____

_____ Chattanooga, Tennessee _____

_____ Encyclopedia Britannica _____

_____ Saskatoon, Saskatchewan _____

_____ Philadelphia, Pennsylvania _____

_____ Vancouver, British Columbia _____

_____ Nuclear Regulatory Commission _____

Form 14-3.

Identifying Apraxia

Name: _____ Age: _____ Date: _____

Examiner's Name: _____

Instructions: Evaluate each behavior in automatic speech, spontaneous speech, and oral reading. Mark a plus (+) if the client has no difficulty. Use the severity scale if the client does exhibit problems with production. Add comments on the right-hand side as needed.

    1 = Mild difficulties

    2 = Moderate difficulties

    3 = Severe difficulties

Oral Reading	Automatic Speech	Spontaneous Speech	
_____	_____	_____	Phonemic anticipatory errors (e.g., *kreen crayon* for *green crayon*) _____
_____	_____	_____	Phonemic perseveratory errors (e.g., pe*p* for pe*t*) _____
_____	_____	_____	Phonemic transposition errors (e.g., A*rifca* for *Africa*) _____
_____	_____	_____	Phonemic voicing errors (e.g., *b*en for *p*en) _____
_____	_____	_____	Phonemic vowel errors (e.g., m*oa*n for m*a*n) _____
_____	_____	_____	Visible or audible searching _____
_____	_____	_____	Numerous and varied off-target attempts _____
_____	_____	_____	Highly inconsistent errors _____
_____	_____	_____	Errors increase with phonemic complexity _____
_____	_____	_____	Fewer errors in automatic speech _____
_____	_____	_____	Marked difficulties initating speech _____
_____	_____	_____	Intrudes a schwa sound _____
_____	_____	_____	Abnormal prosodic features _____
_____	_____	_____	Aware of errors but difficult to correct _____
_____	_____	_____	Receptive-expressive language gap _____

Adapted from Subtest 6: Inventory of Articulation Characteristics of Apraxia, *Apraxia Battery for Adults* (ABA-2), by B. Dabul, 2000, Austin, TX: Pro-Ed.

MOTOR SPEECH DISORDERS

Chapter 15

ASSESSMENT
OF DYSPHAGIA

Many of the muscles used for speech production are also used for chewing and swallowing. Because speech-language pathologists are knowledgeable about oral and pharyngeal anatomy and physiology, clinicians frequently evaluate and treat dysphagia (chewing or swallowing dysfunction), even when a client does not have a communicative disorder. This chapter describes the normal swallow function and procedures for evaluating a client with a possible swallowing impairment. Assessment procedures unique to tracheostomized clients are also included.

It is critical to exercise caution when completing any evaluation with a client with suspected dysphagia; it is a life-threatening disorder. For example, aspiration pneumonia, which can be caused by food or liquid in the lungs, can lead to death. Speech-language pathologists will need to work closely with physicians, nurses, and other medically related personnel to provide safe client care.

OVERVIEW OF ASSESSMENT

History of the Client

    Procedures

        Written Case History

        Information-Getting Interview

        Information from Other Professionals

    Contributing Factors

        Medical Diagnosis

        Pharmacological Factors

        Age

        Intelligence, Motivation, and Levels of Concern

Orofacial Examination

Assessment of Dysphagia

    Procedures

        Screening

        Clinical Evaluation

        Instrumental Evaluation

        Blue-Dye Test

    Analysis

        Type of Dysphagia

        Oral Feeding Feasibility and Safety

Cognitive Assessment

Speech Assessment

Language Assessment

Hearing Assessment

Determining the Diagnosis

Providing Information (written report, interview, etc.)

OVERVIEW OF A NORMAL SWALLOW

Before evaluating a client for a swallowing disorder, it is important to understand the dynamics of a functional swallow. The normal swallow occurs in four phases, each described in the following list. The client with dysphagia will exhibit difficulties within one or more of these phases.

1. *Oral Preparatory Phase*: The food or liquid is manipulated in the oral cavity, chewed (if necessary), and made into a bolus, which is sealed with the tongue against the hard palate. In infants, sucking occurs during the oral preparatory phase.

2. *Oral Phase*: The tongue moves the food or liquid toward the back of the mouth (toward the anterior faucial pillars). To achieve this, the tongue presses the bolus against the hard palate and squeezes the bolus posteriorly. The oral-preparatory and oral phases are voluntary, not reflexive, actions.

3. *Pharyngeal Phase*: During this phase, the swallow reflex is triggered and the bolus is carried through the pharynx. These simultaneous actions occur: (a) the velopharyngeal port closes; (b) the bolus is squeezed to the top of the esophagus (cricopharyngeal sphincter); (c) the larynx elevates as the epiglottis, false vocal folds, and true vocal folds close to seal the airway; and (d) the cricopharyngeal sphincter relaxes to allow the bolus to enter the esophagus.

4. *Esophageal Phase*: During this fourth and final phase, the bolus is transported through the esophagus into the stomach.

The first three phases are of most interest for speech-language pathologists. Problems with the fourth phase (esophageal phase) are treated medically. Figure 15-1 depicts the first three stages of a normal swallow.

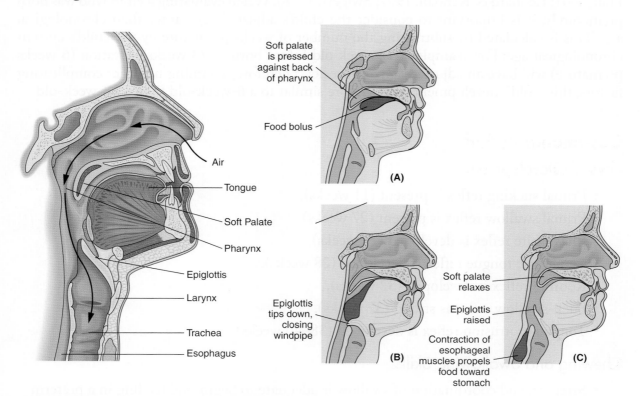

FIGURE 15-1.   Stages of a Normal Swallow

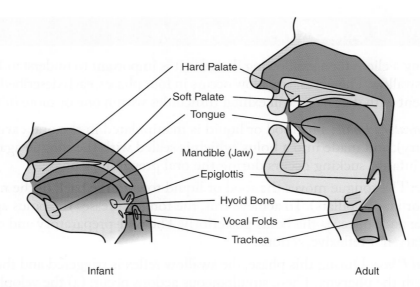

FIGURE 15-2. Anatomical Structures Involved in Swallowing

Anatomical structures involved in swallowing are presented in Figure 15-2. The illustration highlights differences between an adult and an infant. Individual structures change and mature at different rates. Logically, when evaluating pediatric clients it is necessary to consider the child's age and stage of maturation.

A sequence of normal development related to feeding and swallowing is presented next. The developmental milestones include physical changes, refinement of oral motor skills, and social behaviors that influence feeding and swallowing (data from Arvedson & Brodsky, 2002; Hall, 2001; Leonard & Kendall, 1997; Swigert, 1998). When evaluating a child who was born prematurely, it is important to consider the child's adjusted age rather than chronological age. This is calculated by subtracting the number of weeks premature by the child's current chronological age. For example, a 12-week old infant born at 34 weeks' gestation (6 weeks premature) will have an adjusted age of 6 weeks. Therefore, assuming no other complicating factors, this child's development will be more similar to a 6-week-old than a 12-week-old.

Gestational Period

Physical Development

- Primal sucking reflex is present (11 weeks).
- Primal swallow reflex is present (27 weeks).
- Phasic bite reflex is developed (28 weeks).
- Transverse tongue reflex is developed (28 weeks).
- Rooting reflex is developed (32 weeks).
- Suck-swallow reflex is strong (37 weeks).
- Tongue protrusion reflex is developed (38–40 weeks).

Chewing and Swallowing Skills

- Strength and coordination of swallow is adequate to begin oral feeding in a preterm infant at 34–35 weeks' gestation.

At Birth

Physical Development

- The hard palate is broad and short (approximately 2.3 cm long) with only a slight arch.
- The tongue fills the oral cavity and is located only in the oral cavity.
- Fatty tissue (sucking pads) fills the lateral sulci.
- The larynx is high and short (approximately 2 cm long, one-third its eventual adult size); it is located at C3 or C4.
- The pharynx is approximately 4 cm long.
- The esophagus is approximately 8–10 cm long.
- The epiglottis is large and makes contact with the soft palate.
- Delineation between the nasopharynx and oropharynx is obscure.
- There is little to no space between the hyoid bone and the thyroid cartilage.
- The trachea is approximately 4 cm long; it is located at C6 and remains there through adulthood; its diagonal-posterior slope straightens during the first 2 years.
- Infant weighs an average of 7 pounds and is approximately 19 inches long.
- Primitive reflexes are present.

Oral Motor Skills

- Tongue, lips, and jaw move in unison.
- Sucking pads provide sucking stability.
- The larynx and hyoid bone are elevated while eating, enabling nasal breathing.
- Incomplete lip closure around nipple causes some spillage.

Feeding and Social Behaviors

- Infant receives all nourishment through nipple feedings of breast milk or formula.
- When awake, the infant is usually feeding.
- Infant cues for feeding include crying, rooting, sucking, and arousal (0–3 months).

1 Month

Physical Development

- Infant voluntarily brings hands to mouth.
- Lips usually move in unison with other facial structures.

Oral Motor Skills

- Uses a suckle-swallow pattern.
- Tongue may protrude slightly past the bottom lip while feeding.

Feeding and Social Behaviors

- Infant consumes 2–6 ounces of liquid per meal, with six or more feedings per day.
- Pattern for hunger and satiety begins to develop.

- Infant pauses during feedings for burping or satiety.
- Infant prefers being held, and maintains eye contact with feeder.

2 Months

Physical Development

- Lips continue to move in unison with other facial structures.

Feeding and Social Behaviors

- Infant opens mouth in anticipation of feeding.

3 Months

Physical Development

- Cessation of Babkin reflex.
- Head control is significantly improved, with minimal head bobbing.
- Sucking pads begin to diminish as facial muscles are developed.

Feeding and Social Behaviors

- Infant consumes 7–8 ounces of liquid per meal, with four to six feedings per day.
- Infant anticipates feedings.
- Feedings become more social; infant does more smiling and laughing.

4 Months

Physical Development

- Sucking pads continue to diminish as facial muscles are developed.
- Cessation of palmomental reflex.

Oral Motor Skills

- Good coordination of suck-swallow-breathe pattern; sequences 20 or more sucks.
- Sucking becomes less reflexive and more volitional.
- Tongue may protrude and push some food out due to suckle pattern.

Feeding and Social Behaviors

- Feedings are completed within 30 minutes.
- Spoon feeding may be introduced; thin infant cereal may be added to the diet.
- Infant may stop feeding if distracted by activity in the room.

5 Months

Physical Development

- Sucking pads continue to diminish as facial muscles are developed.

Oral Motor Skills

- Infant may involuntarily spit food out.
- Infant may gag on new textures.
- Increased lip and cheek activity while sucking.
- Phasic bite-release pattern is used.

Feeding and Social Behaviors

- Spoon feeding may be introduced (or further refined if introduced in fourth month).
- Diet consists of breast milk, formula, and thin baby cereal.

6 Months

Physical Development

- Cessation of rooting, asymmetric tonic neck, palmar grasp, tongue thrust, and moro reflexes.
- Strength of gag reflex diminishes significantly.
- Sucking pads have diminished.
- First teeth may erupt (6–12 months).
- Head control is established.

Oral Motor Skills

- Munching pattern begins; jaw movement is a vertical up-and-down motion.
- Infant uses rhythmic phasic bite-release pattern on soft cookie; may revert to sucking cookie instead of biting; unable to bite through cookie.
- Infant demonstrates good lip closure around a spoon or nipple. Loss of liquid may occur only at the beginning or end of a feeding.
- Lower lip is used as a stabilizer.
- Sucks liquid from a spouted cup.

Feeding and Social Behaviors

- Diet may consist of breast milk or infant formula, thin baby cereal, and pureed baby foods.
- Infant consumes 9–10 ounces of food or liquid per meal, with four to six feedings per day.
- Infant cues for feeding by calling for attention.
- Infant uses facial expressions to convey likes and dislikes.
- Mealtimes begin to become predictable and linked to the family schedule.

7 Months

Physical Development

- Infant sits unsupported.
- First teeth may erupt (6–12 months).
- Infant skillfully moves objects from hand to hand.

Oral Motor Skills

- Tongue and jaw move up and down in a munching pattern.
- Infant is able to hold the bolus over the molars for chewing using lip closure and cheek action.
- Jaw and tongue are quiet and relaxed when waiting to accept spoon.

Feeding and Social Behaviors

- Infant may express excitement or eagerness when he or she knows a feeding is about to occur.
- Infant can hold the bottle independently.
- Assisted cup drinking may be introduced.
- Thicker pureed foods may be introduced.

8 Months

Physical Development

- First teeth may erupt (6–12 months).
- Infant can hold and control his or her own bottle.

Oral Motor Skills

- Drooling is associated with teething only.
- Vertical munching continues.
- Infant skillfully removes food from a spoon by moving the head forward and clearing the spoon with the lips.
- Infant uses tongue to lateralize food in the oral cavity.
- Infant can maintain long sequences of suck-swallow-breathe pattern.
- Infant may take too much liquid from a cup, resulting in loss of liquid, coughing, or choking.

Feeding and Social Behaviors

- Infant begins self-feeding using hands and fingers; finger foods are added to the diet.
- Mealtimes are noisy and playful.

9 Months

Physical Development

- Sucking behavior replaces suckling behavior.
- First teeth may erupt (6–12 months).

Oral Motor Skills

- Tongue is sensitive enough to detect which foods can and cannot be mashed.
- Lower lip is used as an effective stabilizer for cup drinking.
- Difficulty with suck-swallow-breathe pattern may persist during cup drinking.

Feeding and Social Behaviors

- Infant deliberately reaches for spoon and assists with feeding.
- Infant can bring the bottle or foods to the mouth for self-feeding.

10 Months

Physical Development

- First teeth may erupt (6–12 months).
- The two halves of the mandible begin to fuse.

Oral Motor Skills

- Less up-and-down jaw movement when drinking from a cup.

Feeding and Social Behaviors

- Infant may become impatient during mealtime if caregiver is slow presenting food.
- Infant may turn head in refusal or throw food when full (10–11 months).

11 Months

Physical Development

- First teeth may erupt (6–12 months).

Oral Motor Skills

- Loss of food while eating is rare.
- Infant uses controlled, graded bite on soft cookie (10–12 months).

Feeding and Social Behaviors

- Infant demonstrates good pincer grasp for finger feeding.
- Infant may prefer self-feeding with fingers over assisted feeding with spoon.
- Cup drinking increases; nipple feeding decreases.

12 Months

Physical Development

- Cessation of suckle reflex.
- First teeth may erupt (6–12 months).
- Molars erupt (12–24 months).
- Jaw and tongue work independently (12–24 months).

Oral Motor Skills

- Infant demonstrates excellent control and precision of tongue for eating.
- Infant chews with both rotary and up-and-down movements.
- Pocketing of food is minimal to absent.

- Infant readily bites through soft foods or foods that dissolve quickly; may show some struggle when biting through hard foods (e.g., hard cookie).
- Suck-swallow pattern greatly improved during cup drinking, although some coughing may persist if liquid is flowing too quickly.
- Infant uses lips while chewing.
- Lips are closed while swallowing liquids and solids.
- Infant places tongue beneath cup to help stabilize it.

Feeding and Social Behaviors

- Mealtimes are consistent and linked to the family schedule.
- Cup drinking increases; nipple feeding decreases.
- Infant can grasp the spoon handle with the whole hand, but does not have good control for self-feeding.
- Infant can hold a cup with two hands and take four to five continuous swallows without choking.
- Diet may include coarsely chopped table foods.

13–18 Months

Physical Development

- Molars erupt (12–24 months).
- Coordination for breathing, phonating, and swallowing is fully mature.
- The two halves of the mandible are fused.
- Jaw and tongue work independently (12–24 months).

Oral Motor Skills

- Chewing transitions from up-and-down pattern to rotary pattern.
- Child can tolerate and manage most food textures without difficulty.
- Child uses the tongue to clean lips or upper teeth to clean lower lip.
- Inconsistently chews with lips closed.
- No difficulties with coordination for cup drinking.
- Child uses controlled bite on hard cookie.
- Child opens mouth wider than necessary to bite foods of varying thicknesses.
- Suck-swallow-breathe pattern is coordinated during long drinking sequences.
- Child stabilizes cup by biting cup edge.
- Child closes upper lip around the edge of a cup to provide better seal for drinking.

Feeding and Social Behaviors

- Cup drinking increases; nipple feeding decreases.
- Child feeds self using utensils with increasing skill and coordination.
- Straw drinking may be introduced.

19–24 Months

Physical Development

- Molars erupt (12–24 months).
- The soft palate elongates and thickens.
- Sucking behavior decreases significantly.
- Jaw and tongue work independently (12–24 months).

Oral Motor Skills

- The jaw and tongue work independently.
- Child can bite through most foods without struggle.
- Child effectively manages varying food textures at the same time.
- Child skillfully swallows liquid from a cup with no loss of liquid.
- Child modifies degree of jaw opening for receiving foods of varying thicknesses.
- Child licks lips clean.

Feeding and Social Behaviors

- Nipple feeding is replaced by cup feeding.
- Child effectively feeds self using utensils.
- Child feeds self most of the time.
- Child distinguishes between finger foods and spoon foods.

3 Years

Physical Development

- All 20 deciduous teeth are present.
- The tongue begins to descend and grow in a posterior-inferior direction.
- The larynx slowly elongates and descends (24–48 months).

Oral Motor Skills

- Coordination for chewing and swallowing continues to improve.
- Child uses the tongue to clean areas between gums and cheeks.

Feeding and Social Behaviors

- Child can hold a cup with one hand and drink from an open cup without spillage.
- Child can drink through a straw.
- Child is an independent feeder; diet matches that of the family's.

4–5 Years

Physical Development

- The tongue continues to descend and grow in a posterior-inferior direction.
- The larynx has descended to C6 and is approximately 6 cm long.

- Elongation of the soft plate is complete.
- Delineation of the nasopharynx and oropharynx is more defined and forms an oblique angle.

Oral Motor Skills

- Coordination for chewing and swallowing continues to improve.

Feeding and Social Behaviors

- Child may have strong food likes and dislikes.

6–10 Years

Physical Development

- Descent of the tongue into the pharynx is complete; it forms part of the anterior pharyngeal wall.
- Deciduous teeth start to fall out and are replaced by permanent teeth.

Oral Motor Skills

- Chewing and swallowing are fully mature.

Feeding and Social Behaviors

- Child may continue to have strong food likes and dislikes.

11–18 Years

Physical Development

- Deciduous teeth continue to fall out (through 13th year) and are replaced by permanent teeth.
- Wisdom teeth erupt (17–21 years).
- Oral structures are fully mature.

Feeding and Social Behaviors

- Child continues to explore new foods and develop adult-like preferences.

CLINICAL ASSESSMENT OF PEDIATRIC DYSPHAGIA

We cannot overstate the importance of specific training and study of dysphagia prior to administering a pediatric dysphagia assessment. The information and forms presented in this manual are basic procedures for evaluating pediatric clients. The specific and complex needs of individual children cannot be presented in a text of this nature; therefore we caution against using this text as a sole source of information for evaluating children with this potentially life-endangering disorder. Materials recommended in the "Sources of Additional Information" at the end of this chapter are a few of the many resources available for increasing knowledge and skill in this area.

The assessment of pediatric dysphagia necessarily begins with a thorough case history. Knowing the child's history and current status will lay the foundation for the remainder of the clinical assessment. Forms 15-1, "Pediatric Dysphagia Case History Form and Caregiver Questionnaire—Infant 0–6 Months," and 15-2, "Pediatric Dysphagia Case History Form and Caregiver Questionnaire," are provided to guide this data collection. The first form is appropriate for infants who have not transitioned to solid foods (0 to 4–6 months of age). The second form can be used for all children (ignore irrelevant sections according to child's age and situation). Either form can be completed by a caregiver prior to the assessment or the data can be collected during an information-gathering interview. Information about the infant's or child's current status can also be obtained by reviewing the client's medical records and consulting other professionals involved in the child's care. Specifically:

- *Identify the child's medical status.* For example, was the child born prematurely? Are there neurological concerns? Are there craniofacial abnormalities? Does the child have a history of aspiration pneumonia? Has the child been losing weight?

- *Identify the child's feeding status.* For example, what is the child's typical diet? How is the child positioned during meals? Does the child use adaptive equipment? Has the child been refusing to eat? Does the child self-feed?

- *Be aware of dietary restrictions.* For example, does the child have food allergies? Is the child diabetic? Be careful not to present food or liquids that could be harmful to the child.

- *Converse with caregivers.* For example, learn about the child's feeding/swallowing problems from the caregiver's point of view. Discern the social aspects of mealtimes in the home. Ask the caregiver to bring feeding equipment (chairs, bottles, spoons, etc.) that the child typically uses. Interview the child's pediatrician, nurses, or dietitian to obtain critical information.

Form 15-3, "Pediatric Dysphagia Clinical Evalution," will help with the completion of the clinical portion of the evaluation. A majority of the clinical assessment involves observation of current physical and feeding status. The clinician should also stimulate for improved feeding and swallowing ability by introducing various compensatory techniques. In many instances, the case history and clinical assessment are sufficient for informed diagnostic decisions and recommendations. In other situations, instrumental assessment will also be necessary. Methods of instrumentally assessing swallowing function are described later in this chapter.

Administration and Interpretation

Pediatric clients who are being assessed for dysphagia vary widely in age, medical and physical status, and feeding status. Clients served may be premature babies, older school-age children, or somewhere in between; therefore the assessment process will necessarily be modified depending upon the age and diagnosis of each child. The assessment worksheet provided in this manual can be adapted for varying situations and needs.

Observing alertness is particularly important when assessing infants. Alertness measures provide information about the infant's ability to prepare for and attend to feeding. Six states of consciousness identified by pediatrician T. Berry Brazelton (Als et al., 1977; Brazelton & Nugent, 1995) are widely used to define levels of alertness. They are:

1. *Deep sleep*: Respiratory patterns are deep and regular; the eyes are closed with no rapid eye movements. The body is completely relaxed. The infant may startle, but will not rouse. The infant is relatively "unreachable."

2. *Active sleep*: Respiratory patterns alternate between regular and irregular. The eyes are closed, although rapid eye movements may be noted under the eyelids and the infant may open and close the eyes on occasion. Random spontaneous movements of the limbs may occur. Facial movements may be observed.

3. *Drowsy/in-between state*: A dazed expression is observed, with fully or partially open eyes. Smooth movements of the limbs may occur. Respiration is regular. Infant arouses quickly to stimulation.

4. *Awake/alert*: Eyes are alert and bright. The infant's body is mostly still and the face is attentive. The infant responds predictably to auditory and visual stimuli.

5. *Alert agitated*: Eyes are alert. The body is active. Movements are often disorganized and jerky. The infant is fussy, although readily soothed, in this state. Fussing may escalate to the next state, crying.

6. *Crying*: Intense crying with difficulty comforting. The face may redden and limbs may exhibit tremor-like shaking.

In addition to alertness, physiologic status is also very important to observe when assessing for dysphagia. Physiologic status includes respiratory rate, oxygen saturation levels, and heart rate. Respiratory problems are among the most common causes of dysphagia in young children (Hall, 2001). Observing respiratory patterns, particularly noting changes that occur during and after feeding, provides information about the child's ability to coordinate breathing and eating. A child who is unable to breathe adequately or protect the airway during oral intake will need to be tube fed. Problematic breathing patterns include:

- *Apnea*: Sporadic cessation of breathing
- *Belly breathing*: Extreme abdominal movement (Note: This may be a normal pattern for infants 0–5 months of age.)
- *Reverse breathing*: Abdomen expands on exhalation and compresses on inhalation
- *Thoracic breathing*: Extreme upper chest movement
- *Irregular breathing*: Absence of a normal pattern
- *Shallow breathing*: Minimal movement
- *Gulping*: Rapid and short inhalations with slight backward head movement

Other aspects of physiologic status such as oxygen saturation levels, heart rates, and respiratory rates can also be noted when the child is hooked up to monitors. Nursing staff can assist in reading monitors and interpreting results. Note changes that coincide with or follow oral feeding. Table 15-1 presents normal physiologic data for full-term and preterm infants.

TABLE 15-1   Physiologic Norms for Newborns

	FULL-TERM INFANT	PRETERM INFANT
Resting Heart Rate*	120–140 beats/minute	160–180 beats/minute
Respiratory Rate	30–60 breaths/minute	30–60 breaths/minute
Respiratory Rate While Feeding	40–50 breaths/minute	40–50 breaths/minute
Oxygen Saturation (SaO$_2$)	>95%	≥90%

*Normal heart rate increases during activity and decreases during sleep.
Source: *Swigert (1998).*

Observing sucking is another important procedure when evaluating infants for dysphagia. Non-nutritive sucking (NNS) is a normal and important infant behavior; it is a prerequisite for normal nutritive sucking. NNS occurs in a rhythmic, organized pattern called a burst. Typically, an infant will suck non-nutritively in bursts of six to eight sucks in 3–4 seconds, swallow, then pause for 6–7 seconds to breathe and rest before repeating the sequence. Cycles that deviate from this may indicate poor endurance or poor coordination of the suck-swallow-breathe pattern. An infant who demonstrates respiratory difficulties during NNS is likely to show even greater struggle during nutritive sucking. The infant's suck strength can be assessed by placing a gloved finger in the mouth, pad side down. Note how well the tongue cups the finger, whether lip closure is obtained, and the strength of the suck.

The nutritive sucking (NS) pattern is slower than the NNS pattern. NNS is usually two sucks per second, while NS is one per second. A newborn will suck once, swallow once, and breathe once per burst. The number of sucks per burst will increase to two to three sucks in the first few months as the oral cavity enlarges. The infant will maintain this pattern for 60–80 continuous seconds before pausing to rest. As the infant becomes satiated and fatigued, the pattern usually slows down, with fewer sucks and longer pauses by the end of the feeding. It may be difficult to assess strength and efficiency of the suck during nutritive sucking, especially if the infant is breast feeding. Generally, if the infant has to work hard to express fluid or if the infant is unable to maintain an organized sucking pattern, he or she may need supplemental feeding and/or a bottle with a modified nipple.

Several infantile reflexes should be present at birth. These primitive reflexes cease during the first several months of life. The absence of one or more of these reflexes, or their persistence beyond the age of normal cessation, may indicate neurological impairment. Table 15-2 highlights primitive reflexes that affect feeding and swallowing. Methods of eliciting the reflex, as well as the normal age of cessation, are included. Keep in mind that some reflexes are necessary for proper feeding and swallowing development, whereas others interfere and have a negative impact. Points of clinical significance are described as follows:

- *Asymmetric tonic neck reflex* (also called *tonic neck reflex* or *fencing reflex*): The presence of this reflex may interfere with hand-to-mouth feeding.
- *Babkin* (also called *hand-mouth reflex*): The hand-to-mouth action may aid the ability to receive food into the mouth.
- *Gag reflex*: The gag reflex may or may not be related to swallowing. A hyperactive or hypoactive gag may indicate neurological impairment.
- *Moro reflex* (also called *startle reflex*): Presence of this reflex may interfere with head control, attention, or hand-to-mouth action for feeding.
- *Palmar grasp*: Presence of this reflex may aid early finger feeding and ability to hold a bottle, cup, or spoon.
- *Phasic bite reflex*: This reflex may assist with the development of the early munching patterns.
- *Rooting reflex*: Rooting helps the infant's mouth find the nipple in early feeding. The infant will continue to root until he or she latches on.
- *Sucking or suckling reflex*: This reflex is important for early breast or bottle feeding and later for spoon feeding and cup drinking. The infant instinctively and rhythmically compresses the nipple and draws liquid out, or draws food from a spoon or cup. The term *sucking* is often generically used to refer to both sucking and suckling. The

TABLE 15-2   Normal Primitive Reflexes

REFLEX/ BEHAVIOR	DESCRIPTION	ELICITATION	CESSATION
Babkin	Hand moves to mouth; infant begins to suck on fist or finger	Apply firm pressure to the infant's palm	3 months
Rooting	Movement of the head toward stimulation	Lightly stroke the area around the infant's mouth	3–6 months
Phasic Bite	Rhythmic up-and-down movement of the jaw, limited in power	Apply pressure to the infant's gums	3–6 months
Asymmetric Tonic Neck	"Lancer's position"; arm and leg straightens on the side in which head is turned while the opposite arm and leg flex	Turn the infant's head to one side	4–6 months
Palmar Grasp	Tight-fisted hold on any object placed in the infant's palm	Gently press index finger in infant's palm	4–6 months
Tongue Thrust	Protrusion of tongue from the mouth	Touch the tip of the infant's tongue	4–6 months
Moro/ Startle	Arms, elbows, wrists, and fingers abduct, followed by adduction of arms and flexion of elbows	Drop head backwards suddenly	5–6 months
Suckle	Infant sucks on anything that touches the roof of the mouth. Tongue, lower lip, and jaw work in unison; tongue moves forward and backward while jaw moves up and down	Place nipple in the infant's mouth and stroke the tongue or touch the hard palate	6–12 months
Suck	Infant sucks on anything that touches the roof of the mouth. Up-and-down tongue movement; jaw moves less and more independently than during suckling	Place nipple in the infant's mouth and stroke the tongue or touch the hard palate	2+ years
Gag	Tongue retracts and pharyngeal muscles contract	Touch the back of the infant's tongue or the pharynx	No cessation in most people
Swallow	Bolus of food passes through the pharynx and enters the esophagus	Gently blow in the infant's face*	No cessation

*Santmyer swallow reflex: effective with infants or severely neurologically disabled children.
Note: Reflexes are listed in order of expected cessation.

primary difference between sucking and suckling is the motion of the tongue, which moves forward-back during suckling and up-down during sucking.

- *Swallow reflex* (also called *pharyngeal swallow*): This reflex is triggered when a bolus of food enters the pharynx. The reflex protects the airway and propels the bolus into the esophagus.
- *Tongue thrust reflex*: This reflex provides protection against choking in the early months. Introduction of spoon feeding of solids cannot productively occur until the tongue thrust reflex has ceased.

Abnormal reflexes may also be observed during a dysphagia assessment. Presence of one or more of these reflexes may indicate neurological damage; some are common among children with cerebral palsy. Abnormal reflexes include:

- *Palmomental reflex*: When the palm of the infant's hand is scratched at the base of the thumb, the chin and corner of the mouth contract unilaterally on the same side as the stimulation. This reflex diminishes by 4 months of age.
- *Tonic bite reflex*: The jaw clamps down when teeth or gums are stimulated, and the child may have difficulty releasing it. Firm pressure applied bilaterally to the temporomandibular joints may release the bite. Presence of this reflex interferes with appropriate oral feeding and manipulation of a nipple, cup, or utensil in the oral cavity.
- *Jaw thrust*: The lower jaw is forcefully extended down and appears to be stuck open. It causes difficulty in receiving and keeping food in the mouth.
- *Tongue retraction*: The tongue is pulled back into the hypopharynx, while the tip of the tongue may be held against the hard palate. The child will have difficulty removing food from a utensil and using the tongue for chewing and swallowing.
- *Tongue thrust*: Strong abnormal, and sometimes repetitive, protrusion of the tongue in response to oral stimulation. It interferes with transport of food and liquid to the pharynx. The reflex is abnormal if present after 18 months of age. It should not to be confused with the normal primitive tongue thrust reflex that diminishes by 6 months of age.
- *Lip retraction*: Lips are tightly pulled back in a horizontal line. The child will have difficulty sucking from a nipple, removing food from a spoon, cup drinking, and keeping food in the mouth while chewing.
- *Nasal regurgitation*: Swallowed bolus flows back through the nose. It is associated with abnormal function of the velopharynx.

The assessment of the child's orofacial structures focuses primarily on behaviors or deficits that may impair the child's ability to safely feed, chew, or swallow. With infants, this portion of the assessment is done primarily through observation of the structures at rest. Function can be more readily assessed in older children who are capable of imitating oral movements or responding to directives. Clinical significance of findings include the following:

- Structural abnormalities often impair feeding or swallowing ability. For example, clefts of the soft or hard palate usually interfere with sucking ability. Cleft lip may result in poor labial seal. Abnormalities such as a tracheoesophageal (TE) fistula and esophageal atresia preclude safe oral feeding.
- Oral-motor weakness and/or incoordination may result in poor sucking ability and oral control of the bolus. For example, food or liquid may spill out of the child's

mouth or pool in the mouth after swallowing. The child may be unable to latch onto a nipple or achieve adequate intra-oral pressure for sucking.

- Abnormal muscle tone may impair oral awareness, sucking ability, manipulation of the bolus, or self-feeding. For example, flaccid tone may result in inadequate stability of head or body. The child may be "floppy" and unable to feed, chew, or swallow. Tension may cause difficulty bringing the hand to the mouth. Abnormal reflexes are likely to be noted, such as jaw thrust, tonic bite, and tongue retraction.

- Reduced or abnormal movement of oral structures may impair chewing and swallowing ability. For example, restricted range of jaw movement may cause difficulty latching onto a nipple or biting into solid foods.

- Facial and oral sensitivity may impair a child's ability to feed, chew, or swallow. Reduced sensitivity may reduce awareness and control of food on the face or in the oral cavity. A child who is hypersensitive may refuse to eat.

- Coughing, choking, or wet vocal quality indicate penetration of food or liquid into the airway.

An infant begins eating solid foods usually between 4 and 6 months of age. Once that milestone is met, it is necessary to make observations about feeding, chewing, and swallowing ability with solid foods, and later with cup drinking. Clinical expectations vary depending on the child's age, medical status, and physical maturity. We recommend referring to the sequence of normal development presented earlier in this chapter to enlighten this portion of the assessment. Assess the child's ability to chew and swallow different textures, progressing from the least to most difficult to manage. Note chewing efficiency, oral motor strength and coordination, control of bolus, and pharyngeal behaviors for each texture presented. Also observe the child's posture, attention, and ability to self-feed. When assessing older children, it may be appropriate to refer to the adult clinical assessment of dysphagia section of this chapter for additional diagnostic information.

When appropriate, clinicians should attempt to stimulate improved feeding and swallowing as part of the assessment process. Compensatory or facilitative techniques may include:

- *Modify posture*: For example, incline or recline the head, put the child in a prone position, or have the child positioned fully upright. Any of these may improve jaw stability or reduce clenching, or minimize tongue or jaw thrusting or retraction. It may improve lip motion and seal, or eliminate nasopharyngeal reflux. It also may improve airway protection or improve head control.

- *Manually support jaw, lips, or cheeks*: This may improve a weak suck, assist with labial seal, or minimize jaw or tongue thrusting or retraction. Strategically placed support or pressure can also minimize clenching, reduce anterior loss of food, or reduce pooling.

- *Provide adaptive equipment*: For example, a modified nipple may assist suck, improve organization of suck, or enable desired respiratory function. A maroon spoon (flat-bowled) may inhibit a tonic bite reflex. A child with poor orofacial strength may be able to drink successfully from a straw. An angle-neck bottle may allow a more desirable feeding posture.

- *Alter food*: For example, thicker liquids and foods may improve oral control of the bolus or reduce reflux. Some children may respond better to bland foods with neutral smells, whereas others may do better while eating spicy or tart foods with stronger smells. Modifying food temperature may also improve swallowing.

- *Alter feeding environment*: For example, dimming the lights and playing quiet and calming music or a repetitive noise may calm a child who is alert but unfocused. A calm environment may also help improve an infant's suck-swallow-breathe organization and feeding endurance. Less frequently, but occasionally, a child may require a more stimulating environment to attain a desired level of alertness.

- *Manipulate pace of feeding*: For example, pull or tip the nipple to interrupt flow. Allow frequent pauses to allow the child to rest, reorganize, and maintain respiratory safety.

- *Modify food placement*: For example, touching the lower lip with the spoon before placing it into the mouth may inhibit a tonic bite reflex.

- *Stimulate the face or oral structures*: For example, massaging the cheeks may minimize lip retraction, heighten facial sensitivity, or calm the child. Oral stimulation may increase the child's readiness for feeding or improve lip closure.

CLINICAL ASSESSMENT OF ADULT DYSPHAGIA

Form 15-4, "Adult Bedside Dysphagia Evaluation" will help with the completion of an adult client (bedside) assessment of dysphagia. The form is divided into two segments. The first involves information gathering and an orofacial evaluation specific to dysphagia. The second involves presentation of foods or liquids.[1] It is not necessary to administer both segments with all dysphagic clients. If the client is not alert or if the type of dysphagia is already known, complete the evaluation without presenting food or liquids. If food or liquid are administered orally, and the client exhibits signs of aspiration after swallowing (i.e., choking, coughing, wet voice quality), discontinue the evaluation. Then notify the physician to modify or discontinue oral feeding. Proceed with therapy or refer the client for a radiographic examination to diagnose the disorder more specifically. Be aware that silent aspiration can occur. In this case, the client does not exhibit the outward signs of aspiration. If silent aspiration is suspected, a radiographic study will be necessary to confirm or rule out dysphagia.

Administration and Interpretation

Before beginning the direct assessment, gather thorough information about the client's current status. The best way to obtain this information is to consult with the client's physician or nurse or review the client's medical records. Sometimes a family member or the client can provide this information. Specifically:

- Identify the client's neurological and medical status. For example, was there a recent stroke? Does the client have Parkinsonism? Are there any neurological indicators? Does the client have a history of aspiration pneumonia? Does the client wear dentures?

- Identify the client's feeding status. For example, is the client on a regular diet? Puree diet? Fed via a nasogastric tube? Has the client been losing weight or refusing to eat? Has the client been experiencing backflow, reflux, or vomiting after meals? Is the client fed by someone else? Who will feed the client after discharge from a hospital?

---

1. Caution: Do not administer the feeding portion of the evaluation without some prior training and experience or without the direct supervision of a trained and knowledgeable professional.

- Be aware of dietary limitations. For example, does the client have food allergies? Is the client diabetic? Obtain this information so that foods or liquids are not presented that could be detrimental to the client.
- Identify the client's cognitive status. For example, is the client alert? Is the client able to follow commands? Is there dementia? Will the client be able to cooperate in therapy if treatment is indicated?

Once this preliminary information has been gathered, assess the integrity of the oral mechanism. This assessment is similar to the orofacial evaluation administered as a standard procedure for most communicative disorders, but for a dysphagic client it is important to make special note of behaviors or deficits that may affect the person's ability to safely chew and swallow.

- Poor oral control may be a result of weak and/or uncoordinated lips, tongue, or jaw, or poor oral sensitivity. The client may have difficulty forming a bolus and manipulating the food for chewing or propelling the food back for swallowing, or difficulty keeping the food in the mouth. If the weakness is unilateral, the food typically leaks from the weaker side.
- Chewing difficulties may be caused by incoordination or weakness of the jaw. Also, normal food textures may not be appropriate for a client if teeth are absent or if the client's dentures do not fit properly.
- Nasal regurgitation may occur if velopharyngeal movement is impaired.
- Penetration of the bolus into the airway or complete aspiration may result from weak or uncoordinated laryngeal musculature. If the larynx does not have normal range of motion or if the laryngeal reflex is slow or delayed, the airway is at risk of being obstructed during swallowing. Also, the client may not be able to productively clear food out of the airway if aspiration does occur.

For the second segment of the bedside dysphagia evaluation, present small bites of different textures of food or liquids in order from the easiest to manage (puree) to the most difficult to manage (liquid). A puree texture (e.g., mashed potatoes or applesauce) easily forms into a cohesive bolus and does not need to be chewed. Soft-texture foods (e.g., chopped meat with gravy, or cooked beans) require some chewing, but are easier to manage than regular textures. Regular-texture foods (e.g., toast or chunks of meat) are the most difficult foods to chew and prepare into a bolus. Liquids are the most difficult to manipulate because swallowing liquids involves the least voluntary and reflexive control. Assess the client's ability to manage liquids presented from a spoon, a straw, and a cup. Do not present liquids at all to a client who has difficulty with puree textures.

Part II of the bedside evaluation form lists behaviors that may be observed during the presentation of foods or liquids. The behaviors are grouped according to the applicable phase of the normal swallow. Suspect dysphagia if the client is having difficulty with one or several of these behaviors.

Oral Preparatory Phase

- Food or liquid spills out of the mouth because of poor labial seal. Normally it leaks from the weaker side of the mouth if unilateral paresis is present.
- Food is not chewed adequately because of reduced mandibular strength, reduced lingual strength and range of motion, or reduced oral sensitivity.

- A proper bolus is not formed because of reduced lingual strength and range of motion or reduced oral sensitivity.
- Residual food is pocketed between the cheeks and tongue (lateral sulcus) after the swallow due to reduced buccal tension.
- Residual food is pocketed under the tongue after the swallow due to reduced lingual strength.

Oral Phase

- Food or liquid spills out of the mouth due to poor labial and lingual seal. Normally, leakage occurs from the weaker side of the mouth if unilateral paresis is present.
- Food or liquid falls over the base of the tongue and may be aspirated because of reduced tongue strength or range of motion, or reduced oral sensitivity.
- Residual food is pocketed between the cheeks and tongue (lateral sulcus) after the swallow due to reduced buccal tension.
- Residual food is pocketed under the tongue after the swallow due to reduced lingual strength.
- Residual food is present on the hard palate after the swallow because of reduced lingual elevation.
- Food is spit out of the oral cavity from tongue thrusting.
- The time taken to move the bolus posteriorly is abnormally slow.
- Excessive tongue movement is noted during the swallow due to lingual incoordination, or as a compensatory strategy due to a delayed or absent swallow reflex.

Pharyngeal Phase

- Coughing, choking, or a wet voice quality occurs when food or liquid enters the airway because of a delayed or absent swallow reflex, reduced laryngeal elevation, reduced laryngeal closure, reduced pharyngeal peristalsis (squeezing), or cricopharyngeal dysfunction. With some clients, these outward symptoms do not occur even when aspiration has taken place.
- Nasal regurgitation occurs due to inadequate velopharyngeal closure.
- Excessive saliva and mucus are present due to aspiration and the body's attempt to clear away the foreign material.

Esophageal Phase

- Coughing, choking, or a wet voice quality occurs when food or liquid enters the esophagus, is partially regurgitated, and then enters the airway because of cricopharyngeal dysfunction.
- Regurgitation occurs due to cricopharyngeal dysfunction.

BEDSIDE ASSESSMENT OF THE TRACHEOSTOMIZED CLIENT

When evaluating a tracheostomized client, the swallowing evaluation is modified somewhat. The presence of a tracheostomy may change the pharyngeal pressures that contribute to a functional swallow. Also, the actual hardware can obscure a client's ability to swallow normally and safely. Due to complicating factors related to the tracheostomy, it is critical that the client's physician and respiratory therapist be consulted prior to administering the swallowing assessment. The client's physician can provide valuable information about the client's history and current medical status, and the respiratory therapist can provide information about the client's respiratory status. If possible, have the respiratory therapist present during portions of the evaluation. He or she can monitor the client's ventilation status, assist with cuff deflation and inflation, and suction as needed.

The first portion of the evaluation is the case history. Review medical records, communicate with other caregivers, and talk to the client to gather as much relevant information as possible. In addition to more traditional case history queries, the clinician will also want to ask:

- Why is the person tracheostomized?
- How long has the tracheostomy been in place?
- What kind of tracheostomy tube is present? Is it cuffed? Is it fenestrated?
- What stage, if any, of weaning is the client in?
- What is the client's medical status?

Next, complete the oral-motor assessment. Apply traditional evaluation techniques for determining lip, tongue, and jaw integrity. Occlude the opening of the tracheostomy briefly and ask the client to say "ah" to see if the client can phonate. If the tracheostomy is cuffed, it will need to be deflated to continue the assessment. It is vitally important that the client's physician authorize cuff deflation. Due to other health issues, cuff deflation may be life threatening. If this is the case, postpone further laryngeal evaluation and presentation of food or liquid until the client is more medically stable. If the client can tolerate cuff deflation, deflate the cuff and continue the assessment of laryngeal function.

The Blue-Dye Test

The blue-dye test is a useful tool for determining whether a client is aspirating. Ideally, a blue-dye test is administered over several sessions and days with only one texture introduced per day. This allows the most accurate assessment of the client's abilities to manage varying textures. Follow these five steps to administer a blue-dye test:

1. Ask a respiratory therapist to suction the mouth, the tracheostomy region, and the lungs. If the cuff is still inflated, deflate it now (with physician approval).
2. Add blue food coloring to food or liquid, preferably testing only one texture at a time.
3. Present small amounts of the blue-dyed food or liquid to the client and occlude the tracheostomy tube during every swallow.
4. Suction again and look for the presence of blue dye in the tracheal region.
5. Repeat suctioning every 15 minutes for the next hour, and monitor the tracheal area for blue dye for the next 24 hours. It is important to let other caregivers know that a blue-dye test is in progress so that they can continue to watch for blue coloring in your absence. Form 15-5, "Blue-Dye Test Worksheet," can be posted at the client's bedside to assist in this process. Interpretation: Any positive identification of blue food coloring in the tracheal region indicates that some degree of aspiration has occurred.

The blue-dye test can also be used to assess a client's management of his or her saliva even if no food or liquid is introduced. Dab a small amount of blue food coloring on the client's tongue and monitor the tracheal region in the same manner as if food or liquid had been introduced.

The blue-dye test is a very useful assessment tool, but we must offer this word of caution concerning its reliability: the *presence* of blue dye in the tracheal region will positively identify aspiration; however, the *absence* of blue dye does not necessarily mean the absence of aspiration (Dikeman & Kazandjian, 2003). For this reason, do not use the blue-dye test exclusively to assess for dysphagia.

GRAPHIC IMAGING

Clinical assessment is often inadequate for diagnosing dysphagia. There are two widely used approaches for graphically viewing swallowing function. These are videofluoroscopy and videoendoscopy. Both approaches allow later in-depth analysis of swallowing ability by way of videotaping the studies.

Videofluoroscopy

A videofluorographic swallowing study (VFSS) is a radiographic examination that provides a motion X-ray of the swallow. The procedure may also be called a modified barium swallow (MBS) or oral pharyngeal motility study (OPMS). During the assessment, the client is presented with barium mixture of varying consistencies (e.g., thin liquid, thick liquid, pudding) and sometimes food coated with barium (e.g., cracker, banana). The client swallows the barium mixture as the examiner observes the progression of the barium through the oral and pharyngeal cavities and into the esophagus.

The test allows the clinician to determine whether a client is aspirating or penetrating the airway. It also helps to identify the specific site of aspiration or penetration, its cause, and possible strategies that will increase swallowing safety for the client, such as changing head positioning or modifying bolus size. Although the examination is administered by a radiologist, the speech-language pathologist should make explicit requests about positioning, food consistencies, and compensatory strategies that need to be included as part of the study. When possible, the clinician should be present during the examination to maximize its diagnostic benefits.

Videofluoroscopy is currently the preferred method of graphic assessment because it provides more complete diagnostic information. However, in many situations videofluoroscopy is not feasible. Videoendoscopy is an acceptable alternative in these situations.

Videoendoscopy

Videoendoscopy uses endoscopic equipment to allow the clinician to view the oral and pharyngeal structures before and after the swallow. The procedure is also called fiberoptic endoscopic examination of swallowing (FEES). During the assessment, a small, flexible scope is passed through the nose down to the level of the soft palate. The scope allows the clinician to view pharyngeal and laryngeal structures before and after swallowing, but not during the swallow. Various food consistencies and textures can be presented, or the clinician can view the client's ability to manage saliva in the absence of food or liquid.

The test allows the clinician to monitor overall condition of the swallow, whether there is adequate airway protection, overall timing of the swallow, whether spillage occurs before the swallow, presence of residue after the swallow, ability to clear residue, presence of reflux, and presence of aspiration. Strategies for improving swallow safety and efficiency by way of postural changes, diet modifications, and swallowing maneuvers can also be identified. Videoendoscopy can be done as a bedside procedure.

CONCLUDING COMMENTS

Although dysphagia is not a disorder of communication, its evaluation and treatment are frequently under the domain of the speech-language pathologist. It is a potentially life-threatening disorder and should be evaluated with caution and a thorough understanding of dysphagia. It is important to communicate regularly with a client's physician and other health care professionals so that the client's health and safety are not jeopardized. A clinical or bedside evaluation is often adequate for making diagnostic conclusions about a client with suspected dysphagia; however, there are cases when a graphic study is necessary for completing a thorough examination.

There are diagnostic procedures unique to tracheostomized clients that are followed when completing a dysphagia evaluation. The client's physician and respiratory therapist are invaluable sources of assistance and information. It is especially important to discuss the assessment protocol with the physician prior to completing the evaluation to determine whether the client is medically stable enough to tolerate the assessment. The blue-dye test can be administered to detect aspiration in a tracheostomized client.

SOURCES OF ADDITIONAL INFORMATION

Print Sources

Arvedson, J. C., & Brodsky, L. (2002). *Pediatric swallowing and feeding: Assessment and management* (2nd ed.). Clifton Park, NY: Cengage Learning.

Cichero, J., & Murdoch, B. (Eds.) (2006). *Dysphagia: Foundation, theory and practice.* Indianapolis: Wiley.

Corbin-Lewis, K., Liss, J. M., & Sciortino, K. L. (2005). *Clinical anatomy and physiology of the swallow mechanism.* Clifton Park, NY: Cengage Learning.

Leonard, R., & Kendall, K. (2013). *Dysphagia assessment and treatment planning: A team approach* (3rd ed.). San Diego, CA: Plural.

Murry, T., & Carrau, R. (2012). *Clinical management of swallowing disorders* (3rd ed.). San Diego, CA: Plural.

Swigert, N. B. (2007). *The source for dysphagia* (3rd ed.). East Moline, IL: LinguiSystems.

Swigert, N. B. (2009). *The source for pediatric dysphasia* (2nd ed.). East Moline, IL: LinguiSystems.

Electronic Sources

American Speech-Language-Hearing Association:
http://www.asha.org

Dysphagia Online:
http://www.dysphagiaonline.com

National Foundation of Swallowing Disorders:
http://swallowingdisorderfoundation.com/

"Aspiration Disorders" app by Blue Tree Publishing. Inc.

"Dysphagia" app by Northern Speech Services

Form 15-1.

Pediatric Dysphagia Case History Form
and Caregiver Questionnaire—Infant 0–6 months

General Information

Name: _____ Date of birth: _____

Chronological age: _____ Adjusted age: _____

Birth weight: _____ Current weight: _____

Home address: _____

City: _____ Zip code: _____

Does the child live with both parents? _____

Mother's name: _____ Home phone: _____

Business phone: _____ Cell phone: _____

Father's name: _____ Home phone: _____

Business phone: _____ Cell phone: _____

Referred by: _____

Address: _____

Reason for referral: _____

Primary care physician: _____ Phone: _____

Address: _____

Other physicians or specialists treating child: _____

_____

Brothers and sisters (include names and ages): _____

_____

_____

_____

Prenatal and Birth History

Mother's general health during pregnancy (illnesses, accidents, medications, etc.):

List any medications taken during the pregnancy.

(continues)

Form 15-1. continued

Length of pregnancy: _____   Length of labor: _____

General condition: _____

Apgar scores (if known): _____

Circle type of delivery: head first   feet first   breech   Caesarian

Were there any unusual conditions that may have affected the pregnancy?

Were there any complications during the delivery?

Were there any complications immediately after the birth?

Child's Medical History

List medical diagnoses.

List any medications the child has taken, or is currently taking.

Has the child had any surgeries? If yes, describe.

Form 15-1. continued

Describe any major accidents or hospitalizations.

Has the child had any breathing problems, either occasional, recurring, or continuous? If yes, please describe.

Has the child experienced any illnesses (e.g., ear infection, allergy, high fever, seizure, pneumonia, other)?

Child's Feeding and Swallowing History

Was the child breast-fed? If yes, for how long? Were there any difficulties?

When was the child first given a bottle? Were there any difficulties?

Was the child ever fed through a feeding tube? If yes, why? What type of tube? For how long?

(continues)

Form 15-1. continued

Current Feeding and Swallowing Status

How is the child normally positioned during a meal (e.g., lying down, held with head slightly elevated, etc.)?

Describe nutritional intake in a typical day. Include time of day, duration of meal (in minutes), and amount consumed per meal.

Does the child receive supplemental tube feedings? If yes, how often? Duration of meal? Bolus size? Type of tube used?

How does the child let you know he or she is hungry?

How does the child let you know he or she is full?

Form 15-1. continued

Please check behaviors you have observed during or immediately after a meal.

Struggle swallowing _____   Struggle breathing _____   Reflux _____

Fussiness _____   Falling asleep _____   Spitting food_____

Refusal to eat _____   Gurgly voice _____   Vomiting _____

Food/liquid coming out of nose _____

Please provide further description of all items checked.

In general, are mealtimes a pleasant experience? If no, explain.

Please describe any additional observations or concerns about the child's feeding and swallowing status.

Person completing form:_____

Relationship to child: _____

Signed: _____ Date: _____

Form 15-2.

Pediatric Dysphagia Case History Form and Caregiver Questionnaire

General Information

Name: _____   Date of birth: _____

Chronological age: _____   Adjusted age: _____

Birth weight: _____   Current weight: _____

Home address: _____

City: _____   Zip code: _____

Does the child live with both parents? _____

Mother's name: _____   Home phone: _____

Business phone: _____   Cell phone: _____

Father's name: _____   Home phone: _____

Business phone: _____   Cell phone: _____

Referred by: _____

Address: _____

Reason for referral: _____

Primary care physician: _____   Phone: _____

Address: _____

Other physicians or specialists treating child: _____

_____

Brothers and sisters (include names and ages): _____

_____

_____

_____

Prenatal and Birth History

Mother's general health during pregnancy (illnesses, accidents, medications, etc.):

List any medications taken during the pregnancy.

(continues)

Form 15-2. continued

Length of pregnancy: _____   Length of labor: _____

General condition: _____

Apgar scores (if known): _____

Circle type of delivery: head first   feet first   breech   Caesarian

Were there any unusual conditions that may have affected the pregnancy?

Were there any complications during the delivery?

Were there any complications immediately after the birth?

Child's Medical History
List medical diagnoses and concerns.

Form 15-2. continued

List any medications the child has taken, or is currently taking.

Has the child had any surgeries? If yes, describe.

Describe any major accidents or hospitalizations.

Has the child had any breathing problems, either occasional, recurring, or continuous? If yes, please describe.

Has the child experienced any illnesses (e.g., ear infection, allergy, high fever, seizure, pneumonia, other)?

(continues)

Form 15-2. continued

Child's Developmental History

Provide the approximate age at which the child began to do the following activities:

Crawl _____ Sit _____ Stand _____

Walk _____ Feed self _____ Dress self _____

Use toilet _____ Use single words _____ Sleep through night _____

Does the child have difficulty walking, running, or participating in other activities that require small or large muscle coordination?

Does the child have difficulty with speech production?

Do you have any concerns about the child's development to date?

Child's Educational History

School: _____ Grade: _____

Teacher: _____

How is the child doing academically?

Form 15-2. continued

How does the child interact with others (e.g., shy, aggressive, uncooperative)?

Does the child receive special services? If yes, describe.

Has an individualized education plan (IEP) been developed? If yes, please describe the most important goals.

Child's Feeding and Swallowing History

Was the child breast-fed? If yes, for how long? Were there any difficulties?

Was the child ever fed through a feeding tube? If yes, why? What type of tube? For how long?

(continues)

Form 15-2. continued

Provide the approximate age at which the child began to do the following activities:

Drink from a bottle _____ Eat solid foods _____

Eat from a spoon _____ Self-feed with fingers _____

Self-feed with spoon _____ Drink from a cup _____

Discontinue bottle _____ Discontinue pacifier _____

Current Feeding and Swallowing Status

Describe nutritional intake in a typical day. Include time of day, duration of meal (in minutes), food consumed, and amount consumed per meal.

How is the child normally positioned during a meal (e.g., high chair, lying down, infant seat, etc.)?

Is any adaptive equipment used?

List food likes/dislikes.

Form 15-2. continued

List foods that the child has difficulty eating or drinking. Describe difficulty.

Does the child take nutritional supplements? If yes, describe.

Does the child drool? If yes, how often?

How does the child let you know he or she is hungry?

How does the child let you know he or she is full?

(continues)

Form 15-2. continued

Please check behaviors you have observed during or immediately after a meal:

Choking _____ Gagging _____ Crying _____

Struggle swallowing _____ Struggle breathing _____ Reflux _____

Fussiness _____ Falling asleep _____ Spitting food _____

Refusal to eat _____ Gurgly voice _____ Vomiting _____

Food/liquid coming out of nose _____

Please provide further description of all items checked.

In general, are mealtimes a pleasant experience? If no, explain.

Form 15-2. continued

Please describe any other observations or concerns about the child's feeding and swallowing status.

Person completing form: _____

Relationship to child: _____

Signed: _____ Date: _____

Form 15-3.

Pediatric Dysphagia Clinical Evaluation

Name: _____ DOB: _____

Chronological age: _____ Adjusted age: _____

Summary of Medical History: _____

_____

_____

Summary of Current Feeding Status: _____

_____

_____

Examiner's Name: _____ Date: _____

Make a check (✓) or fill in the appropriate information for the items below. The clinician can circle one of several possible features seen with some items. Comments of any observations can be next to various items.

Alertness

Before feeding	During feeding	After feeding	
_____	_____	_____	Deep sleep
_____	_____	_____	Light sleep
_____	_____	_____	Drowsy/semi-dozing
_____	_____	_____	Quiet alert
_____	_____	_____	Active alert
_____	_____	_____	Alert agitated
_____	_____	_____	Crying

Difficulty waking child? yes/no

Physiologic Status

Before feeding	During feeding	After feeding	
_____	_____	_____	Heart rate (HR)
_____	_____	_____	Oxygen saturation (SaO$_2$)
_____	_____	_____	Respiratory rate (RR)

(continues)

Form 15-3. continued

Describe respiratory pattern before feeding.

Describe respiratory pattern after feeding.

Apnea? yes/no

Primitive Reflexes

_____ Asymmetric tonic neck: present/absent

_____ Babkin: present/absent

_____ Gag: present/absent/overactive

_____ Moro: present/absent

_____ Palmar grasp: present/absent

_____ Phasic bite: present/absent

_____ Rooting: present/absent

_____ Suckling/Sucking: present/absent

_____ Swallow: present/absent

_____ Tongue thrust: present/absent

Abnormal Reflexes

Note abnormal reflexes observed during feeding:

_____ Tonic bite: absent/present/able to stimulate opening of jaw

_____ Jaw thrust: lower jaw is extended down and appears to be stuck open

_____ Tongue retraction: tongue is pulled back into the hypopharynx; the tip of the tongue may be held against the hard palate

Form 15-3. continued

Physical Strength, Stability, and Posture

_____ General muscle tone: normal/flaccid/tense/fluctuating

_____ Head control/stability: good/poor/emerging

_____ Head/neck/trunk alignment: good/hyperextension of neck

_____ Shoulder alignment: good/elevated/retracted/adducted

_____ Pelvic stability: good/poor/emerging

_____ Trunk stability: good/poor/emerging

Orofacial Structures

Jaw

_____ Size: normal/large/small

_____ Position at rest: normal/protruded/retracted/clenched

_____ Movement: normal/reduced on right/reduced on left/restricted/thrust

_____ Strength: normal/weak

_____ Teeth present: no/yes

Additional comments:

Cheeks

_____ Position at rest: normal/asymmetrical

_____ Tone: normal/flaccid/tense

_____ Strength: normal/weak

Additional comments:

(continues)

Form 15-3. continued

Lips

_____ Position at rest: normal/asymmetrical/open

_____ Tone: normal/flaccid/tense

_____ Strength: normal/weak

_____ Movement: normal/reduced on right/reduced on left

_____ Structural deviance: none/cleft/scar

_____ Drooling: none/mild/moderate/excessive

Additional comments:

Tongue

_____ Size: normal/large/small/atrophy

_____ Tone: normal/flaccid/tense

_____ Position at rest: normal/protruded/retracted/flat/thick/bunched

_____ Movements at rest: none/tremor/fasciculation

_____ Strength: normal/weak

_____ Protrusion: normal/restricted/thrust/reduced on right/reduced on left

_____ Lateralization: normal/reduced on right/reduced on left/thrusting

_____ Elevation: normal/restricted

Additional comments:

Palate

_____ Position at rest: normal/asymmetrical

_____ Cleft: none/hard palate/soft palate/cleft type: _____

Additional comments:

Form 15-3. continued

Pharynx/Larynx

_____ Vocal quality: normal/wet/gurgly

_____ Gag: normal/absent/hyperactive

Additional comments:

Facial Sensitivity

_____ Face: normal/hypersensitive/hyposensitive

_____ Mouth: normal/hypersensitive/hyposensitive

Additional comments:

Feeding Presentation

_____ Method: breast/bottle/bottle type: _____

_____ Position: supine/head slightly elevated/prone/on side

Additional comments:

Stress Cues During Feeding

Mild-Moderate Stress Cues

_____ Change in facial expression: glassy/stare/panic/worry/smile/grimace/averted gaze

_____ Crying: silent/weak/strong

_____ Change in body movement: squirm/twitch/tremor/excessive movements

_____ Change in muscle tone: flaccid/tense/hypertonic/hypotonic

_____ Gasping: silent/audible

_____ Sweating

(continues)

Form 15-3. continued

Severe Stress Cues

_____ Gagging

_____ Coughing

_____ Choking: silent/audible

_____ Reflux: spit up/vomit

_____ Change in skin color: flushed/blue/grey/mottled/paling around nostrils

_____ Change in respiration: rate increase/irregular/struggle/apnea/noisy

_____ Change in heart rate: bradycardia/tachycardia

_____ Change in oxygen saturation levels: decrease/increase

Additional comments:

Sucking Observations

Non-nutritive Sucking

_____ Burst cycles: _____

_____ Endurance: normal/reduced/total time (from onset to fatigue): _____

_____ Labial seal on finger/nipple: adequate/weak

_____ Lingual cupping: present/absent

_____ Suck strength: adequate/weak

_____ Respiration: normal/uncoordinated/struggle (describe): _____

Additional comments:

Form 15-3. continued

Nutritive Sucking

_____ Burst cycles at onset: _____ Pattern of decline: normal/too rapid

_____ Endurance: normal/reduced/total time (from onset to finish): _____

_____ Amount consumed: _____

_____ Fluid loss at seal: normal/none/excessive

_____ Lingual cupping: present/absent

_____ Suck strength: adequate/weak

_____ Suckle/swallow ratio: at beginning _____ at end _____

_____ Fluid expression: good/fair/poor

_____ Respiration: normal/uncoordinated/struggle (describe) _____

_____ Swallow reflex: normal/delayed/absent/multiple swallows

_____ Pharyngeal response: none/cough/gag/wet voice/wet breathing

Additional comments:

Spoon Feeding Observations

_____ Food presented: thick puree/thin puree/ground/chopped

_____ Fed by: caregiver/self

_____ Removal: suckle/suck

_____ Clearance of food with lips: all/most/some/none

_____ Loss of food: none/minimal/excessive

_____ Mandibular movement: normal/thrust

_____ Lingual movement: normal/thrust/retracted/residue after swallow

_____ Amount consumed: _____ Time taken: _____

Additional comments:

(continues)

Form 15-3. continued

Cup Feeding Observations

_____ Liquid presented: thin/thick

_____ Cup type: normal/cut-out/free-flow lid/suck-release lid

_____ Cup stabilization: tongue under cup/bite

_____ Fed by: caregiver/self

_____ Removal: suckle/suck

_____ Lingual movement: normal/thrust/retracted/pooling after swallow

_____ Loss of liquid: none/minimal/excessive

_____ Mandibular movement: normal/thrust

_____ Amount consumed: _____ Time taken: _____

Additional comments:

Bite/Chew Observations

_____ Food presented: chopped/chewy/soft/hard

_____ Loss of food: none/minimal/excessive

_____ Lingual control: good/reduced

_____ Mandibular movement: rotary/up-down

_____ Labial movement: coordinated/uncoordinated

_____ Amount consumed: _____ Time taken: _____

Additional comments:

Swallow Observations

_____ Pharyngeal swallow: normal/delayed/absent/multiple swallows

_____ Pharyngeal response: cough/gag/choke

_____ Vocal quality after swallow: normal/wet/gurgly

Additional comments:

Stimulability

List compensatory strategies attempted. Describe response.

Recommendations

Food type(s):

Position:

Presentation:

Feeding schedule:

Adaptive equipment:

Further assessment:

Other:

Form 15-4.

Adult Bedside Dysphagia Evaluation

Name: _____ Age: _____ Date: _____

Examiner's Name: _____

PART I

Current medical/neurological status: _____

Current medications: _____

Current feeding status: _____

Dietary limitations: _____

Cognitive status: _____

Ask the client to do the following. Model as necessary. Make a check (✓) in the left-hand column and circle any observations.

Jaw

_____ Open and close mouth: normal/incomplete/deviates right/deviates left

_____ Open and close mouth against mild pressure: normal/weak

Is the client groping?

Look at the client's dentition. Make a note of abnormal occlusion or missing teeth.

Does the client wear dentures or partials? If yes, do they fit properly?

(continues)

Form 15-4. continued

Lips

_____ Pucker the lips: normal/reduced excursion

_____ Smile: normal/droops right/droops left/droops bilaterally

_____ Protrude tongue: normal/droops right/droops left/droops bilaterally

_____ Say "mamamamama": normal/poor labial seal

_____ Hold air in the cheeks: normal/poor labial seal/nasal emission

Is the client drooling? If yes, from which side?

Brush the lips lightly with hot, cold, sweet, and lemon-flavored cotton-tip swabs. How does the client respond to the different stimuli?

Tongue

Lick lips: normal/incomplete excursion

_____ Protrude tongue: normal/deviates right/deviates left

_____ Elevate tongue: normal/incomplete excursion

_____ Say "lalalalala": normal/slow/poor alveolar contact

_____ Say "gagagagaga": normal/slow/poor velar contact

Is the client's articulation normal? Is dysarthria present?

Brush the tongue lightly with hot, cold, sweet, and lemon-flavored cotton-tip swabs. How does the client respond to the different stimuli?

Form 15-4. continued

Pharynx

_____ Sustain "ah" (observe velopharyngeal movement): normal/absent/weak on right/weak on left/hypernasal

Is a gag reflex present? If yes, is it abnormal? Describe the reflex (e.g., hypoactive, hyperactive, delayed).

Larynx

_____ Say "ah" for 5 seconds: normal/unable to sustain

_____ Clear your throat: normal/weak/absent

_____ Cough: normal/weak/absent

_____ Swallow (feel laryngeal movement): larynx elevates normally/reduced excursion

_____ Change pitch upward: normal/reduced range

_____ Say "ah" and get louder: normal/no intensity change

_____ Say "ah" (note voice quality): normal/wet/breathy/hoarse

PART II

Check the behaviors the client exhibits for each texture presented. Also note whether the client is aware of difficulties and is able to compensate appropriately. *Caution: Do not administer the feeding portion of this evaluation without some prior training and experience, or without the direct supervision of a trained and knowledgeable professional.*

	Puree	Chopped	Regular	Liquid
Food falls out of mouth (indicate side)	_____	_____	_____	_____
Food is pushed out of mouth	_____	_____	_____	_____
Struggle while chewing	_____	_____	_____	_____
Unable to form bolus	_____	_____	_____	_____
Unable to move bolus side-to-side	_____	_____	_____	_____

(continues)

Form 15-4. continued

	Puree	Chopped	Regular	Liquid
Unable to move bolus back to pharynx	_____	_____	_____	_____
Pocketing of food (indicate location)	_____	_____	_____	_____
Multiple attempts to swallow	_____	_____	_____	_____
Residual food on tongue	_____	_____	_____	_____
Residual food on hard palate	_____	_____	_____	_____
Unable to suck liquid through a straw	_____	_____	_____	_____
Difficulty grasping cup with lips	_____	_____	_____	_____
Difficulty holding straw with lips	_____	_____	_____	_____
Nasal regurgitation	_____	_____	_____	_____
Swallow too rapid	_____	_____	_____	_____
Swallow delayed (indicate seconds)	_____	_____	_____	_____
Laryngeal elevation absent	_____	_____	_____	_____
Laryngeal elevation delayed (indicate seconds)	_____	_____	_____	_____
Laryngeal elevation incomplete	_____	_____	_____	_____
Coughing after swallow	_____	_____	_____	_____
Throat clearing after swallow	_____	_____	_____	_____
Wet voice quality after swallow	_____	_____	_____	_____
Excessive saliva and mucus present	_____	_____	_____	_____
Oral regurgitation	_____	_____	_____	_____

Was the client aware of difficulties?

What did the client do to compensate for chewing or swallowing problems?

Form 15-5.

Blue-Dye Test Worksheet

<u>Attention</u>

A 24-hour Blue-Dye Test is in progress

Date: _____ Start time: _____

Please indicate below if blue coloring is suctioned or observed in the tracheal region.

Time: _____ Location of blue coloring: _____
Observed by: _____
Other comments: _____
_____

Time: _____ Location of blue coloring: _____
Observed by: _____
Other comments: _____
_____

Time: _____ Location of blue coloring: _____
Observed by: _____
Other comments: _____
_____

Please consult the speech–language pathologist as needed for further explanation or comments.

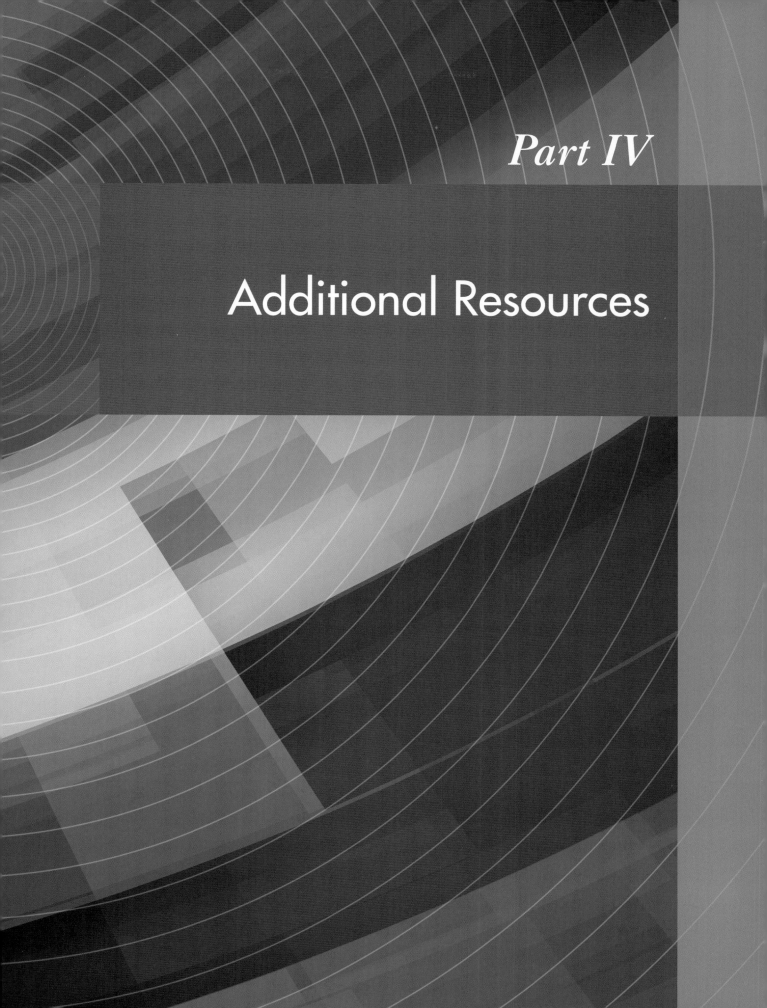

Part IV

Additional Resources

Chapter 16

HEARING CONSIDERATIONS

The assessment of hearing is within the professional province of the audiologist, not the speech-language pathologist. However, the speech-language clinician is interested in clients' hearing abilities since hearing loss directly affects the development or maintenance of optimal communicative skills. Specifically, we are interested in the effects of hearing impairment on:

• The assessment of communicative development and abilities
• The development or maintenance of a communication disorder
• Treatment recommendations and the selection of appropriate treatment procedures and target behaviors
• Academic, social, or vocational development

Even though speech-language pathologists are limited to screening a client's hearing, it is important for clinicians to understand hearing loss, audiological assessment procedures, interpretation of findings Clinicians, and implications of hearing loss on speech and language development.

OVERVIEW OF COMMON HEARING PATHOLOGIES

There are three types of hearing loss: conductive, sensorineural, and mixed. In addition, it is helpful for speech-language pathologists to have basic knowledge of auditory processing disorder and retrocochlear pathology. These conditions are described in this section. To help with foundational understanding of ear anatomy in relation to these pathologies, a pictorial representation of the ear is presented in Figure 16-1.

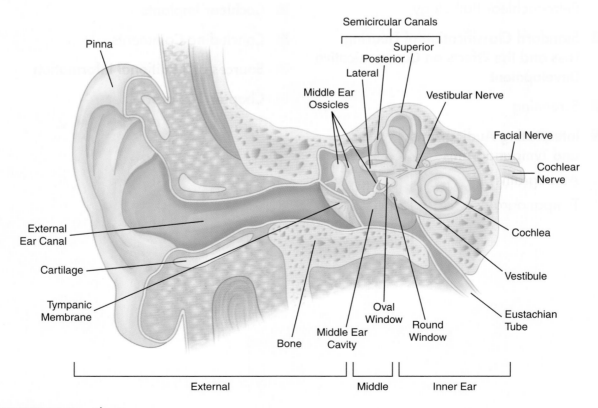

FIGURE 16-1. The Ear

Conductive Hearing Loss

A conductive hearing loss occurs when the transmission of sound is interrupted. This occurs in the outer ear or, more frequently, in the middle ear. In children, the most common cause of middle ear dysfunction is otitis media, or middle ear infection. (See "Medical Conditions Associated with Communicative Disorders" in Chapter 17 and the Glossary for descriptions of otitis media.) In adults, the most common cause of conductive hearing impairment is otosclerosis, a disease of the middle ear ossicles that may cause the footplate of the stapes to attach to the oval window. The most common cause of conductive hearing impairment among the geriatric population is ear canal collapse. Other less common causes of conductive hearing loss are aural atresia (closed external auditory canal), stenosis (narrow external auditory canal), and external otitis (infected and swollen external auditory canal; also known as "swimmer's ear").

Sensorineural Hearing Loss

A sensorineural hearing loss occurs when the hair cells of the cochlea or the acoustic nerve (CN VIII) are damaged. The impairment is associated with the loss of hearing through bone conduction, and it is considered a permanent impairment. Causes of sensorineural hearing loss include:

- Ototoxicity, or damage from drugs (including certain antibiotics)
- Infections, such as meningitis or maternal rubella
- Genetic factors, such as certain birth defects that result in partially developed or missing parts of the cochlea or auditory nerve
- Anoxia or syphilis contracted during the birth delivery
- Presbycusis associated with the effects of aging
- Ménière's disease, a unilateral disease that is characterized by vertigo (dizziness) and tinnitus (noise in the ear)

Mixed Hearing Loss

Mixed hearing losses involve a combination of a conductive and sensorineural loss. Both air and bone conduction pathways are involved so the hearing loss is partially conductive and partially sensorineural, but the hearing by bone conduction is typically the better of the two. The sensorineural component of a mixed hearing loss determines the amount of speech sound distortion that is present. Thus, bone conduction audiograms are the best indicators of the degree of difficulty a client will have recognizing and discriminating speech, even if it has been amplified.

Auditory Processing Disorder

Auditory processing disorder (APD), also called *central auditory processing disorder* (CAPD), is a neurological condition that stems from problems in the auditory center of the brain. Hearing acuity and intelligence are normal, yet the client is unable to process auditory information normally. Clients with APD may have difficulties detecting or localizing sound or discriminating speech. Noisy or highly distracting environments tend to worsen the difficulties. Tinnitus may also be present.

Children with APD often struggle academically. They may be unable to follow complex verbal directions, exhibit spelling and reading deficits, have difficulty engaging in class discussions, or have difficulty focusing and completing assignments. The symptoms of APD are similar to those of other conditions, such as dyslexia, attention deficit disorder, autism spectrum disorder, or specific language impairment. It is important to differentiate APD from other disorders, and to be aware that APD may coexist with these other conditions. Although the assessment and diagnosis of APD is primarily the responsibility of an audiologist, a speech-language pathologist may participate as a member of a diagnostic team.

Retrocochlear Pathology

Retrocochlear pathology involves damage to the nerve fibers along the ascending auditory pathways from the internal auditory meatus to the cortex. This damage is often, but not always, the result of a tumor. Depending on the pathology, a hearing loss may or may not be detected when hearing is tested with pure tones. However, many clients with retrocochlear pathology perform poorly on speech-recognition tasks, particularly when the speech signal is altered by filtering, adding noise, and so forth. Several speech-recognition tests as well as auditory brainstem response (ABR) tests and other auditory evoked potentials help identify the presence of retrocochlear pathology. Such testing is clearly beyond the province of the speech-language pathologist and, depending on their training and the equipment available to them, some audiologists as well.

STANDARD CLASSIFICATION OF HEARING LOSS AND THE EFFECTS ON COMMUNICATIVE DEVELOPMENT

Hearing losses vary in severity from individual to individual. A frequently used standard classification system for describing severity levels of hearing loss is presented in Table 16-1. The classifications described are related to average hearing levels obtained during pure tone audiometry. Because hearing losses vary immensely, their influence on speech and language development also varies. Logically, the greater the severity of the hearing loss, the greater its potential negative impact on speech and language. You can easily see this relationship in Table 16-2, which presents the rehabilitative and communicative effects of hearing loss at different severity levels. Keep in mind that the guidelines are general. Hearing loss affects individuals differently, regardless of severity, and specific intervention is dependent on such factors as:

- The type of loss
- The dB levels and frequencies affected
- Age of onset

TABLE 16-1   Description of Hearing Loss Severity by Decibel Levels

HEARING LEVEL (IN DB)	SEVERITY OF HEARING LOSS
−10 to 15	Normal hearing
16 to 25	Slight hearing loss
26 to 40	Mild hearing loss
41 to 55	Moderate hearing loss
56 to 70	Moderately severe hearing loss
71 to 90	Severe hearing loss
91+	Profound hearing loss

TABLE 16-2   Effects of Hearing Loss on Communication and Types of Habilitative Intervention with Children

Minimal hearing loss (16- to 25-dB HL)	At 15 dB a student can miss up to 10% of the speech signal when a teacher is at a distance greater than 3 feet and when the classroom is noisy.
Mild hearing loss (26- to 40-dB HL)	With a 30-dB loss, a student can miss 25–40% of a speech signal. Without amplification, the child with 35-to 40-dB loss may miss at least 50% of class discussion.
Moderate hearing loss (41- to 55-dB HL)	Child understands conversational speech at a distance of 3 to 5 feet (face to face) only if structure and vocabulary are controlled. Without amplification, the amount of speech signal missed can be 50–75% with a 40-dB loss, and 80–100% with a 50-dB loss.
Moderate to severe hearing loss (56- to 70-dB HL)	Without amplification, conversation must be very loud to be understood. A 55-dB loss can cause a child to miss up to 100% of speech information.
Severe hearing loss (71- to 90-dB HL)	Without amplification, the child may hear loud voices about 1 foot from the ear. When amplified optimally, children with hearing ability of 90 dB or better should be able to identify environmental sounds and detect all the sounds of speech.
Profound hearing loss (>90-dB HL)	Aware of vibrations more than tonal patterns. May rely on vision rather than hearing as the primary avenue for communication and learning.
Unilateral hearing loss (normal hearing in one ear with the other ear exhibiting at least a mild permanent loss)	May have difficulty hearing faint or distant speech. Usually has difficulty localizing sounds and has greater difficulty understanding speech in background noise.

Source: Elena Plante and Pelagie Beeson, *Communication and Communication Disorders: A Clinical Introduction.* (p. 268)

- The client's age when the loss was diagnosed
- Previous intervention (e.g., therapy or educational placement, type of intervention, communication mode)
- Medical intervention (e.g., ongoing, sporadic)
- The client's intelligence
- The client's motivation
- The client's general health
- Care and stimulation provided by caregivers (For example, caregivers may provide speech and language stimulation in the home, learn sign language, learn how to "troubleshoot" hearing aid problems, or include the client in family activities.)

Figure 16-2 shows phonemes plotted on an audiogram according to frequency and loudness during normal conversational speech. Because of the shape of the speech zone, this is often referred to as the *speech banana*. Speech-language pathologists sometimes use the speech banana

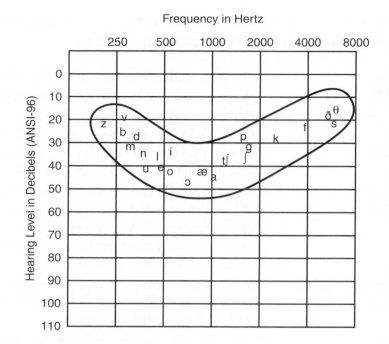

FIGURE 16-2 The Speech Banana

when counseling clients or caregivers on the effects of hearing loss on speech and language development. A client's audiological findings can also be superimposed over the speech banana audiogram to show which phonemes the individual may and may not be able to perceive.

SCREENING

Speech-language pathologists often provide a hearing screening as part of the complete diagnostic evaluation to identify a potential peripheral hearing loss that may affect a client's communicative development or abilities. When a client fails a screen, he or she should be referred to an audiologist for further evaluation.

Screens are typically administered at 20 or 25 dB for the frequencies 1000 Hz, 2000 Hz, and 4000 Hz. For some clients, particularly children, it is common to use more conservative criteria—15 dB at 500 Hz, 1000 Hz, 2000 Hz, 4000 Hz, and 8000 Hz—to reduce the risk of missing someone with a mild hearing loss. Form 16-1, the "Hearing Screening Form," is useful for recording findings.

INTERPRETING AUDIOGRAMS AND TYMPANOGRAMS

The audiologist is responsible for the complete evaluation and diagnosis of hearing impairment. However, the speech-language pathologist needs to understand hearing, how it is tested, how to interpret assessment results, and how the results apply to individual clients. The reference materials in this section are designed to help the speech-language pathologist more thoroughly understand a client's hearing impairment and its impact on the communicative disorder, diagnosis, treatment program, and referral process.

Audiograms are used to record the results of audiological testing. The symbols used on an audiogram are listed in Table 16-3. These symbols may be presented in differentiating

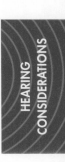

TABLE 16-3   Audiometric Symbols

Response

Recommended set of symbols for those cases when thresholds are measured.

MODALITY	EAR		
	LEFT	UNSPECIFIED	RIGHT
AIR CONDUCTION—EARPHONES			
UNMASKED	✗		◯
MASKED	☐		◁
BONE CONDUCTION—MASTOID			
UNMASKED	>	<	∨
MASKED	⌐		⌐
BONE CONDUCTION—FOREHEAD			
UNMASKED	⌐	>	⌐
MASKED			
AIR CONDUCTION—SOUND FIELD			
	✗	S	∅
ACOUSTIC—REFLEX THRESHOLD			
CONTRALATERAL	⌐		Y
IPSILATERAL	⊥		T

No Response

Recommended set of symbols for those cases when no responses are elicited.

MODALITY	EAR		
	LEFT	UNSPECIFIED	RIGHT
AIR CONDUCTION—EARPHONES			
UNMASKED	✗↙		◯↘
MASKED	☐↙	↔	◁↘
BONE CONDUCTION—MASTOID			
UNMASKED	↗	↦	↙
MASKED	⌐↗	↦	⌐↘
BONE CONDUCTION—FOREHEAD			
UNMASKED	⌐↙		⌐↘
MASKED			
AIR CONDUCTION—SOUND FIELD			
	✗↙	S↦	∅↘
ACOUSTIC—REFLEX THRESHOLD			
CONTRALATERAL	⌐↗		⌐↘
IPSILATERAL	⌐↗		⌐↘

Source: "Guidelines for Audiometric Symbols", *ASHA* (April 1991, Supplement No. 2), 32(4), 25–30. Copyright 1991 by the American Speech-Language-Hearing Association. Reprinted with permission.

colors to denote sidedness. If color is used, red represents the right side, and blue represents the left side.

Audiograms

The audiograms in Figures 16-3 through 16-9 illustrate several basic patterns of hearing loss. Exact configurations vary across individuals and according to the type, frequencies, and decibel levels of the loss. The hearing losses in these examples are bilateral (involving both ears), although unilateral hearing losses are also common.

The Three Basic Patterns (Conductive, Sensorineural, and Mixed Losses)

Figures 16-3 through 16-5

Various Patterns of Hearing Losses

Figures 16-6 through 16-9

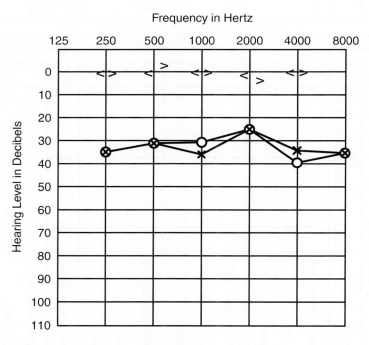

FIGURE 16-3 Audiogram of a Conductive Hearing Loss. (Note the airbone gap.)

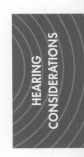

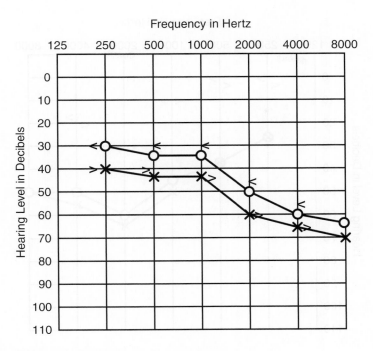

FIGURE 16-4   Audiogram of a Sensorineural Hearing Loss

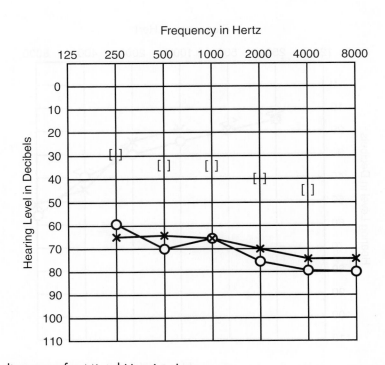

FIGURE 16-5   Audiogram of a Mixed Hearing Loss

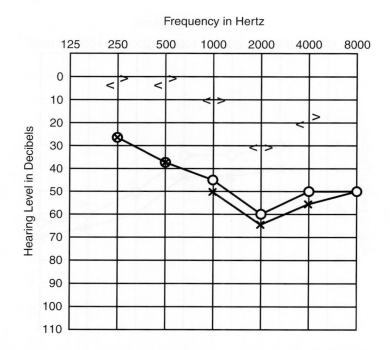

FIGURE 16-6   Audiogram of a Conductive Hearing Loss Caused by Otosclerosis. (Note the Carhart notch in bone conduction.)

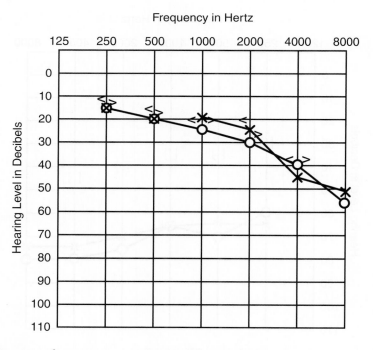

FIGURE 16-7   Audiogram of a Hearing Loss Caused by Presbycusis

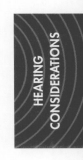

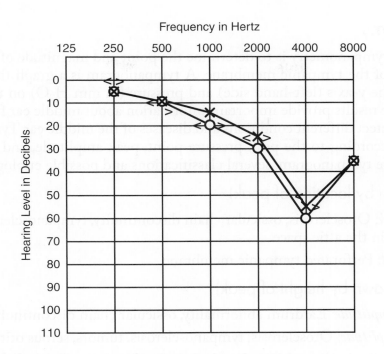

FIGURE 16-8 Audiogram of a Noise-Induced Sensorineural Hearing Loss

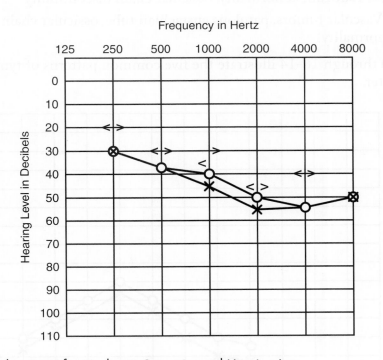

FIGURE 16-9 Audiogram of a Moderate Sensorineural Hearing Loss

Tympanograms

The purpose of tympanometry is to determine the point and magnitude of greatest compliance (mobility) of the tympanic membrane. A tympanogram is a graph that illustrates the compliance on the y-axis (left-hand side) and pressure (in mm H_2O) on the x-axis (across the bottom). The results provide important information about middle ear function and help diagnosticians detect different conditions and diseases of the middle ear. Tympanograms can be interpreted according to the peak pressure point, peak amplitude, and shape. Based on dimensions of the tympanogram, several classifications and possible etiologies are:

Pressure (shown by location of peak)

- *Normal peak*: Otosclerosis, ossicular chain discontinuity, tympanosclerosis, cholesteatoma in the attic space
- *No peak/flat*: Perforated tympanic membrane

Compliance (shown by height of peak)

- *Increased amplitude*: Eardrum abnormality, ossicular chain discontinuity
- *Reduced amplitude*: Otosclerosis, tympanosclerosis, tumors, serous otitis media
- *Normal amplitude*: Eustachian tube blockage, early acute otitis media

Shape (shown by slope)

- *Reduced slope*: Otosclerosis, ossicular chain fixation, otitis media with effusion, tumor
- *Increased slope*: Eardrum abnormality, ossicular chain discontinuity
- *Not smooth*: Vascular tumors, patulous eustachian tube, ossicular chain discontinuity, eardrum abnormality

Figures 16-10 through 16-14 illustrate the five common patterns of tympanograms that clinicians encounter.

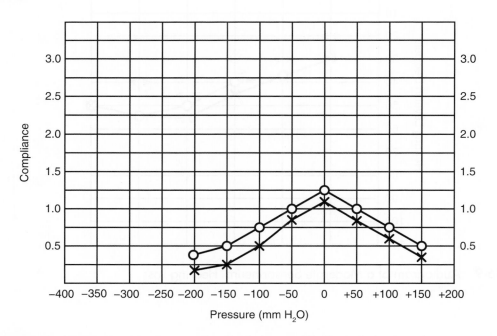

FIGURE 16-10   Type A Tympanogram—Normal Pressure and Compliance Functions

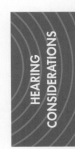

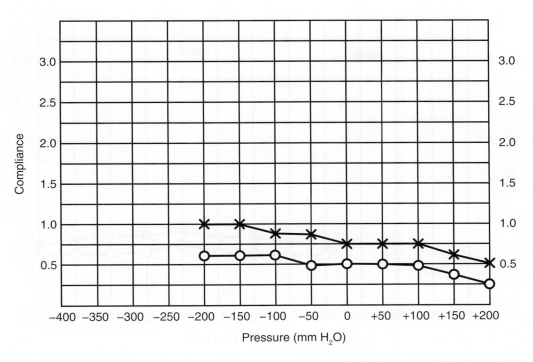

FIGURE 16-11 Type B Tympanogram—Fluid in the Middle Ear (flat). This May Indicate Otitis Media

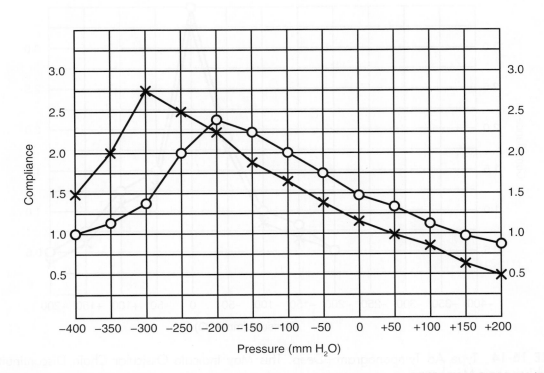

FIGURE 16-12 Type C Tympanogram—Retracted Tympanic Membranes (Shift to Negative Side). This May Indicate Eustachian Tube Blockage or Otitis Media

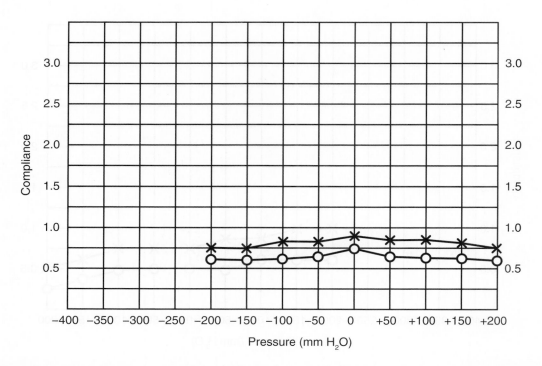

FIGURE 16-13 Type As Tympanogram—Shallow. This May Indicate Otosclerosis or Tympanosclerosis

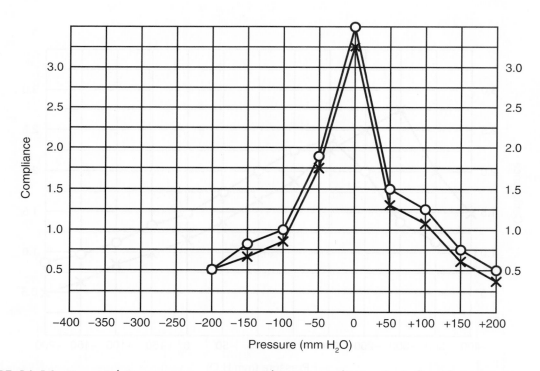

FIGURE 16-14 Type Ad Tympanogram—Deep. This May Indicate Ossicular Chain Discontinuity or Flaccid Tympanic Membrane

SPEECH AUDIOMETRY

Speech audiometry evaluates a client's ability to hear and understand speech. It can also be useful for assessing the effects of amplification. Two important speech audiometric findings are *Speech Reception Threshold* (SRT) and *Speech Recognition* scores. An SRT indicates the lowest decibel level at which a client can correctly identify a standard list of two-syllable words (called *spondees*) 50% of the time. *Cupcake*, *baseball*, and *hotdog* are examples of spondee words. A normal SRT is within plus or minus 6 dB from the pure tone average (average of pure tone thresholds at 500 Hz, 1000 Hz, and 2000 Hz).

The speech recognition score reveals the client's ability to recognize words. The test is administered at a comfortable decibel level above the SRT. The client is asked to select the correct word from similar-sounding pairs (*cat-bat*, *beach-peach*, etc.), or to repeat back single words (*day*, *cap*, etc.). A normal score is 90–100% correct.

ENVIRONMENTAL NOISE LEVELS

Table 16-4 lists several environmental noises that occur at different decibel levels. This information is useful for counseling clients or their caregivers about hearing loss and its effect on communication.

TABLE 16-4   Environmental Noise Levels

dB LEVEL	ENVIRONMENTAL NOISE	dB LEVEL	ENVIRONMENTAL NOISE
0 dB	Barely audible sound	50 dB	Moderate rainfall Moderate restaurant clatter Inside a typical urban home
10 dB	Normal breathing Soft rustle of leaves	60 dB	Normal conversation (50–70 dB) Background music Department store
20 dB	Whisper at 5 feet away Watch ticking	70 dB	Television Freeway traffic Vacuum cleaner Bus Noisy restaurant
30 dB	Whisper at 15 feet away	80 dB	Doorbell Telephone ring Alarm clock Noisy restaurant Police whistle Garbage disposal Blow dryer
40 dB	Quiet office Library Birds chirping out the window Refrigerator		

continued on the next page

Table 16-4, continued from the previous page

dB LEVEL	ENVIRONMENTAL NOISE	dB LEVEL	ENVIRONMENTAL NOISE
90 dB	Lawnmower Shop tools Shouted conversation Subway Busy urban street Food blender	120 dB	Thunderclap Hammering nails Ambulance siren Live rock concert
100 dB	Snowmobile School dance Tympani and bass drum rolls Chain saw Pneumatic drill Jackhammer	130 dB	Jackhammer Power drill Percussion section of symphony orchestra Stock car race
110 dB	Shouting in ear Baby crying Squeaky toy held close to the ear Power saw Leaf blower Motorcycle Busy video arcade Symphony concert Car horn	140 dB	Jet engine at takeoff Firecracker Toy cap gun Firearms Air raid siren
		150 dB	Artillery fire at 500 feet Firecracker Rock music at peak
		160 dB	Fireworks at 3 feet
		170 dB	High-powered shotgun
		180 dB	Rocket launching from pad

Sources: American Speech-Language Hearing Association (2007), Johnson (2005), League for the Hard of Hearing (2007b).

HEARING AIDS

There are three basic styles of hearing aids:

1. In-the-ear (ITE) hearing aids fit completely inside the outer ear. They are commonly recommended for mild to severe hearing loss, and are worn primarily by adults. Some include a telecoil (T) that allows the user to receive sound through the circuitry of the hearing aid instead of the microphone.

2. Behind-the-ear (BTE) hearing aids are worn behind the ear and connect to a plastic earmold that is worn inside the outer ear. They are used for mild to profound hearing loss. Although they are appropriate for individuals of any age, children most commonly use them; this is because the earmolds need to be replaced regularly to accommodate the changing shape of the child's outer ear.

3. Canal hearing aids are very small and fit tightly in the ear canal. In-the-canal (ITC) aids are made to fit the size and shape of the user's ear canal. Completely-in-canal (CIC) aids fit deeper in the canal and are almost completely hidden in the ear canal. They are recommended for mild to moderately severe hearing loss and are worn primarily by adults.

Before beginning a diagnostic evaluation of a client with a hearing impairment, do a quick listening check of his or her hearing aid(s). This is important! Imagine making a diagnosis of *moderate articulation disorder* or *mild receptive language impairment* only to discover that the client's malfunctioning hearing aid was impeding his or her typical communication. Do not allow a broken hearing aid to skew diagnostic conclusions and recommendations. Complete a quick listening check by following these six steps. Attach the aid to a stethoscope or your own earmold for Steps 2 through 5.

1. Check the battery. Is it missing? Is it weak?
2. Alternate the on-off switch. Do you hear distortions? Crackling noises? Other unusual sounds? No sound at all?
3. Turn the hearing aid to low volume and gradually increase to maximum volume. Is the transition smooth? Distorted?
4. Produce the sounds /a/, /i/, /u/, /ʃ/, and /s/. Are they audible? Clear?
5. Tap on the case. Do you hear changes in the sound?
6. Check for feedback. Is there a crack somewhere?

Troubleshooting Hearing Aid Problems

Depending on the work setting, the clinician may see clients who are having trouble with their hearing aids. In some cases, the problem will have to be addressed by a trained hearing aid specialist (i.e., audiologist, hearing aid dispenser, hearing aid manufacturer). In other cases, you will be able to identify the problem and possibly correct it. For example, a client may report that the hearing aid is not amplifying anything. On inspection, you may discover that the tubing is twisted, the battery is dead, or the T (telecoil) switch is on. These problems are easily resolved on the spot by untwisting the tubing, replacing the battery, or turning the T switch off. If unable to resolve the problem, refer the client to the hearing aid dispenser or manufacturer if the aid is broken, or to a physician if the trouble is caused by impacted ear wax.

Table 16-5 is a troubleshooting guide for basic hearing aid problems. Refer to this table when encountering a client with hearing aid trouble.

VIBROTACTILE AIDS

Vibrotactile aids are sometimes used by clients with profound hearing losses. Essentially, the vibration of sound is felt through the skin. These vibratory aids are worn on the hand, wrist, stomach, back, arm, or thigh. Depending on the hearing loss, vibrotactile aids may be used together with more traditional amplification or used alone. One primary benefit of vibrotactile stimulation is its capacity to increase speech-reading abilities.

TABLE 16-5   Troubleshooting Hearing Aid Problems

PROBLEM	CAUSE
Hearing aid dead	Bad battery
	Battery in backward
	Battery is wrong size
	Dirty cord contacts
	Broken cord
	Loose cord plug
	Tubing twisted
	Earmold plugged with cerumen
	Ear canal plugged with cerumen
	Receiver plugged with cerumen
	Switch turned to telecoil (T)
Hearing aid weak	Bad battery
	Earmold partially plugged with cerumen
	Microphone opening plugged with dirt or foreign object
	Moisture in the earmold
	Cracks in the earmold
	Ear canal plugged with cerumen
	Receiver plugged with cerumen
Intermittency	Dirty cord contacts
	Broken cord
	Loose cord plug
	Plastic tube collapsed
	Sweat in the hearing aid
	Dirty controls
	Telecoil switch is on
Acoustic feedback	Earmold not inserted properly
	Child has outgrown earmold
	Earmold loose from receiver nubbin
	Microphone too close to receiver
	Volume control too high
	Microphone housing loose
	Crack or leak in earmold, plastic tubing, earhook, or opening to earhook
	Ear canal blocked with cerumen
Distorted or muffled sound	Weak battery
	Earmold partially plugged with cerumen
	Amplifier no longer working correctly
	Dirty microphone
	Ear canal plugged with cerumen

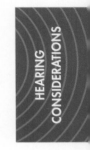

PROBLEM	CAUSE
Noise in the sound	Dirty or frayed cord
	Loose receiver cap
	Loose microphone housing
	Volume control worn
	Moisture in the aid
	Dirty microphone
	Poor battery contacts
	Telecoil switch is on
	Earmold blocked with cerumen
	Receiver plugged with cerumen

COCHLEAR IMPLANTS

Cochlear implants may be an appropriate alternative to conventional amplification for some clients. Candidates include children and adults with severe hard of hearing or profound deafness. The implant bypasses damaged portions of the ear and directly stimulates the auditory nerve, which the brain interprets as sound. The implant consists of an external unit that sits behind the ear and an internal unit that is surgically placed under the skin. The external unit has a microphone that collects sound and a speech processor that arranges the sound picked up by the microphone. The signal is then received by the internal transmitter/stimulator and converted to electrical impulses that are sent to different parts of the auditory nerve.

A cochlear implant does not restore normal hearing. Adults receiving implants after loss of functional hearing must relearn how to interpret sounds. Children receiving implants must also participate in a post-implantation therapy program to help them acquire speech and language skills. The benefits people receive from cochlear implantation vary and are dependent upon several factors. These include:

- The length of time the person was deaf or severely hearing impaired
- The extent of the person's prior hearing experience
- The number of functioning auditory nerve fibers present
- The motivation of the user, and the user's parents if a child
- The availability of auditory skills development programs to assist in hearing training or retraining

CONCLUDING COMMENTS

Hearing is an extremely important factor in the development and maintenance of communicative abilities. A hearing loss can contribute to or even be the single cause of many communicative disorders. The audiologist is responsible for evaluating and diagnosing hearing loss. The speech-language pathologist is responsible for understanding the audiological assessment results and their impact on a client's speech and language. A client's best interests are clearly served when audiologists and speech-language pathologists pool their knowledge, abilities, and clinical skills on the client's behalf.

SOURCES OF ADDITIONAL INFORMATION

Print Sources

Bess, F. H., & Humes, L. E. (2008). *Audiology: The fundamentals* (4th ed.). Baltimore: Lippincott Williams & Wilkins.

Clark, J. G., & Martin, F. N. (2011). *Introduction to audiology* (11th ed.). Needham Heights, MA: Allyn and Bacon.

DeBonis, D. A., & Donohue, C. L. (2008). *Survey of audiology: Fundamentals for audiologists and health professionals* (2nd ed.). Needham Heights, MA: Allyn and Bacon.

Roeser, R. J., Valente, M. J., & Hosford-Dunn, H. (2007). *Audiology diagnosis* (2nd ed.). New York: Thieme.

Tye-Murray, N., & Clark, W. W. (2014). *Foundations of aural rehabilitation: Children, adults, and their family members* (4th ed.). Clifton Park, NY: Cengage Learning.

Electronic Sources

American Speech-Language-Hearing Assocuation:
http://www.asha.org

Center for Hearling and Communication:
http://www.chchearing.org

Hearing Loss Association of America:
http://www.hearingloss.org

National Institute on Deafness and Other Communication Disorders:
http://www.nidcd.nih.gov

Form 16-1

Hearing Screening Form

Name: _____ Age: _____ Date: _____

Address or School: _____

Patient History

_____ Family history of hearing loss _____

_____ Ear infections _____

_____ Earaches _____

_____ Tinnitus _____

_____ Surgery _____

_____ Hearing aid _____

_____ Medications _____

_____ Diseases associated with hearing loss _____

_____ Exposure to noise _____

_____ Other relevant information _____

Previous Hearing Evaluations (date, place, findings): _____

_____

Evaluation

X or ✓ = Responded appropriately

O or − = Did not respond

CTN   = Could not test (specify reason)

dB level _____

	500 Hz	1000 Hz	2000 Hz	4000 Hz	8000 Hz
Right:	_____	_____	_____	_____	_____
Left:	_____	_____	_____	_____	_____

Conclusions

Passed screen

Failed screen

Recommendations

MEDICAL DIAGNOSES ASSOCIATED WITH COMMUNICATIVE DISORDERS

- ■ Diseases and Conditions
- ■ Syndromes
- ■ Concluding Comments
- ■ Sources of Additional Information

There are hundreds of medical diagnoses that can impact a client's communicative abilities. This chapter provides a brief description of many of the most common diseases, conditions, and syndromes, and highlights their clinical significance. Keep in mind that most illnesses or conditions have potential implications for the development of a speech-language disorder. For example, a person prone to frequent illness, whether or not each incident is long lasting or serious, is also more prone to a communicative disorder. This is especially true for children who have had multiple hearing losses due to otitis media during the crucial period of speech-language acquisition, or those who have frequently missed school due to illness and now lag behind their peers in communicative, social, and educational development.

A disease condition acquired by a pregnant woman may also influence the normal growth of her unborn child. Specific disruptions in fetal development are related to the time during gestation that the illness was acquired. First trimester illnesses impose the greatest developmental risks on the growing baby. Many congenital disorders have associated speech and language impairments.

DISEASES AND CONDITIONS

Adenoidectomy

An adenoidectomy is a partial or complete surgical removal of the adenoid tissue. This procedure is usually performed when a child's adenoids enlarge and block the nasopharynx or eustachian tubes. The blockage often results in breathing difficulties or frequent bouts of otitis media.

Clinical Significance

- The child may have experienced a prolonged period of hearing loss due to otitis media prior to the adenoidectomy.
- Velopharyngeal incompetence resulting in hypernasality may occur in rare cases.

Allergies

Allergies are physical hypersensitivities to substances that are eaten, inhaled, injected, or brought into contact with the skin. Symptoms of an allergy attack often include headache, shock, excessive mucus production, constriction of bronchioles, and skin conditions such as redness, swelling, and itching.

Clinical Significance

- Fluid buildup in the middle ear can occur, possibly resulting in hearing loss and associated speech and language difficulties.

Asthma

Asthma is characterized by periodic attacks of wheezing, tightness in the chest, and breathing difficulties. It can be triggered by allergies, emotional stress, infection, drug use, inhalation of irritants, vigorous exercise, or a psychosomatic disorder. Asthma is relatively common among school-age children, and there is a tendency to outgrow the condition over time. Asthma can usually be kept under control with medical assistance.

Clinical Significance

- Successive and severe attacks can result in reduced oxygen supply to the body and permanent disability.

Cerebrovascular Accident

See Stroke.

Chickenpox (Varicella)

Chickenpox is a mild, infectious disease caused by a herpes virus. The primary symptom is a rash that appears mostly on the skin and the lining of the mouth and throat. Chickenpox primarily affects children between the ages of 5 and 9. It is less common in adolescents and adults. In children, recovery is usually fast (7 to 10 days); adolescents and adults are more prone to complications and a slower recovery period. Immunization is available for individuals over the age of 12 months.

Clinical Significance

- Chickenpox is usually a mild illness. However, in rare cases, it is associated with severe complications, such as Reye's syndrome, pneumonia, encephalitis, and even death.
- If the chickenpox eruptions occur in the ears, there may be a toxic effect that results in bilateral hearing loss.

Colds

The common cold is usually caused by a viral infection of the nose and throat, although the larynx and lungs may also be involved. Symptoms include nasal congestion, runny nose, sneezing, mild sore throat, watery eyes, hoarseness, abdominal pain, and coughing. A temporary conductive hearing loss may also be present. Colds usually occur in winter months, and children are most prone to acquiring them. Immunity to cold viruses increases as a child grows older; therefore, the frequency of infection and severity are reduced over time.

Clinical Significance

- Colds are not serious in most cases, although infections can spread to the middle ears, sinuses, larynx, trachea, or lungs. This can result in secondary bacterial infections with complications such as laryngitis, bronchitis, otitis media, and sinusitis.

Convulsions

See Seizures.

Croup

Croup is a viral disorder characterized by a barking-like cough, hoarseness, respiratory distress, and inhalatory stridor resulting from swelling of the larynx and trachea. In most cases, it is a complication of influenza or a cold. It can also be caused by an allergic reaction.

Croup is a childhood disorder, primarily affecting children between the ages of 3 months and 3 years (although it can affect children up to 7 years of age). Attacks usually occur at night and subside after a few hours, and the condition may continue for several days. It is most common in the fall and winter months.

Clinical Significance

- Severe croup is an indication of epiglottitis, which can be fatal.
- In rare cases, there may be reduced oxygen supply to the body and permanent disability. An emergency tracheostomy may be necessary.

Dizziness

Dizziness is a sensation of spinning, either within the person or in the person's environment. It is a symptom of several types of neurological or aural disturbances. The person with dizziness may also feel nauseated, vomit, and have reduced control of balance. Dizziness can occur as a result of a severe blow to the head. It may also be an indication of a stroke, transient ischemic attack, subdural hemorrhage or hematoma, or brain tumor.

The term *vertigo* is often used interchangeably with dizziness, but they are not the same. Vertigo is dizziness experienced secondary to a middle ear pathology such as Ménière's disease, otitis media, labyrinthitis, or ototoxicity.

Clinical Significance

- A middle ear pathology may be present.
- Because dizziness is associated with balance problems, a person could fall down and suffer a head injury, although this is rare.

Draining Ear

Draining ear is not a disease condition, but is a common symptom of certain disorders. A greenish-yellow discharge from the ear canal may be an indication of otitis externa, otitis media, or mastoiditis. The infected person may also experience pain in the ear during head movement.

Clinical Significance

- Complications associated with draining ear must be evaluated according to the etiology of the condition.
- When the drainage obstructs the outer ear canal, a temporary hearing loss may occur.

Encephalitis

Encephalitis is an inflammation of the brain cells. Symptoms of mild encephalitis are similar to those of most viral infections, including fever, headache, and a loss of energy and appetite. Other symptoms and complications include irritability, restlessness, drowsiness (which may deepen into a coma in severe cases), loss of muscular power in the arms or legs, double vision, brain dysfunction, and impairment of speech and hearing. Babies and the elderly are at the highest risk for such complications.

Clinical Significance

- In severe cases, permanent brain damage can occur.
- Speech and language impairments may result.
- Recovery from a severe episode of encephalitis may be very slow, requiring long-term rehabilitation.

Flu

See Influenza.

German Measles (Rubella)

German measles is a contagious viral disease that is similar to, but milder than, common measles. It is characterized by a rash of small, flat, reddish-pink spots that appear on the face and neck and spread to the trunk and limbs. German measles is most common among children. Immunization is available for children over the age of 12 months.

Clinical Significance

Developing fetuses of pregnant women who have contracted the disease or received a vaccine within the three months preceding conception are at great risk for serious birth defects. These defects include:

- Malformations, microcephaly, hydrocephaly, and meningoencephalitis
- Heart defects and vision defects
- Mental retardation
- Deafness
- Behavior problems such as hyperactivity, impulsivity, poor attention span, and sleep disturbances
- Delayed speech and language development

Headaches

Headaches occur because of increased strain on muscles of the face, neck, and scalp (called tension headaches), or because of increased swelling of the blood vessels in the head (called vascular headaches). The resulting pain is located in the meninges, not the brain tissues. Many factors can lead to headaches, including stress, alcohol consumption, overeating, exposure to noise, eyestrain, poor body posture, and head injury. They can also be a symptom of another medical condition, such as a viral infection or a hemorrhage. Common headaches should be differentiated from migraine headaches, which are much more intense and incapacitating.

Clinical Significance

- A headache may be a symptom of more serious medical conditions, such as a central nervous system disorder or a hemorrhage.

High Fever

A high fever is a rise in body temperature above 100°F (37.8°C). It is usually a symptom of an infection. Other causes include severe trauma, reaction to medication or immunization, and certain types of cancer. In young children, a high fever can lead to febrile seizures. If the fever is very high, up to 107°F (41.6°C), permanent brain damage can result.

Clinical Significance

- Clinical is usually dependent upon the etiology of the high fever.
- In rare cases, hearing loss can occur if a high fever generates damaging toxins.

Human Immunodeficiency Virus (HIV)

See Acquired Immunodeficiency Syndrome (AIDS) under Syndromes later in this chapter.

Influenza (Flu)

Influenza is a viral disease that is characterized by chills, high fever, muscular pains, headache, sore throat, and sneezing. A dry, hacking cough, possible chest pains, and runny nose follow these symptoms. Complete recovery typically occurs within 1 to 2 weeks. The disease is highly contagious and usually occurs in epidemics, especially in the winter and spring months. Complications include bronchitis, bacterial pneumonia, viral pneumonia, otitis media, febrile seizures, skin rash, Reye's syndrome, and Guillain-Barré syndrome. Infants, the elderly, and people with suppressed immune systems or certain chronic diseases are most susceptible to complications.

Clinical Significance

- Conditions that occur as complications of influenza may be associated with speech and language difficulties.

Mastoiditis

Mastoiditis is an inflammation of all or part of the mastoid process. It occurs most commonly when a middle ear infection spreads to the mastoid. Symptoms include intense pain behind the ear, fever, a rapid pulse rate, discharge from the affected ear, swelling behind the affected ear, and a pronounced hearing loss. A mastoidectomy (partial or complete removal of the mastoid) may be necessary in severe cases.

Clinical Significance

- Speech and language difficulties associated with hearing loss may be present.

Measles (Rubeola)

Measles is a viral disease that primarily affects the skin and respiratory tract. Symptoms include nasal congestion, runny nose, cough, fever, and a characteristic rash. Measles is a highly contagious and potentially dangerous disease. Complications include hearing loss, otitis media, bronchitis, pneumonia, learning disabilities, encephalitis, meningitis, permanent brain damage, mental retardation, vision problems, seizures, and death. A pregnant woman who contracts measles is at risk for premature labor or spontaneous abortion. Her newborn baby may have a low birth weight and, if the disease was contracted during the first trimester of fetal development, congenital malformation.

Measles often occurs in epidemics, but because immunization is available for children over 12 months old, it is not common. It should not be confused with German measles (rubella), which is much less serious, except during pregnancy.

Clinical Significance

- Speech and language difficulties associated with hearing loss may be present.
- The client may exhibit learning disabilities.
- Neurological problems may be present.

Ménière's Disease

Ménière's disease is a condition of the middle ear. Characteristic symptoms of Ménière's disease include tinnitis, rotational vertigo, a feeling of fullness in the middle ear, and sensorineural hearing loss. These symptoms are episodic, progressive, and fluctuate in intensity and frequency. The disease usually begins as a unilateral condition but it eventually becomes bilateral.

Clinical Significance

- Complete deafness in one or both ears can occur.
- In severe cases of vertigo, a person could fall and suffer a head injury.

Meningitis

Meningitis is an inflammation of the meninges (the membranous coverings of the brain and spinal cord). Bacteria or viruses can spread to these membranes through the bloodstream or cavities and bones of the skull, or from a skull fracture. Symptoms include fever, headache, chills, nausea, vomiting, irritability, a stiff neck, confusion, and photophobia (inability to tolerate bright light). A deep red or purplish skin rash occurs in some cases.

The viral form of meningitis usually imposes no associated complications. Meningitis stemming from a bacterial infection, however, is a very serious condition requiring aggressive medical treatment. Complications associated with bacterial meningitis include convulsions, coma, permanent deafness, permanent blindness, mental deterioration, or death. Babies and the elderly are especially prone to these complications.

Clinical Significance

- Brain damage can occur in severe cases.
- Speech and language problems associated with hearing loss or neurological problems may be present.

Mumps

Mumps is a contagious viral infection of the salivary glands, particularly of the parotid glands located just anterior to the ears. The infected person may experience difficulty opening the mouth, dryness of the mouth, pain during swallowing, fever, diarrhea, vomiting, and general feelings of illness. Once the mumps virus has entered the body, it can pass through the bloodstream to many different glands and to the brain. Mumps can occur at any age, but it is most common in children between the ages of 5 and 15. Immunization is available for children over the age of 12 months.

Clinical Significance

- Meningitis, encephalitis, pancreatitis, febrile seizures, respiratory tract infections, or ear infections can occur as a complication.
- A mild to severe hearing loss can occur. The hearing loss is typically (but not exclusively) unilateral.

Otitis Media

Otitis media is an infection of the middle ear. The infection may be viral or bacterial, and it usually spreads from the nose and throat to the ear through the eustachian tube. The infection can also enter the middle ear through a ruptured eardrum. The symptoms of acute otitis media include a feeling of fullness in the affected ear that is followed by pain, fever, and hearing loss. If untreated, the acute condition may lead to chronic otitis media, which is much more serious and permanently damaging. Otitis media is very common among children, particularly those under 6 years of age.

Clinical Significance

- Otitis media is nearly always associated with a temporary hearing loss. This can directly influence speech and language development because repeated infections are common among children during the critical years of speech and language acquisition.
- Middle ear pressure from pus buildup may cause the eardrum to burst.
- Permanent hearing impairment can occur in chronic cases.

Parkinson's Disease

Parkinson's disease is a degenerative condition caused by gradual deterioration of nerve centers in the brain. This deterioration disrupts the brain's normal balance of dopamine and acetylcholine, resulting in progressive loss of control of movement. One of the first symptoms of Parkinson's disease is a rhythmic tremor of the hands and head, often accompanied by involuntary rubbing together of the thumb and forefinger. As the condition progresses, automatic physical movements associated with walking, writing, and speaking also become impaired. Other symptoms include excessive salivation, abdominal cramps, and, in the latest stages of the disease, deterioration of memory and thought processes. It most often affects people who are late middle age and older. Parkinson's disease is sometimes medically controlled with carbidopa/levodopa which can significantly reduce the severity of the condition.

Clinical Significance

- Parkinson's disease can result in mild to profound communication and swallowing impairments, depending on the individual and the stage of progression of the disease.
- Dysphagia and hypokinetic dysarthria are characteristic.
- As deterioration increases, cognitive function may be impaired.

Pneumonia (Pneumonitis)

Pneumonia is a general term for inflammation of the lungs. The several types of pneumonia are differentiated by their origins and severity. Most cases are viral or bacterial in origin although fungi; inhalation of food, vomit, or pus; or inhalation of poisonous gas can also cause pneumonia. Symptoms vary according to the type of pneumonia. Symptoms include nasal congestion, cough, fever, chills, shortness of breath, bluish skin, chest pain, sweating, blood in the phlegm, or possible mental confusion. Severity varies considerably from mild and uncomplicated to extremely dangerous and life threatening.

Clinical Significance

- Pneumonia, particularly aspiration type, may indicate dysphagia.

Rubella

See German Measles (Rubella).

Rubeola

See Measles (Rubeola).

Seizures

Seizures, also called *convulsions*, are uncontrollable muscle contractions caused by abnormal electrical activity in the brain. They vary considerably in severity. During a generalized *tonicoclonic seizure*, also called a *grand mal seizure*, the person loses consciousness and exhibits jerking movements of the whole body. The seizure may last only seconds or several minutes before the person regains consciousness and then often falls into a deep sleep. Most febrile convulsions (those associated with a fever) are of this type.

Absence seizures, also called *petit mal seizures*, are much less severe. The person may exhibit a blank stare and appear to be daydreaming for several seconds. After the seizure is over, he or she does not remember that it happened. This type of seizure can occur many times in one day.

A *psychomotor seizure*, also called a *temporal lobe attack*, occurs when a person exhibits violent behavior, laughs, or cries for no apparent reason. The seizure lasts for a few minutes. Afterward, he or she is not aware that it occurred.

Infantile spasms are sudden episodes in which a baby or toddler drops his or her head to his or her chest and doubles up at the waist. Afterward the child may fall asleep. These convulsions last only a second to a few seconds and can occur several times a day.

Seizures occur most often in children and are often outgrown by adulthood. People prone to seizures usually have idiopathic epilepsy or a minor fever-causing infection. Other causes include meningitis, encephalitis, hypoglycemia, brain damage, cerebral palsy, or a brain tumor.

Clinical Significance

- A head injury can occur during a seizure, although this is rare.
- Neurological problems related to speech, language, and swallowing may be present.

MEDICAL DIAGNOSES

Sinusitis

Sinusitis is an inflammation or infection of the sinuses (the moist air spaces behind the bones of the upper face). Symptoms include coughing, a greenish discharge through the nose, increased nasal congestion, fever, and a general feeling of illness. Facial pain may also be present in the area(s) of the inflamed sinus or sinuses. Sinusitis is common. Some people have repeated attacks nearly every time they have a cold. The condition can also be acquired through damage to the nasal bones, nasal obstruction by a foreign object, or a nasal deformity.

Clinical Significance

• Untreated sinusitis can spread to the bones or into the brain.

Stroke (Cerebrovascular Accident)

A cerebrovascular accident (CVA), commonly known as a *stroke*, occurs when part of the brain is damaged because its blood supply is disrupted. There are three etiologies of a stroke. A cerebral *hemorrhage* occurs when an artery bursts or leaks and blood seeps into the brain tissue. A cerebral *thrombosis* occurs when a clot forms in an artery and eventually grows until it partially or completely blocks the flow of blood at that point. A cerebral *embolism* occurs when foreign material is carried through the bloodstream and becomes caught, obstructing the flow of blood to the brain. The result of a stroke is dependent on the area of the brain affected and the severity of the damage. Symptoms of a stroke include headache, blurred or double vision, confusion, dizziness, slurred speech or an inability to talk, weakness or numbness on only one side of the body, difficulty swallowing, and loss of consciousness. These symptoms persist for a period of at least 24 hours and usually significantly longer (unlike a transient ischemic attack).

Clinical Significance

• Depending on the severity of the stroke, the consequent deficits can be mild to profound. Speech, language, swallowing, and cognition can be affected, resulting in dysarthria, aphasia, apraxia, dysphagia, or cognitive-linguistic impairments.

Tinnitus

Tinnitus is an unwanted noise in the ear that varies in quality and pitch among people with the condition. Various descriptions of tinnitus have included a buzzing sound, a highpitched whistle, a grinding noise, or a low-pitched roar. Some people experience the condition continuously, while others report intermittent attacks of tinnitus. Tinnitus is usually associated with ear problems such as earwax buildup, Ménière's disease, age-related hearing loss, trauma from loud noises, or trauma from a sudden change in barometric pressure. Stress, a virus, diet, thyroid problems, hypertension, head trauma, drug intake, and dental problems can also trigger it.

Clinical Significance

• Tinnitus can be an early symptom of progressive hearing loss, meningitis, encephalitis, ototoxicity (loss of hearing from medications), or an acoustic neuronoma (a tumor in the ear).

Tonsillitis

Tonsillitis is an inflammation of the tonsils caused by a bacterial or viral infection. Symptoms include sore throat, pain when swallowing, headache, chills, fever, swollen glands on the neck, and red, inflamed tonsils. Some children experience febrile convulsions. The disease is common among children, especially those between 2 and 6 years of age. Tonsillitis is highly infectious and is often accompanied by an infection of the adenoids, otitis media, and sinusitis. If the condition occurs frequently or is especially severe, a tonsillectomy may be recommended.

Clinical Significance

- Frequent bouts of tonsillitis may be associated with intermittent hearing loss.

Transient Ischemic Attack (TIA)

A transient ischemic attack (TIA) occurs when there is an interference of normal blood flow to the brain. Typically, a foreign material flowing through the bloodstream becomes caught and disrupts the brain's blood supply, much like a cerebral embolism (see *Stroke*). The symptoms are very similar to a stroke and include headache, dizziness, blurred or double vision, confusion, slurred speech, swallowing difficulty, and weakness or numbness on one side of the body. These symptoms, however, are short lived (less than 24 hours) because the foreign material is eventually dislodged or broken up and blood circulation to the brain is restored.

Clinical Significance

- A TIA is usually not complicated because the resulting impairments are temporary, although it is often a warning of an impending stroke.

SYNDROMES

A syndrome is a distinct collection of symptoms that together are characteristic of a specific disease or disorder. The etiology may be viral, bacterial, genetic, chromosomal, teratogenic (a foreign agent causing embryonic or fetal structural abnormalities), or traumatic. Many syndromes have been named and described, yet many more remain unidentified by medical experts. Some of the major syndromes that affect communicative abilities, and therefore may be seen by clinicians for speech, language, or hearing services, are described in this section. Use caution when using this information and consider these factors:

1. *Syndrome severity varies tremendously.* A child diagnosed with a given syndrome may exhibit barely detectable symptoms or may be a "textbook example."

2. *Individual symptoms vary.* For example, a child with mental retardation may be severely intellectually impaired or may have near normal intelligence.

3. *All symptoms associated with a syndrome need not be present.* Syndromes are a collection of many symptoms which appear in varying degrees; some symptoms may not appear at all.

MEDICAL DIAGNOSES

4. *Symptoms that are not described in this section may also be present.* Only the major characteristics of each syndrome have been highlighted. Other less common symptoms may also be observed.

5. *These descriptions are presented only as a starting point of inquiry about syndromes associated with communicative disorders.* We suggest you consult the sources listed under Sources of Additional Information at the end of this chapter for more information.

Acquired Immunodeficiency Syndrome (AIDS)

Acquired immunodeficiency syndrome (AIDS), in which infected particles enter the bloodstream and replicate themselves to the point of outnumbering healthy cells, is caused by the human immunodeficiency virus (HIV). A person infected with HIV may appear healthy for several years or a lifetime before developing AIDS. The virus is transmitted through some infected bodily fluids. An unborn baby will acquire the virus if his or her mother is a carrier. AIDS symptoms include:

- Impaired natural defense mechanism due to the depletion of healthy white blood cells
- High risk for multiple infections (especially pneumonia, swollen lymph glands, fever, and encephalitis), cancer (particularly skin cancer), and neurological illnesses
- In adults: fever, weight loss, swollen glands, general weakness, headaches, drowsiness, confusion, and infections of the mouth, skin, or chest
- In children: low birth weight, developmental delay, upper respiratory infections, pneumonia, ear diseases, and sensorineural hearing loss. Children are prone to more severe infections than adults. Infected children are especially at risk for cancer of the external ear, cancer of the oral cavity, and cortical atrophy.
- Dysphagia associated with generalized weakness
- Language disorders associated with hearing loss
- Articulation disorders associated with hearing loss

Alport's Syndrome

Alport's syndrome is a hereditary syndrome that is more common among males than females. Characteristics include:

- Nephritis (kidney disease)
- Bilateral, sensorineural hearing loss that is progressive and often leads to total deafness
- Language disorders associated with hearing loss
- Speech disorders associated with hearing loss

Apert's Syndrome

Apert's syndrome is a hereditary syndrome. Characteristics include:

- Craniosynostosis (premature fusion of the cranial sutures) resulting in a tall head shape with a small head diameter and underdeveloped midfacial features

- Class III malocclusion and irregular tooth placement
- Strabismus (vision problems)
- Syndactyly (webbing) or synostosis (joining of bones) of the hands or toes, usually affecting the second through fourth digits
- Conductive hearing loss
- Cleft palate
- Mouth breathing
- Difficulty eating
- Hyponasality and a forward posturing of the tongue
- Articulation problems related to structural abnormalities and hearing loss
- Language difficulties associated with mental retardation and hearing loss

Asperger's Syndrome

Asperger's syndrome is a developmental, neurobiological disorder that is part of the autism spectrum. It is most common among boys. Characteristics include:

- Impaired social skills
- Obtuseness, limited interests, and unusual preoccupations
- Preference for sameness in routines or rituals; difficulties with transitions
- Speech and language difficulties, particularly in the areas of pragmatics and prosody
- Limited facial expressions apart from anger or misery
- Excellent rote memory and musical ability
- Difficulty reading nonverbal communications (body language)
- Poor awareness of personal body space
- Clumsy and uncoordinated motor movements
- Extreme sensitivity to sounds, tastes, smells, and sights

Brachman–de Lange Syndrome

See Cornelia de Lange Syndrome.

Branchio-Oto-Renal (BOR) Syndrome

Branchio-oto-renal (BOR) syndrome is a genetic syndrome characterized by:

- Ear deformities, including ear pits or tags on the outer ear, cupping of the outer ear, a malformed exterior auditory canal, and ossicular bone abnormalities
- Abnormal kidney development
- Cysts and fistulas on the neck
- Mild to profound conductive, sensorineural, or mixed hearing loss
- Language disorders associated with hearing loss
- Articulation disorders associated with hearing loss

MEDICAL DIAGNOSES

Cornelia de Lange Syndrome

This syndrome is also called the *de Lange* or *Brachman–de Lange syndrome*. It is a congenital syndrome characterized by:

- Short stature, infantile posture, microcephaly, small extremities, and contracted elbows
- Small and dysmorphic nose, thin and down-turned upper lip
- Synophrys (abundant eyebrows joined at the midline)
- Congenital heart failure; possible failure to thrive
- Cleft palate
- Hearing loss
- Severe speech and language problems
- Feeding difficulties
- Severe mental retardation

Cri du Chat Syndrome

Cri du chat syndrome is a chromosomal disorder resulting from a deletion of the short arm of the fifth chromosome. Characteristics include:

- An infant's characteristic cry that resembles a crying cat (thus the French name *cri du chat*, or "cry of the cat")
- Narrow oral cavity, laryngeal hyperplasia, and low-set ears
- Mental retardation and behavioral problems
- Delayed motor development
- Language difficulties associated with mental retardation

Crouzon Disease

Crouzon disease is a genetic syndrome characterized by:

- Craniosynostosis (premature fusion of the cranial sutures) resulting in an oddly shaped head with a short front-to-back distance and a tall forehead
- Midfacial and maxillary hypoplasia (underdevelopment), a "beak-shaped" or "parrot-like" nose, and hypertelorism (increased distance between the eyes)
- Brachydactyly (shortness of fingers)
- Ptosis (drooping of the eyelids)
- Class III malocclusion
- Shallow oropharynx, high palatal arch, long and thick soft palate
- In some cases, a hearing loss that is usually conductive, but occasionally sensorineural
- Hyponasality
- Articulation disorders resulting from structural abnormalities in the oral cavity and hearing loss

de Lange Syndrome

See Cornelia de Lange Syndrome.

Down Syndrome (Trisomy 21 Syndrome)

Down syndrome is the most common and well-known disorder resulting from a chromosomal abnormality. Its name, trisomy 21, refers to a triplicate (rather than the normal duplicate) of chromosome 21, which results in a total of 47 rather than the usual 46 chromosomes. This chromosomal distinction is present in about 95% of all patients with Down syndrome. Its major characteristics include:

- Generalized hypotonia
- Open-mouth posture with tongue protrusion
- A flat facial profile and brachycephaly (shortened front-to-back diameter of the skull)
- Small nose, ears, and chin
- Mental retardation or developmental delay
- Cardiac malformations in about 40% of cases
- Unilateral or bilateral hearing loss; most commonly, a mild-moderate conductive impairment
- Delayed speech development, complicated by orofacial abnormalities
- Delayed language and language disorders, particularly syntactic and morphologic problems
- Abnormal voice and resonance features, including hypernasality, nasal emission, and breathiness
- Articulation disorders

Ectrodactyly–Ectodermal Dysplasia–Clefting Syndrome (EEC Syndrome)

Ectrodactyly–ectodermal dysplasia–clefting (EEC) syndrome is a genetic syndrome characterized by:

- Ectrodactyly (absence of one or more fingers or toes) or syndactyly (webbing between digits)
- Sparse hair
- Cleft lip and palate; dental abnormalities
- Maxillary hypoplasia (underdevelopment)
- Chronic serous otitis media in early childhood often resulting in conductive hearing loss
- Articulation and resonance problems associated with cleft lip, cleft palate, velopharyngeal incompetence, and dental/maxillary abnormalities
- Language problems associated with hearing loss

Facio-Auriculo-Vertebral Spectrum

See Goldenhar Syndrome.

Fetal Alcohol Syndrome (FAS)

Fetal alcohol syndrome (FAS), caused by maternal consumption of alcohol, is the leading cause of birth defects and the third leading cause of mental retardation in the United States. The syndrome may result even if the mother is a light, "social" drinker. Characteristics vary depending, at least in part, on the amount of alcohol consumed and the developmental stage of the fetus. Common features include:

- Significant growth retardation
- Short palpebral fissures (slits of the eyes); a short, upturned nose; and ears that rotate posteriorly
- Maxillary hypoplasia and micrognathia (underdeveloped upper and lower jaw); a thin upper lip, and microcephaly
- Hypotonia
- Congenital heart abnormalities and kidney disorders
- Poor motor coordination
- Irritability during infancy and hyperactivity during childhood
- Abnormalities of the outer ear may be present, but hearing is generally normal
- Cleft palate and small teeth
- Intellectual disability
- Articulation disorders
- Language disabilities, including deficits in syntax, semantics, and pragmatics
- Fluency disorders
- Voice disorders

First and Second Branchial Arch Syndrome

See Goldenhar Syndrome.

Fragile X Syndrome

This syndrome is the second most common cause of genetically based intellectual disability (second to Down syndrome). It occurs when there is a fragile spot on the long arm of the X chromosome (technically, Xq27). Characteristics include:

- A large head, a prominent forehead, a large jaw, and large ears
- Intellectual disability
- Psychiatric and behavioral problems
- Delayed speech and motor development
- Jargon, echolalia, perseveration, and inappropriate language
- Absence of nonverbal communications that typically accompany speech
- Voice problems
- Articulation disorders

Goldenhar Syndrome

This syndrome has also been referred to as hemifacial microsomia, facio-auriculo-vertebral spectrum, ocular-auriculo-vertebral dysplasia, and first and second branchial arch syndrome. It is characterized by:

- Mandibular hypoplasia (underdeveloped lower jaw) resulting in facial asymmetry (usually unilateral, but it may be bilateral)
- Facial palsy, microtia (underdeveloped ears), atresia, and hemifacial microsomia (portions or all of the head are small)
- Cleft palate, velar asymmetry, velar paresis, or other oral structural malformations
- Congenital heart disease and kidney disease
- Articulation and resonance disorders resulting from oral structural abnormalities
- Hearing loss that is usually conductive, but occasionally sensorineural
- Language disorders in some cases
- Intellectual disability is not characteristic.

Hemifacial Microsomia

See Goldenhar Syndrome.

Hunter Syndrome

See Mucopolysaccharidosis Syndromes.

Hurler Syndrome

See Mucopolysaccharidosis Syndromes.

Maroteaux-Lamy Syndrome

See Mucopolysaccharidosis Syndromes.

Moebius Syndrome

Moebius syndrome is a genetic syndrome characterized by:

- Facial and hypoglossal (and trigeminal in some cases) nerve disturbances causing bilabial paresis (partial paralysis or weakness) and difficulties lateralizing, elevating, depressing, or protruding the tongue
- Facial diplegia (bilateral paralysis) resulting in an expressionless, mask-like facial appearance, and unilateral or bilateral loss of abductor muscles. The upper face is affected more than the lower face. The eyelids may not fully close.
- Cleft palate, hypoplasic (underdeveloped) mandible, and hypoplasic limbs
- Intellectual disability in about 10–15% of all cases
- Conductive hearing loss in some cases

- Feeding difficulties in infancy
- Articulation disorders due to limited strength, range of motion, and speed of movement of the articulators
- Language development problems, presumably due to early hospitalizations for aspiration, lack of early growth due to feeding problems, and reduced parental expectations for development

Mohr Syndrome

See Orofaciodigital Syndromes.

Morquio Syndrome

See Mucopolysaccharidosis Syndromes.

Mucopolysaccharidosis (MPS) Syndromes (Including Hurler, Scheie, Hunter, Sanfilippo, Morquio, Maroteaux-Lamy, and Sly Syndromes)

The mucopolysaccharidosis (MPS) syndromes are a group of rare disorders (perhaps 100–700 occurrences per year in the United States). Common characteristics include:

- Excessive storage of complex carbohydrates (mucopolysaccharidoses) in the body
- Progressive physical and mental deterioration
- Hearing loss
- Thick hair and eyebrows
- Speech, language, and hearing problems: these occur in all of the MPS disorders, but there is limited documentation about specific communication impairments associated with each syndrome.

The most common MPS syndromes are Hurler and Hunter syndromes. The differential diagnosis of Hunter syndrome is essential because it is a recessively inherited syndrome that carries a 25% chance of subsequent recurrence. Other MPS syndromes include Sanfilippo, Morquio, Maroteaux-Lamy, and Sly syndromes.

Neurofibromatosis Type 2 (NF-2)

Neurofibromatosis Type 2 (NF-2) is a genetic syndrome characterized by:

- Benign tumor growth, primarily in the brain and spinal cord. Tumor growth on both auditory nerves is particularly common, resulting in severe hearing loss or total deafness.
- Possible tumor growth on cranial nerves associated with swallowing, speech, eye movements, and facial sensations, and on the spinal nerves going to the limbs
- Language disorders associated with hearing loss
- Speech disorders associated with hearing loss
- Dysphagia

Noonan Syndrome

Noonan syndrome is a genetic syndrome characterized by:

- Congenital heart disease
- Short stature, narrow chest, and webbing of the neck
- Hypertelorism (increased distance between the eyes), and ptosis (drooping of the eyelids). The ears may be abnormally shaped, have prominent pinnae, and be set low with a slight posterior rotation.
- Intellectual disability in some cases
- Articulation disorders
- Delayed language and limited expressive language skills
- Hypernasality

Oculo-Auriculo-Vertebral Dysplagia

See Goldenhar Syndrome.

Orofaciodigital Syndromes (Including Mohr Syndrome)

There are about seven orofaciodigital syndromes. The most common is orofaciodigital syndrome Type II, or Mohr syndrome. This syndrome is characterized by:

- Short stature and digital abnormalities, such as short digits and polydactyly (extra fingers or toes). Both feet have two big toes.
- Cleft lip and palate
- Tongue malformations, such as partial clefting at midline and nodules
- Absent central incisors
- Mandibular hypoplasia (underdeveloped jaw); short labial frenulum
- Conductive hearing loss, usually resulting from atresia, ossicular chain malformation, or chronic otitis media (particularly subsequent to cleft palate)
- Varying intellectual abilities from extreme disability to normal intelligence
- Articulation disorders resulting from orofacial abnormalities, intellectual disability, and hearing loss
- Language problems related to intellectual disability

Oto-Palatal-Digital (OPD) Syndrome (Taybi Syndrome or Rubinstein-Taybi Syndrome)

This syndrome is also known as *Taybi syndrome* or *Rubinstein–Taybi syndrome*. It is characterized by:

- Bone dysplagia (abnormal tissue development), which may result in short and broad finger or toe tips and limited ability to bend the elbows
- Micrognathia (small or recessed chin) and missing teeth

- Small stature and a short torso
- Mild hypertelorism (increased distance between the eyes)
- Cleft palate
- Chewing, sucking, and swallowing difficulties
- Bilateral conductive hearing loss, malformations of the ossicular chain, frequent otitis media
- Intellectual disability
- Articulation and resonance problems associated with hearing loss and cleft palate
- Language problems and learning disabilities associated with intellectual disability

Pendred Syndrome

This syndrome is a recessively inherited genetic disorder characterized by:

- Defective thyroid metabolism; goiter (enlarged thyroid) in middle childhood
- Characteristic profound hearing loss, although mild–moderate losses occur occasionally. Conductive, sensorineural, or mixed hearing losses have been reported and may be progressive in some cases.
- Speech and language difficulties associated with hearing impairment

Pierre Robin Sequence (or Syndrome)

Pierre Robin sequence is not a true syndrome because it is a combination of several clinical findings caused by one or many etiologies. It may also be called *Pierre Robin syndrome*, *Robin sequence*, or *Robin deformation sequence*. Characteristics include:

- Mandibular hypoplasia (underdevelopment) and glossoptosis (downward displacement of the tongue)
- Cleft of the soft palate. The cleft is typically U-shaped (rather than the more common V-shape) or in the form of a bifid uvula, which is most clearly seen during phonation of "ah."
- Respiratory problems resulting from the medical diagnosis of failure to thrive and hypoxic (lack of oxygen) brain damage are reported in some cases.
- Low-set ears, deformed pinnae, an unusual angle of the ear canal, and ossicular defects
- Conductive hearing loss associated with otitis media, cleft palate, and ear abnormalities
- Articulation and resonance problems related to cleft palate
- Language disorders and learning disabilities related to hearing loss and post-hypoxic brain damage

Prader-Willi Syndrome

This genetic syndrome is sometimes referred to as *Prader-Labhart-Willi syndrome*. Symptoms include:

- Hypotonia (poor muscle tone) and small stature
- Obesity, especially after the second year of life. Excessive appetite and weight gain are long-term problems that must be managed.
- Hypogonadism (underdeveloped genitals)
- Slow motor development
- Intellectual disability ranging from mild to severe. In some cases intelligence is normal.
- Feeding difficulties related to hypotonia
- Delayed language and language disorders
- Dysarthria and apraxia in some cases; nasal emissions. Articulation disorders range from mild to severe. Speech may be unintelligible.

Refsum Disease

Refsum disease is a genetic syndrome characterized by:

- Chronic polyneuritis (inflammation of the peripheral nerves)
- Cerebellar ataxia (disturbed balance)
- Retinitis pigmentosa (a deteriorating condition involving inflammation and pigment infiltration in the retina) and night blindness
- Heart disease in about 50% of the cases
- Skeletal abnormalities such as spondylitis (vertebral inflammation) and kyphoscoliosis (backward and lateral curvature of the spinal column) in about 75% of the cases
- Progressive sensorineural hearing loss in about 50% of cases, often beginning in early adulthood
- Articulation disorders associated with hearing loss
- Ataxic dysarthria, with its characteristic errors of articulation, voice, rate, and prosody

Reye's Syndrome

Reye's syndrome is an acute disease that sometimes develops when a person is recovering from a viral illness, such as influenza or chickenpox. It primarily affects children. Pressure within the brain increases significantly and abnormal fat accumulates in the liver and other organs. The disease progresses quickly. Death is common. If it is not treated in its earliest stages, irreversible brain damage can occur. Residual effects can include:

- Eating and sleeping disturbances
- Anxiety, depression, and social withdrawal
- Fine or gross motor skills deficits

- Problems with attention, concentration, and memory
- Speech and language problems
- Learning disabilities

Rett Syndrome

Rett syndrome is an autistic-like genetic syndrome that affects girls almost exclusively. It is characterized by:

- Seemingly normal development in the first 6 to 18 months before changes in mental and social behavior are apparent
- Loss of muscle tone
- Breathing difficulties
- Disrupted sleep patterns
- Habitual wringing or rubbing of hands negates functional hand use
- Severe limb, oral, and verbal apraxia
- Loss of speech between 1 and 4 years of age
- Extreme social anxiety
- Seizures

Robin Sequence (or Syndrome)

See Pierre Robin Sequence.

Rubinstein-Taybi Syndrome

See Oto-Palatal-Digital (OPD) Syndrome.

Sanfilippo Syndrome

See Mucopolysaccharidosis Syndromes.

Scheie Syndrome

See Mucopolysaccharidosis Syndromes.

Shprintzen Syndrome (VCFS)

See Velo-Cardio-Facial Syndrome (VCFS).

Sly Syndrome

See Mucopolysaccharidosis Syndromes.

Stickler Syndrome

Stickler syndrome is a genetic syndrome characterized by:

- Midfacial hypoplasia (underdevelopment) and micrognathia (underdeveloped chin)
- Visual problems, including cataracts and retinal detachments and severe myopia

- Long and thin extremities often with prominent ankle, knee, or wrist joints
- Hypotonia
- Cleft palate, submucosal cleft, or bifid uvula
- Malformed ears in some cases
- Intellectual disability is not characteristic.
- Conductive, sensorineural, or mixed hearing loss, and chronic serous otitis media
- Feeding, sucking, and swallowing problems in infancy
- Language and learning disorders related to hearing loss and cleft palate
- Articulation disorders, nasal emission, and hypernasality related to cleft palate

Taybi Syndrome

See Oto-Palatal-Digital (OPD) Syndrome.

Treacher Collins Syndrome

Treacher Collins syndrome is a genetic syndrome characterized by:

- Facial abnormalities, including mandibular and maxillary hyperplasia (underdeveloped upper and lower jaw), malar hypoplasia (underdeveloped cheeks) and a beakshaped nose
- Overt or submucosal cleft palate, high hard palate, short and immobile soft palate, and downward slanting palpebral fissures
- Coloboma (clefting defect) of the lower eyelids
- Dental malocclusion, hyperplasia (underdevelopment) of the teeth, and an open bite
- Upper respiratory problems that affect breathing may be present
- Atresia, malformations of the pinnae, and middle ear structural abnormalities. Inner ear malformations, such as enlarged cochlear aqueducts or absent horizontal canals, occur in severe cases.
- Conductive (in most) or sensorineural (in some) hearing loss
- Early childhood problems with chewing, sucking, and swallowing
- Language-learning problems associated with hearing loss
- Articulation disorders associated with hearing loss and orofacial abnormalities

Townes-Brocks Syndrome (TBS)

Townes-Brocks syndrome (TBS) is a genetic syndrome characterized by:

- Anorectal malformations such as skin-covered anus, anal stenosis, and rectovaginal or rectoperineal fistulae. Medical conditions of the urinary and renal tracts are typical.
- Hand and foot malformations such as digit deformities, syndactyly (webbing), and polydactyly (extra digits)
- External ear malformations such as "lop"-shaped ears, microtia, and ear tags or pits
- Mild to profound sensorineural hearing loss

- Cleft lip and palate in some cases
- Microcephaly, hypoplastic mandible, incomplete closure of the left side of the mouth
- Intellectual disability in about 10% of cases
- Heart problems in about 10% of cases
- Swallowing difficulties
- Language disorders associated with hearing loss and intellectual disability if present
- Speech disorders associated with hearing loss and cleft palate if present

Trisomy 21 Syndrome

See Down Syndrome.

Turner Syndrome

This genetic syndrome, also called *XO syndrome*, is a chromosomal disorder that affects only females. It occurs when there is a missing X chromosome (most common) or an abnormality of an X chromosome (less common). It is characterized by:

- Short stature, outward angle of the elbows, excessive skin or webbing of the neck, congenital swelling of the foot, neck, and hands
- Sexual infantilism, amenorrhea (absence of the menstrual cycle), and infertility
- Heart problems
- Pigmented skin lesions
- Narrow maxilla and palate and micrognathia (underdeveloped chin)
- Cleft palate and high arched palate in some cases
- External ear deformities, including long, low-set, and cupped ears and thick earlobes
- Sensorineural hearing loss, usually noticed after age 10. Some authorities report that the hearing loss is congenital, whereas others suggest that it is degenerative. Otitis media is common in infancy and early childhood.
- Intellectual disability
- Right-hemisphere dysfunction
- Language problems related to hearing loss
- Articulation disorders resulting from hearing loss and structural abnormalities of the face

Usher Syndrome

Usher syndrome is the leading cause of combined deafness-blindness in the United States. It is a congenital syndrome characterized by:

- Severe to profound congenital sensorineural hearing loss associated with incomplete development or atrophy at the basal end of the organ of Corti in the cochlea. High frequencies are usually more affected than low frequencies, which is consistent with cochlear involvement. Vestibular problems are also very common.

- Retinitis pigmentosa (progressive retinal atrophy and migration of pigmentation); night blindness in early childhood, progressing to limited peripheral vision; eventual total blindness
- Language problems associated with deafness
- Articulation and resonance disorders associated with deafness

Van der Woude Syndrome

Van der Woude syndrome is a genetic syndrome characterized by:

- Congenital pits (fistulae) or mounds on the lower lip in all cases. They are typically bilateral and directly inferior to the nares.
- Cleft lip or palate in most cases. The upper lip may have a wide Cupid's bow or "gull-wing" appearance. Velopharyngeal incompetence is common, especially if there is a deep pharynx and submucosal or overt clefting.
- Conductive hearing loss and otitis media
- Chewing, sucking, and swallowing problems in early childhood
- Language disorders related to hearing loss
- Hypernasality and nasal emission associated with cleft palate
- Articulation disorders associated with hearing loss. The lip pits do not normally cause speech problems because bilabial closure is not affected.

Velo-Cardio-Facial Syndrome (VCFS)

Velo-Cardio-Facial syndrome (VCFS), also called *Shprintzen syndrome*, is caused by a deletion of the long arm of chromosome 22. It is characterized by:

- Cleft palate
- Heart defects
- Short stature, curvature of the spine (scoliosis), tapered fingers
- Microcephaly, retrognathia (retruded lower jaw), facial asymmetry
- Small and almond-shaped eyes, strabismus, puffy eyelids, cataracts
- Prominent nasal bridge, bulbous nasal tip that may appear slightly bifid, narrow nostrils and nasal passages
- Small and asymmetric ears, narrow external ear canals
- Muscular weakness
- Learning difficulties that may not become apparent until the school-age years
- Borderline normal intellect, occasional intellectual disability
- Feeding difficulties with possible failure to thrive; nasal regurgitation
- Frequent otitis media
- Conductive and sensorineural hearing loss
- Unilateral vocal cord paresis
- High-pitched voice, hoarseness, and velopharyngeal insufficiency

- Articulation deficits related to cleft, glottal stop substitutions
- Mild language impairment

Waardenburg Syndrome

Waardenburg syndrome is a genetic syndrome characterized by:

- Pigment abnormalities such as heterochromia iridis (different colors of the iris), vitiligo (unpigmented, pale patches of skin), and the most noticeable feature—a white forelock in the hair (which may be masked if the entire scalp turns white prematurely)
- Short palpebral fissures, cleft lip or palate, and a prognathic (markedly projected) mandible
- Profound sensorineural hearing loss that is unilateral or bilateral
- Language disorders associated with congenital hearing loss
- Hypernasality and nasal emission in cases occurring with a cleft palate
- Articulation disorders associated with clefting, palatal insufficiency, a prognathic mandible, and hearing loss

XO Syndrome

See Turner Syndrome.

CONCLUDING COMMENTS

This chapter described many medical conditions, diseases, and syndromes that have a potential impact on speech-language development and function. The information provided here is simplified and non-exhaustive. Further research is recommended, especially when working with a client diagnosed with a particular diagnosis. An accurate assessment for a speech-language disorder depends upon thorough knowledge of associated medical diagnoses.

SOURCES OF ADDITIONAL INFORMATION

Print Sources

Gerber, S. E. (2001). *Handbook of genetic communicative disorders*. Burlington, MA: Academic Press.

Shprintzen, R. J. (2000). *Syndrome identification for speech–language pathology*. Clifton Park, NY: Cengage Learning.

Venes, D., & Tabor, C. W. (Eds.). (2013). *Taber's cyclopedic medical dictionary* (22nd ed.). Philadelphia: F.A. Davis.

Electronic Sources

MedicineNet.com:
http://medicinenet.com

U.S. National Library of Medicine:
http://www.nlm.nih.gov

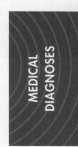

MEDICAL DIAGNOSES

Chapter 18

QUICK REFERENCES AND CAREGIVER HANDOUTS

- **Speech, Language, and Motor Development**

- **Suggestions for Increasing Speech and Language Development in Children**

- **Speech Sounds and Normal Development**

  Phonetic Symbols of the English Language

- **Reading and Writing Development**

- **Theory of Mind**

- **Communication Options for Laryngectomees**

- **Impact of Hearing Loss in a Classroom Environment**

- **Environmental Noise Levels**

- **Images for Conveying Information**

- **Sources of Additional Information**

The materials in this section are quick reference materials useful for personal review or caregiver handouts. Some materials are presented in other parts of the text and repeated here in a format that is easy to copy and present to a caregiver.

SPEECH, LANGUAGE, AND MOTOR DEVELOPMENT

The following information provides a general summary of the developmental sequence of speech, language, and motor skills in normal children. Because children develop at different rates, avoid strictly applying age approximations. The time intervals are provided only as a general guideline for age appropriateness. Cultural considerations should also be made.

0–6 Months
Speech and Language Skills

- Frequently coos, gurgles, and makes pleasure sounds
- Uses a different cry to express different needs
- Smiles when spoken to
- Recognizes voices
- Localizes to sound
- Listens to speech
- Uses the phonemes /b/, /p/, and /m/ in babbling
- Uses sounds or gestures to indicate wants
- Responds to *no* and changes in tone of voice

Motor Skills

- Smiles
- Rolls over from front to back and back to front
- Raises head and shoulders from a face-down position
- Establishes head control
- Sits while using hands for support
- Reaches for objects with one hand but often misses
- Visually tracks people and objects
- Watches own hands

7–12 Months
Speech and Language Skills

- Understands *no* and *hot*
- Responds to simple requests
- Understands and responds to own name
- Recognizes words for common items (e.g., *cup, shoe, juice*)

- Babbles using long and short groups of sounds
- Uses a large variety of sounds in babbling
- Imitates some adult speech sounds and intonation patterns
- Uses speech sounds rather than only crying to get attention
- Listens when spoken to
- Uses sound approximations
- Begins to change babbling to jargon
- Uses speech intentionally for the first time
- Uses nouns almost exclusively
- Has an expressive vocabulary of one to three words
- Uses characteristic gestures or vocalizations to express wants

Motor Skills

- Crawls on stomach
- Stands or walks with assistance
- Stands momentarily without support
- Puts self in a sitting position
- Sits unsupported
- Drinks from a cup
- Pulls self up to stand by furniture
- Holds own bottle
- Has poor aim and timing of release when throwing
- Uses a primitive grasp for writing, bangs crayon rather than writes
- Transfers objects from hand to hand
- Explores objects with index finger

13–18 Months

Speech and Language Skills

- Imitates individual words
- Uses adult-like intonation patterns
- Uses echolalia and jargon
- Omits some initial consonants and almost all final consonants
- Produces mostly unintelligible speech
- Follows simple commands
- Receptively identifies one to three body parts
- Has an expressive vocabulary of 3 to 20 or more words (mostly nouns)
- Combines gestures and vocalization
- Makes requests for more of desired items

Motor Skills

- Walks without assistance
- Walks up and down stairs with assistance
- Runs, but falls frequently
- Imitates gestures
- Removes some clothing items (e.g., socks, hat)
- Attempts to pull zippers up and down
- Uses common objects appropriately
- Uses smooth and continuous reach to grasp objects
- Builds a simple tower of three to four blocks

19–24 Months

Speech and Language Skills

- Uses words more frequently than jargon
- Has an expressive vocabulary of 50–100 or more words
- Has a receptive vocabulary of 300 or more words
- Starts to combine nouns with verbs and nouns with adjectives
- Begins to use pronouns
- Maintains unstable voice control
- Uses appropriate intonation for questions
- Is approximately 25–50% intelligible to strangers
- Asks and answers "What's that?" questions
- Enjoys listening to stories
- Knows five body parts
- Accurately names a few familiar objects
- Understands basic categories (e.g., toys, food)
- Points to pictures in a book when named

Motor Skills

- Walks sideways and backwards
- Uses pull toys
- Strings large beads
- Picks up objects from the floor without falling
- Kicks a ball
- Jumps in place
- Climbs and stands on a chair
- Reaches automatically with primary concern on manipulation of object
- Walks up and down stairs

- Stands on one foot with help
- Seats self in a child's chair
- Makes a tower of four or more blocks high
- Scribbles in circles

2–3 Years
Speech and Language Skills

- Speech is 50–75% intelligible
- Understands *one* and *all*
- Verbalizes toilet needs (before, during, or after act)
- Requests items by name
- Identifies several body parts
- Follows two-part commands
- Asks one- to two-word questions
- Uses two- to four-word phrases
- Uses words that are general in context
- Continues use of echolalia when difficulties in speech are encountered
- Has a receptive vocabulary of 500–900 or more words
- Has an expressive vocabulary of 50–250 or more words (rapid growth during this period)
- Exhibits multiple grammatical errors
- Understands most things said to him or her
- Frequently exhibits repetitions—especially starters, "I," and first syllables
- Speaks with a loud voice
- Increases range of pitch
- Uses vowels correctly
- Consistently uses initial consonants (although some are misarticulated)
- Frequently omits medial consonants
- Frequently omits or substitutes final consonants
- Uses auxiliary *is* including the contracted form
- Uses some regular past-tense verbs, possessive morphemes, pronouns, and imperatives
- Maintains topic over several conversational turns

Motor Skills

- Walks with characteristic toddling movements
- Begins developing rhythm
- Balances on one foot for one second
- Walks on tiptoes

- Turns pages one by one, or two to three at a time
- Folds paper roughly in half on imitation
- Builds a tower of six to eight blocks
- Scribbling resembles writing
- Paints with whole arm movements
- Undresses self
- Takes objects apart and reassembles them
- Climbs well

3–4 Years
Speech and Language Skills

- Understands object functions
- Understands opposites (stop–go, in–on, big–little)
- Follows two- and three-part commands
- Produces simple verbal analogies
- Uses language to express emotion
- Uses four to five words in sentences
- Repeats 6- to 13-syllable sentences accurately
- May continue to use echolalia
- Uses nouns and verbs most frequently
- Is conscious of past and future
- Has a 1,200–2,000 or more word receptive vocabulary
- Has a 800–1,500 or more word expressive vocabulary
- May repeat self often, exhibiting blocks, disturbed breathing, and facial grimaces during speech
- Increases speech rate
- Speech is approximately 80% intelligible
- Appropriately uses *is*, *are*, and *am* in sentences
- Tells two events in chronological order
- Engages in long conversations
- Sentence grammar improves, although some errors still persist
- Uses some contractions, irregular plurals, future-tense verbs, and conjunctions
- Consistently uses regular plurals, possessives, and simple past-tense verbs
- Uses an increasing number of compound or complex sentences

Motor Skills

- Kicks ball forward
- Turns pages one at a time

- Learns to use blunt scissors
- Runs and plays active games with abandonment
- Balances and walks on toes
- Unbuttons, but cannot button
- Uses one hand consistently for most activities
- Traces a square, copies a circle, and imitates horizontal strokes
- Puts on own shoes, but not necessarily on the correct foot
- Rides a tricycle
- Jumps in place with both feet together
- Dresses and undresses self

4–5 Years

Speech and Language Skills

- Imitatively counts to five
- Continues understanding of spatial concepts
- Has a receptive vocabulary of 10,000 or more words
- Counts to ten by rote
- Listens to short, simple stories and can answer questions about them
- Answers questions about function
- Uses adult-like grammar most of the time
- Grammatical errors primarily in irregular forms, reflexive pronouns, adverbial suffixes, and comparative/superlative inflections
- Has an expressive vocabulary of 900–2,000 or more words
- Uses sentences of four to eight words
- Answers complex two-part questions
- Asks for word definitions
- Speaks at a rate of approximately 186 words per minute
- Reduces total number of repetitions
- Significantly reduces number of persistent sound omissions and substitutions
- Frequently omits medial consonants
- Speech is usually intelligible to strangers even though some articulation errors may persist
- Accurately tells about experiences at school, at friends' homes, etc.

Motor Skills

- Pushes, pulls, and steers wheeled toys
- Jumps over 6-inch-high object and lands on both feet together
- Throws ball with direction

- Balances on one foot for 5 seconds
- Pours from a pitcher
- Spreads substances with a knife
- Uses toilet independently
- Skips to music
- Hops on one foot
- Walks on a line
- Uses legs with good strength, ease, and facility
- Grasps with thumb and medial finger
- Holds paper with hand when writing
- Draws circles, crosses, and diamonds
- Draws figures that represent people, animals, objects
- Copies simple block letters
- Dresses and undresses without assistance

5–6 Years

Speech and Language Skills

- Follows instructions given to a group
- Asks *how* questions
- Uses past tense and future tense appropriately
- Uses conjunctions
- Has a receptive vocabulary of approximately 13,000 words
- Sequentially names days of the week
- Counts to 30 by rote
- Continues to drastically increase vocabulary
- Uses sentence length of four to six words
- Reverses sounds occasionally
- Exchanges information and asks questions
- Uses sentences with details
- Accurately relays a story
- Sings entire songs and recites nursery rhymes
- Communicates easily with adults and other children
- Uses appropriate grammar in most cases

Motor Skills

- Walks backward heel-to-toe
- Does somersaults
- Cuts on a line with scissors

- Cuts food with a knife
- Ties own shoes
- Builds complex structures with blocks
- Gracefully roller skates, skips, jumps rope, and rides a bicycle
- Competently uses miniature tools
- Buttons clothes, washes face, and puts toys away
- Catches a ball with hands
- Makes precise marks with crayon, confining marks to a small area
- Draws recognizable people with head, trunk, legs, and arms

6–7 Years

Speech and Language Skills

- Understands *left* and *right*
- Uses increasingly more complex descriptions
- Engages in conversations
- Has a receptive vocabulary of approximately 20,000 words
- Uses a sentence length of approximately six words
- Understands most concepts of time
- Counts to 100 by rote
- Uses most morphologic markers appropriately
- Uses passive voice appropriately

Motor Skills

- Improved coordination and balance for climbing, bike riding, and other sports activities
- Shows reduced interest in writing and drawing
- Draws pictures that are not proportional
- Uses adult-like writing, but it is slow and labored
- Runs lightly on toes
- Walks on a balance beam
- Cuts out simple shapes
- Colors within the lines
- Indicates well-established right- or left-handedness
- Dresses self completely
- Brushes teeth without assistance

SUGGESTIONS FOR INCREASING SPEECH AND LANGUAGE DEVELOPMENT IN CHILDREN

- From birth, talk to your child *a lot*. Bath time, mealtime, and bedtime are perfect opportunities to model language and build vocabulary. Talk about what you are doing, seeing, or thinking, or talk about what is going to happen.
- Provide a good language model. Speak clearly, maintain eye contact, and use natural intonation when talking to your child.
- Acknowledge and expand on what your child says. If he or she says,"Milk," reply with "You want milk? I will get milk for you. Here is your milk."
- Give your child opportunities to communicate. Ask questions that require a choice, such as, "Do you want water or juice?" If your child points to something he or she wants, encourage speech by saying, "Tell me what you want?" Pause after asking questions or making comments to give your child an opportunity to talk.
- Imitate and reinforce sounds and words your child says. If a word is said incorrectly, never criticize. Repeat it back, modeling the correct pronunciation.
- Sing children's songs, especially repetitive songs such as *The Wheels on the Bus* and *If You're Happy and You Know It*. Use hand and body motions to reinforce the words.
- Play with your child frequently. Name objects and colors, count, describe things, make animal sounds, and take turns. Play "let's pretend" and "I'm thinking of . . ." games.
- Read to your child frequently. Name pictures in a book and talk about the story. Rhyming books are especially good for early literacy development.
- With older children, make up stories together with a setting, characters, a plot with a conflict, and a resolution.
- Avoid screen time as a passive activity. Instead, watch or play together. Talk about what you are watching. Make predictions and talk about the characters. Play cognitive and language-building games together on devices such as iPads or tablets. Solo play does not build language and can hinder growth.
- Follow your child's lead. For example, if he or she likes animals, read books about animals; talk about what animals say, where they live, what they eat, what they look like, etc.; visit a zoo together.
- Consult a speech-language pathologist if you are concerned about your child's communicative development.

QUICK REFERENCES

SPEECH SOUNDS AND NORMAL DEVELOPMENT

The following figures and tables are useful for providing information about sounds of the English language and normal consonant development.

Phonetic Symbols of the English Language

This table shows International Phonetic Alphabet (IPA) symbols of English consonants and vowels and their translations.

CONSONANTS				VOWELS			
VOICED		**UNVOICED**				**R-CONTROLLED**	**DIPHTHONGS**
/b/ as in big		/p/ as in pin		/i/ as in meet		/ɝ/ as in sure (stressed)	/aɪ/ as in bye
/d/ as in dog		/t/ as in tie		/ɪ/ as in it			/eɪ/ as in crayon
/g/ as in go		/k/ as in cat		/e/ as in eight		/ɚ/ as in mother (unstressed)	/aʊ/ as in out
/v/ as in vase		/f/ as in far		/ɛ/ as in met			/ɔɪ/ as in boy
/z/ as in zoo		/s/ as in sit		/æ/ as in ask		/ɪɚ/ as in ear	/oʊ/ as in mode
/ð/ as in this		/θ/ as in think		/ə/ as in control (unstressed)		/ɛɚ/ as in hair	
/ʒ/ as in measure		/ʃ/ as in shake				/ɔɚ/ as in or	
/dʒ/ as in jump		/tʃ/ as in chip		/ʌ/ as in country (stressed)		/ɑɚ/ as in car	
/m/ as in mop		/h/ as in hi					
/n/ as in no				/u/ as in too			
/ŋ/ as in sing				/ʊ/ as in book			
/l/ as in light				/o/ as in go			
/r/ as in rake				/ɔ/ as in dog			
/j/ as in yes				/ɑ/ as in saw			
/w/ as in wet							

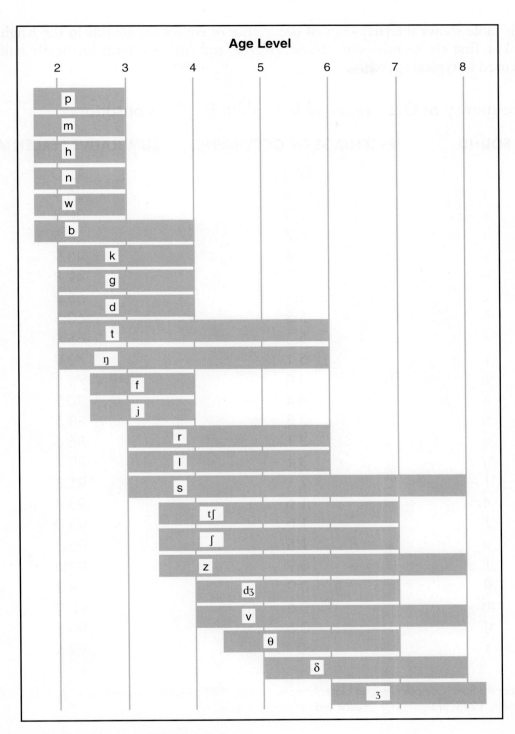

Age Ranges of Normal Consonant Development

Average age estimates and upper age limits of customary consonant production. The bar corresponding to each sound starts at the median age of customary articulation; it stops at an age level at which 90% of all children are customarily producing the sound (data from Templin, 1957; Wellman et al., 1931). From "When Are Speech Sounds Learned?" by E. Sander, 1972, *Journal of Speech and Hearing Disorders, 37*, 55–63. Copyright 1972 by the American Speech-Language-Hearing Association. Reprinted with permission.

This table shows the frequency of occurrence of consonant sounds in the English language. The first six sounds—/n/, /t/, /s/, /r/, /d/, and /m/—account for nearly half of the sounds used in typical speech.

The Frequency of Occurrence of Individual English Consonants

SOUND	PERCENTAGE OF OCCURRENCE	CUMULATIVE PERCENTAGE
n	12.0	12.0
t	11.9	23.9
s	6.9	30.8
r	6.7	37.5
d	6.4	43.9
m	5.9	49.8
z	5.4	55.2
ð	5.3	60.5
l	5.3	65.8
k	5.1	70.9
w	4.9	75.8
h	4.4	80.2
b	3.3	83.5
p	3.1	86.6
g	3.1	89.7
f	2.1	91.8
ŋ	1.6	93.4
j	1.6	95.0
v	1.5	96.5
ʃ	0.9	97.4
θ	0.9	98.3
dʒ	0.6	98.9
tʃ	0.6	99.5
ʒ	<0.1	99.6

Source: Adapted from "Computer-Assisted Natural Process Analysis (NPA): Recent Issues and Data," by L. D. Shriberg and J. Kwiatkowski, 1983, in *Seminars in Speech and Language, 4*, p. 4.

READING AND WRITING DEVELOPMENT

The following information presents the normal sequence of development for reading and writing.

Birth–2 Years

Reading

- From birth, a child is exposed to print (e.g., on household items, billboards, books, etc.).
- Child accumulates knowledge about letters, words, and books.

3 Years

Reading

- Metalinguistic knowledge develops (i.e., knowledge that language consists of discrete phonemes, words, phrases, and sentences).
- Phonological awareness develops, (i.e., awareness that words are made up of sound segments).
- Knowledge of the alphabetic principle begins (i.e., letters in English represent speech sounds).
- Child recognizes words that rhyme (e.g., *hat, rat*) and words that begin with the same sound (e.g., *big ball*).
- Print awareness develops; child understands that print has meaning and structure (e.g., moves from left to right, top to bottom; words are separated by space). Child recognizes trademark logos (e.g., McDonald's®) and the child's own name.

Writing

- Child scribbles, but with no discernable letters.
- Some scribble shows basic knowledge of conventional rules of writing; scribble may occur in lines, may flow from left to right and top to bottom, and may show some conventional spacing.

4 Years

Reading

- Phonemic awareness develops (i.e., awareness that words are made up of specific units of sounds that have distinct features).
- Child says words that rhyme (e.g., *dog, frog*) and words that begin with the same sound (e.g., *cup, cap*).
- Child segments a sentence into separate words (e.g., *The boy jumped* is segmented to *the-boy-jumped*).
- Child counts the number of syllables in words.

Writing

- Writing resembles standard letters and words.
- Child must interpret his or her writing for others.

5 Years (Kindergarten)

Reading

- Child knows when words do not rhyme (e.g., *hog* does not rhyme with *hat*).
- Child recites and names letters of the alphabet and numbers 1–10.
- Child identifies the first sound of a spoken word and separates it from the rime (the first vowel and any following vowels and consonants of a syllable) (e.g., *dog* begins with *d*).
- Child blends the beginning sound with the remaining sounds of a word.
- Child segments multisyllabic words into syllables (e.g., *elephant* is *el-e-phant*).
- Child reads some familiar words by sight.

Writing

- Child knows basic conventional rules of writing; scribble may occur in lines, may flow from left to right and top to bottom, and may show spacing between words.
- Child writes a few meaningful words, usually common nouns and the child's own name.
- Most upper- and lowercase letters are written legibly.

6 Years (First Grade)

Reading

- Phonetic decoding and blending develops; child isolates sounds in short words (e.g., *cat* is *c-a-t*) and can blend two to three sounds to form words (e.g., *b-a-t* is *bat*).
- Child makes up rhymes.
- Child associates sounds with alphabetic symbols (i.e., sound–symbol association).
- Child segments a final consonant from the rest of the word (e.g., separates *bi-* from *-g* in *big*).
- Simple words are sounded out when reading.
- Child matches spoken word with print.
- Child has a sight vocabulary of 100 words.
- Child reads and comprehends grade-level material.

Writing

- Child shows knowledge of the relationship between letters and sounds.
- Mostly uppercase letters are used.
- Child writes strings of letters (not words) with no spacing.

- Only one or some letters in a word are written, usually the first consonant, to represent a whole word or syllable.
- Invented spellings are typical; initial and final consonants are present, although vowels may be omitted.
- Begins sentences with a capital letter and ends sentences with a period.
- Subject matter of writing usually expresses feelings, personal ideas, and memories.
- Sentences are short and simple.
- Grammatical errors are common (e.g., verb tense, regular and irregular plurals).

7 Years (Second Grade)

Reading

- Child counts the number of phonemes in a word.
- Child uses phonetic strategies and orthographic processing (learned spelling patterns and sight words) to read new words.
- Child rereads and self-corrects as needed.
- Contextual clues for comprehension are used (e.g., pictures, titles, headings, etc.).
- Questions are answered by locating information in written material.
- Child has good comprehension of basic story elements.
- Child retells a story.
- Child reads spontaneously.

Writing

- Phonetic spellings decrease and traditional spellings increase; spelling rules are applied more frequently.
- Child correctly uses upper- and lowercase letters, space between words, and basic punctuation.
- Writing is legible.
- Child writes simple fiction and nonfiction based on a model and using a variety of sentence types.
- Writing is organized with a beginning, middle, and end.
- Familiar words are correctly spelled.
- Morphologic structures in the spelling system are better internalized.

8 Years (Third Grade)

Reading

- Basic phonetic patterns are mastered.
- Child segments and deletes consonant clusters.
- Maturing experience with sound–symbol associations allows decoding of more unfamiliar words.

- Child uses word analysis skills when reading.
- Child uses language content and schema knowledge to aid in comprehension.
- What will happen in a story is predicted.
- Child uses reading materials to learn about new topics.
- Child reads grade-level books fluently.

Writing

- Conventional spellings are used primarily, and a dictionary is used to learn new or correct spellings.
- Vowels are used correctly most of the time.
- Letters are transposed in less-frequently-used words.
- Child writes narratives, letters, and simple expository reports.
- Sentence lengths increase and include more complex forms.

9 Years (Fourth Grade)
Reading

- Decoding skills are fully automatic, enabling fluent reading.
- Child reads for pleasure and to learn.
- Child reads and understands a variety of literature types (e.g., fiction, nonfiction, historical fiction, poetry).
- Written instructions are followed.
- Child takes brief notes and uses reference materials.
- Child makes inferences from text.
- Content of text is paraphrased.

Writing

- Child recognizes misspellings and can correctly spell unfamiliar words by using orthographic knowledge.
- Conventions and exceptions in spelling rules are known.
- Child uses narrative and expository writing.
- Child organizes writing by using a beginning, middle, and end to convey a central idea.
- Own work is edited for grammar, punctuation, and spelling.

10 Years (Fifth Grade)
Reading

- Child reads a variety of literary forms.
- Character and plot development is described.

- Child describes characteristics of poetry.
- Lengthier and more complex text is comprehended.

Writing

- Child writes for a variety of purposes using a variety of sentence structures.
- Vocabulary is used effectively.
- Child revises and edits own writing.

11–18 Years (6th–12th Grade)

Reading

- Child reads for learning and entertainment.
- Child becomes a more mature, critical reader.
- Reading skills are applied to obtain new knowledge and specific information.

Writing

- Child writes sentences that are longer than spoken sentences and more linguistically complex.
- Expository writing is used to provide explanations and descriptions.

19+ Years (College)

Reading

- Materials are read for inquiry, critical analysis, and entertainment.
- New ideas are integrated into an existing knowledge base.

Writing

- Persuasive text is written.

This table shows the normal progression of phonemic awareness for the development of reading and writing.

Phonemic Awareness Benchmarks

AGE OF DEVELOPMENT	PHONEMIC AWARENESS SKILLS
3 years	• Familiar with known nursery rhymes (e.g., *Jack and Jill*). • Recognizes alliteration (e.g., the words *my milk* begin with same first sound) • Recognizes words that rhyme (e.g., *cat* and *bat*)
4 years	• Segments a sentence into separate words • Segments multisyllabic words into syllables (e.g., *cowboy* has two parts, *cow* and *boy*) • Says words that rhyme
5 years	• Counts the number of syllables in words • Segments the beginning sound (onset) from the rest of a word (rime) (*b-at*) • Blends the beginning sound with the rest of a word • Identifies a word that does not rhyme with a target (e.g., *dog* does not rhyme with *jam* and *ham*)
6 years	• Makes up rhymes • Matches initial consonants in words (e.g., *big* and *boy* begin with same first sound) • Blends two or three phonemes to make a word (e.g., phonemes /k/ /æ/ /t/ form the word *cat*) • Segments initial consonant blends from the rest of the word (e.g., divides *trick* into *tr-* and *-ick*) • Segments the final consonant from the rest of the word (e.g., divides *make* into *ma-* and *-ke*)
7 years	• Counts the number of phonemes in a word • Blends isolated phonemes to form words • Segments phonemes within words • Spells phonetically • Adds phonemes to, or deletes phonemes from, words
8 years	• Relocates phonemes in a word to make a new word (e.g., moves *t* in *tar* to the end to make *art*) • Segments consonant clusters • Deletes consonant clusters

Sources: Goldsworthy (2003); Justice (2006); Naremore, Densmore, and Harman (2001).

This table presents the normal sequence of development for learning to spell.

Spelling Benchmarks

STAGE	AGE	CHARACTERISTICS
Precommunicative Spellers	3–5 years	• Scribble; no discernable letters • The child interprets the scribble • Some scribble shows basic knowledge of conventional rules of writing: scribble may occur in lines, may flow from left to right and top to bottom, and may show some conventional spacing
Semiphonetic Spellers	5–6 years	• Child shows early knowledge of the relationship between letters and sounds • Child uses mostly uppercase letters • Child often writes in strings of letters (not words) with no spacing • Child writes only one or some letters in a word, usually the first consonant, to represent a whole word or syllable
Phonetic Spellers	6–7 years	• Child can phonetically map out most words; initial and final consonants are present, although vowels may not be • Words are often not recognizable, but can be deciphered using rules of phonetics • Child uses upper- and lowercase letters • Child uses space between words • Child correctly spells words he or she knows
Transitional Spellers	7–8 years	• Child uses less phonetic spelling and more conventional spelling • Vowels used are correct more often • Child transposes letters in less-frequently-used words
Conventional Spellers	8+ years	• Child knows conventional spelling for most familiar words • Child often knows when words don't look right • Child can often correctly figure out how to spell unfamiliar words by using orthographic knowledge • Child has knowledge of conventions and exceptions in spelling rules

Source: Adapted from Gentry (2004).

QUICK REFERENCES

THEORY OF MIND

Theory of Mind (ToM) is the knowledge that other people have thoughts and emotions separate from our own. The following table shows normal developmental expectations of ToM.

Milestones of Metacognitive Knowledge ToM and Emotional Knowledge ToM in Normally Developing Children

AGE OF MASTERY	ToM KNOWLEDGE
Metacognitive Knowledge	
3	Predict uncomplicated behaviors or situations (e.g., Mommy will get a puzzle out of the game closet, because that is where puzzles are stored.)
5	Understand that people can hold false beliefs (e.g., Mom thinks the cookie jar is full; she doesn't know I ate the cookies.)
7	Understand nested beliefs (e.g., "Mom thinks that Dad thinks . . .")
Emotional Knowledge	
5	Relate experiences in which they felt sad, happy, mad, scared, or surprised
7	Relate experiences in which they felt jealous, guilty, or embarrassed

Source: "Autism," by C. Westby and N. McKellar, in *The Survival Guide for School-Based Speech-Language Pathologists* (pp. 263–303), by E. P. Dodge (Ed.), 2000, Clifton Park, NY: Cengage Learning.

COMMUNICATION OPTIONS FOR LARYNGECTOMEES

This table describes the major advantages and disadvantages of the three primary communication options following laryngectomy.

Advantages and Disadvantages of the Three Primary Alaryngeal Communication Options

ARTIFICIAL LARYNX

Advantages:	Easy to use
	Speech is generally intelligible
	Suitable for use immediately after surgery in most cases
	Can be an interim source of communication
Disadvantages:	Mechanical, "robot-like" vocal quality
	Draws attention to the speaker
	Requires good articulation skills
	Requires the use of one hand

ESOPHAGEAL SPEECH

Advantages:	Does not require reliance upon a mechanical device
	Both hands are free while speaking
	Vocal productions are the client's "own voice"
	More natural sounding than electromechanical devices
Disadvantages:	Difficult to learn (approximately one-third of laryngectomees are unable to learn esophageal speech)
	Client may need to learn to habitually speak in shorter phrases
	Vocal intensity is sometimes insufficient
	Client may have a hoarse voice quality
	Potential articulatory errors, excessive stoma noise, "klunking," and facial grimacing need to be overcome during the learning process

TRACHEOESOPHAGEAL SPEECH

Advantages:	Most natural voice quality of all alaryngeal communication options
	Greater pitch and intensity range than esophageal speech
	Easier and faster to learn than esophageal speech
	Clients can effectively produce sentences of normal length
Disadvantages:	Requires additional surgery
	Maintenance of the prosthesis is required
	Manual occlusion of the stoma is required if a tracheostoma valve is not used
	Some risk of aspiration of the prosthesis

IMPACT OF HEARING LOSS IN A CLASSROOM ENVIRONMENT

Effects of Hearing Loss on Communication and Types of Habilitative Intervention with Children

Minimal hearing loss (16- to 25-dB HL)	At 15 dB a student can miss up to 10% of the speech signal when a teacher is at a distance greater than 3 feet and when the classroom is noisy.
Mild hearing loss (26- to 40-dB HL)	With a 30-dB loss, a student can miss 25–40% of a speech signal. Without amplification, the child with 35- to 40-dB loss may miss at least 50% of class discussion.
Moderate hearing loss (41- to 55-dB HL)	Child understands conversational speech at a distance of 3 to 5 feet (face to face) only if structure and vocabulary are controlled. Without amplification, the amount of speech signal missed can be 50–75% with a 40-dB loss, and 80–100% with a 50-dB loss.
Moderate to severe hearing loss (56- to 70-dB HL)	Without amplification, conversation must be very loud to be understood. A 55-dB loss can cause a child to miss up to 100% of speech information.
Severe hearing loss (71- to 90-dB HL)	Without amplification, the child may hear loud voices about 1 foot from the ear. When amplified optimally, children with hearing ability of 90 dB or better should be able to identify environmental sounds and detect all the sounds of speech.
Profound hearing loss (>90-dB HL)	Aware of vibrations more than tonal patterns. May rely on vision rather than hearing as the primary avenue for communication and learning.
Unilateral hearing loss (normal hearing in one ear with the other ear exhibiting at least a mild permanent loss)	May have difficulty hearing faint or distant speech. Usually has difficulty localizing sounds and has greater difficulty understanding speech in background noise.

Adapted from: Elena Plante and Pelagie Beeson, *Communication and Communication Disorders: A Clinical Introduction.* (p. 268)

ENVIRONMENTAL NOISE LEVELS

dB LEVEL	ENVIRONMENTAL NOISE	dB LEVEL	ENVIRONMENTAL NOISE
0 dB	Barely audible sound	90 dB	Lawnmower
10 dB	Normal breathing		Shop tools
	Soft rustle of leaves		Shouted conversation
20 dB	Whisper at 5 feet away		Subway
	Watch ticking		Busy urban street
30 dB	Whisper at 15 feet away		Food blender
40 dB	Quiet office	100 dB	Snowmobile
	Library		School dance
	Birds chirping out the window		Tympani and bass drum rolls
	Refrigerator		Chain saw
50 dB	Moderate rainfall		Pneumatic drill
	Moderate restaurant clatter		Jackhammer
	Inside a typical urban home	110 dB	Shouting in ear
60 dB	Normal conversation		Baby crying
	(50–70 dB)		Squeaky toy held close
	Background music		to the ear
	Department store		Power saw
70 dB	Television		Leaf blower
	Freeway traffic		Motorcycle
	Vacuum cleaner		Busy video arcade
	Bus		Symphony concert
	Noisy restaurant		Car horn
80 dB	Doorbell	120 dB	Thunderclap
	Telephone ring		Hammering nails
	Alarm clock		Ambulance siren
	Noisy restaurant		Live rock concert
	Police whistle	130 dB	Jackhammer
	Garbage disposal		Power drill
	Blow dryer		Percussion section of
			symphony orchestra
			Stock car race

continued on the next page

QUICK
REFERENCES

continued from the previous page

dB LEVEL	ENVIRONMENTAL NOISE	dB LEVEL	ENVIRONMENTAL NOISE
140 dB	Jet engine at takeoff	160 dB	Fireworks at 3 feet
	Firecracker	170 dB	High-powered shotgun
	Toy cap gun	180 dB	Rocket launching from pad
	Firearms		
	Air raid siren		
150 dB	Artillery fire at 500 feet		
	Firecracker		
	Rock music at peak		

Sources: American Speech-Language Hearing Association (2007), Johnson (2005), League for the Hard of Hearing (2007b).

IMAGES FOR CONVEYING INFORMATION

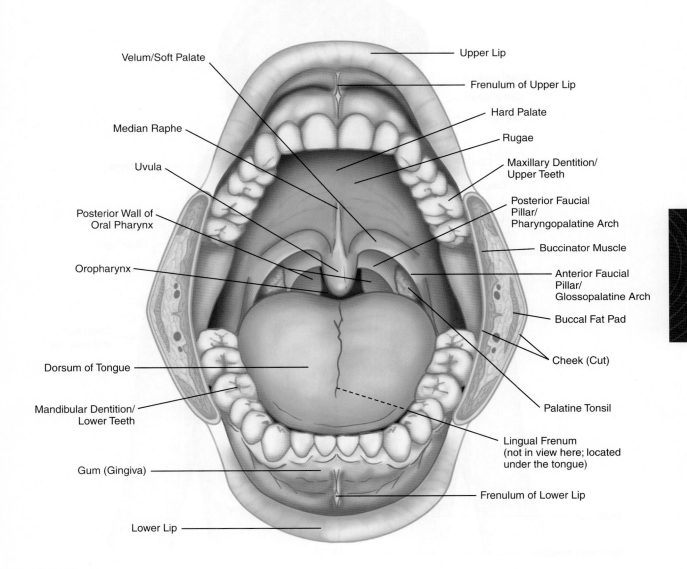

Oral Structures

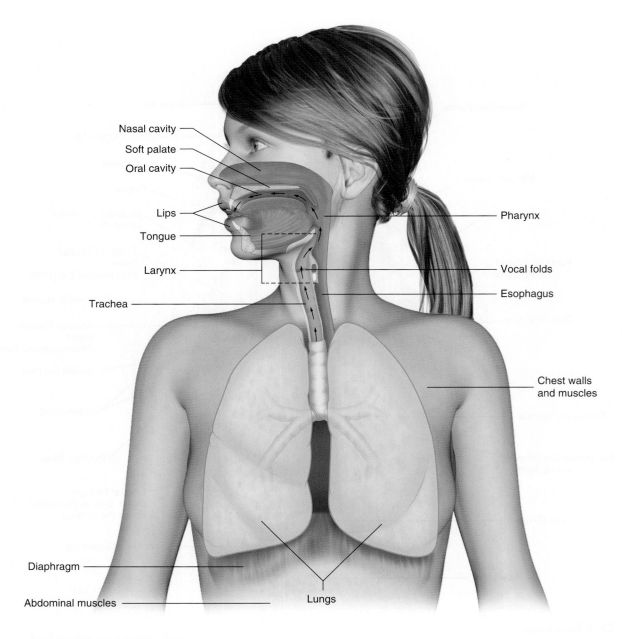

Nasal cavity

Soft palate

Oral cavity

Lips

Tongue

Larynx

Trachea

Diaphragm

Abdominal muscles

Pharynx

Vocal folds

Esophagus

Chest walls and muscles

Lungs

Anatomy of the Vocal Mechanism

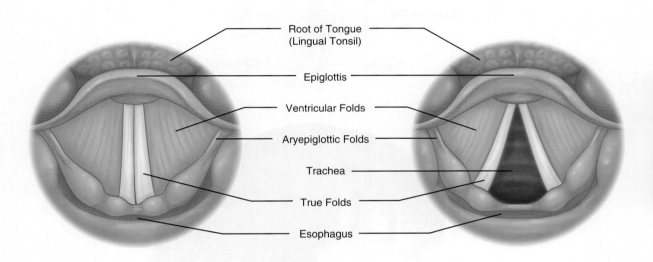

Root of Tongue
(Lingual Tonsil)

Epiglottis

Ventricular Folds

Aryepiglottic Folds

Trachea

True Folds

Esophagus

The Vocal Folds

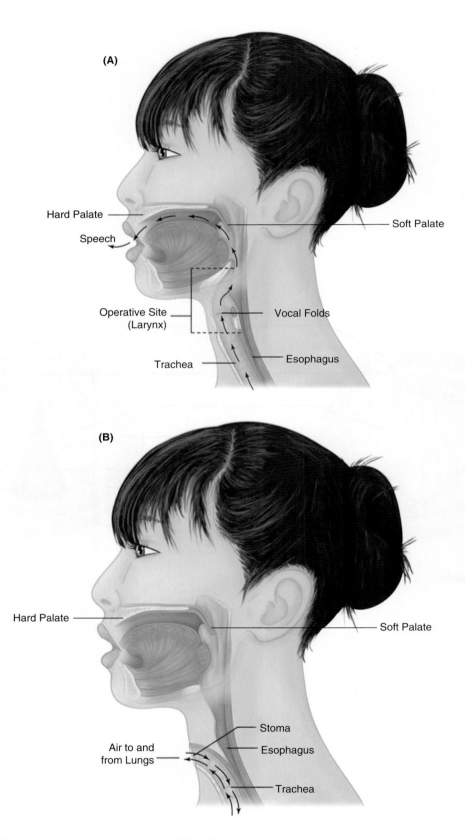

(A)

Hard Palate

Soft Palate

Speech

Operative Site
(Larynx)

Vocal Folds

Trachea

Esophagus

(B)

Hard Palate

Soft Palate

Stoma

Air to and
from Lungs

Esophagus

Trachea

Larynx (a) Before Laryngectomy and (b) After Laryngectomy

Source: Adapted from InHealth Technologies.

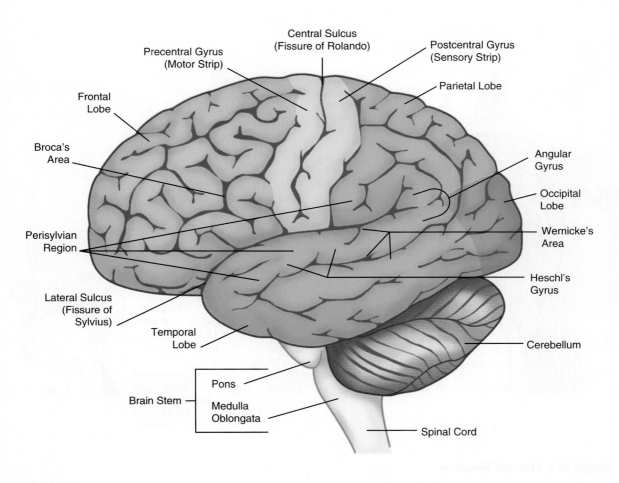

The Brain

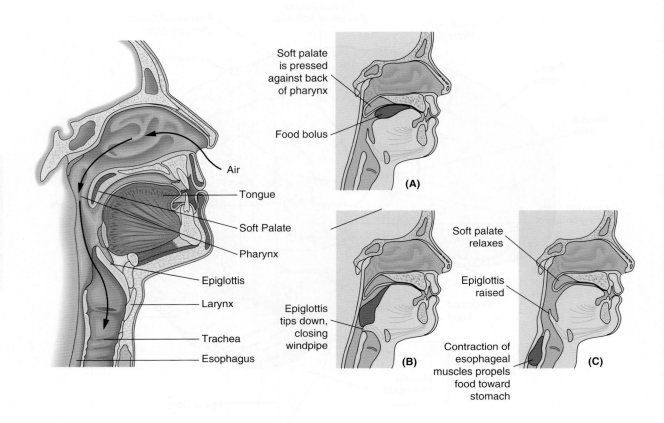

Soft palate
is pressed
against back
of pharynx

Food bolus

Air

Tongue

Soft Palate

Pharynx

Epiglottis

Larynx

Trachea

Esophagus

(A)

Epiglottis
tips down,
closing
windpipe

(B)

Soft palate
relaxes

Epiglottis
raised

Contraction of
esophageal
muscles propels
food toward
stomach

(C)

Stages of a Normal Swallow

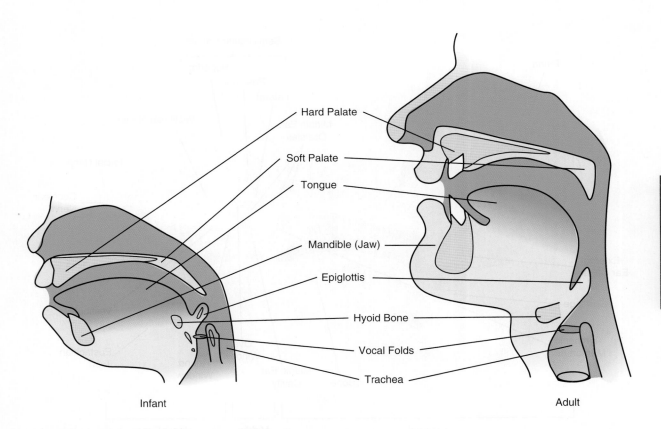

Hard Palate

Soft Palate

Tongue

Mandible (Jaw)

Epiglottis

Hyoid Bone

Vocal Folds

Trachea

Infant

Adult

Anatomical Structures Involved in Swallowing

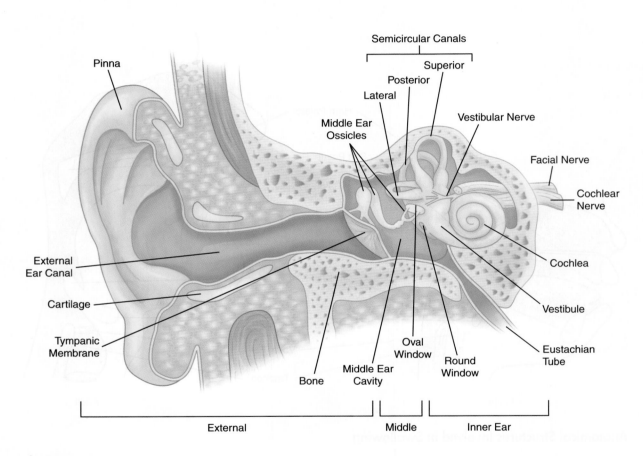

The Ear

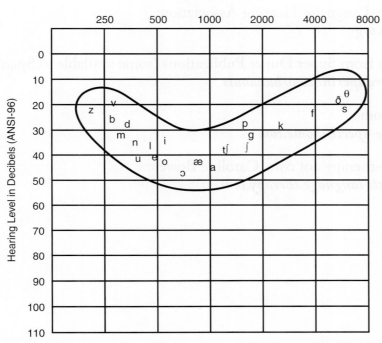

Frequency in Hertz

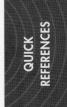

The Speech Banana

SOURCES OF ADDITIONAL INFORMATION

Print Sources

Mawhinney, L., & Scott McTeague, M. (2004). *Early language development: Handouts and activities with bonus CD-ROM*. Greenville, SC: Super Duper Publications.

Electronic Sources

Advance Healthcare Network for Speech and Hearing Patient Handouts:
http://speech-language-pathology-audiology.advanceweb.com/Clinical-Resources/Patient-Handouts/Patient-Handouts.aspx

American Speech-Language-Hearing Association:
http://www.asha.org

Handy Handouts from Super Duper Publications (some available in Spanish):
http://www.superduperinc.com/handouts

Home Speech Home
http://www.home-speech-home.com

Speech-language-therapy dot com, Caroline Bowen:
http://www.speech-language.therapy.com

REFERENCES

Adamovich, B., & Henderson, J. (1992). *Scales of cognitive ability for traumatic brain injury.* Austin, TX: Pro-Ed.

Als, H., Tronick, E., Lester, B. M., & Brazelton, T. B. (1977, September). The Brazelton neonatal behavioral assessment scale (BNBAS). *Journal of Abnormal Psychology, 5*(3), 215–231.

American Speech-Language-Hearing Association. (2002). *Knowledge and skills needed by speech-language pathologists with respect to reading and writing in children and adolescents* [knowledge and skills]. Available from http://www.asha.org/

American Speech-Language-Hearing Association. (2007a). *Childhood apraxia of speech* [technical report]. Available from http://www.asha.org/

American Speech-Language-Hearing Association. (2007b). *Noise and Hearing Loss.* Retrieved from http://www.asha.org/

American Speech-Language-Hearing Association. (2009). *How does your child hear and talk?* Rockville, MD: American Speech-Language-Hearing Association.

Apel, K., & Masterson. J. (1998). *Assessment and treatment of narrative skills: What's the story?* Rockville, MD: American Speech-Language-Hearing Association.

Arvedson, J.C. & Brodsky, L. (2002). *Pediatric swallowing and feeding assessment and management* (2nd ed.). Clifton Park, NY: Thompson Learning.

Bankson, N. W. (1990). *Bankson language test* (2nd ed.). Austin, TX: Pro-Ed.

Bayles, K., & Tomoeda, C. (1993). *Arizona battery for communication disorders of dementia* (ABCD). Tucson, AZ: Canyonlands.

Bayles, K., & Tomoeda, C. K. (1995). *Functional linguistic communication inventory.* Austin, TX: Pro-Ed.

Bayley, N. (2005). *Bayley scales of infant and toddler development* (3rd ed.). San Antonio, TX: Pearson.

Bernthal, J. E., & Bankson, N. W. (2004). *Articulation and phonological disorders* (5th ed.). Needham Heights, MA: Allyn & Bacon.

Blakeley, R. W. (2000). *Screening test for developmental apraxia of speech* (2nd ed.). Austin, TX: Pro-Ed.

Bleile, K. M. (2004). *Manual of articulation and phonological disorders: Infancy through Adulthood* (2nd ed.). Clifton Park, NY: Delmar Learning.

Boehm, A. E. (2001). *Boehm test of basic concepts* (3rd ed.). New York: Psychological Corporation.

Boersma, P., & Weenink, D. (2014). Praat: Doing phonetics by computer (Version 5.4) [Computer program]. Retrieved from http://www.praat.org/

Bolton, S. O., & Dashiell, S. E. (1998). *INteraction CHecklist for augmentative communication: An observational tool to assess interactive behavior (INCH)* (Rev.). Bisbee, AZ: Imaginart.

Bowers, L., Huisingh, R., LoGiudice, C., & Orman, J. (2002). *Test of semantic skills—primary*. East Moline, IL: LinguiSystems.

Bray, M. A., Kehle, T. J., Lawless, K. A., & Theodore, L. A. (2003). The relationship of self-efficacy and depression to stuttering. *American Journal of Speech-Language Pathology, 12*, 425–431.

Brazelton, T. B., & Nugent, J. K. (1995). *The neonatal behavioral assessment scale*. Mac Keith Press, Cambridge.

Brookshire, R. H. (2003). *An introduction to neurogenic communication disorders* (6th ed.). St. Louis: Mosby-Year Book.

Brookshire, R. H., & Nicholas, L. E. (1997). *Discourse comprehension test* (2nd ed.). Albuquerque, NM: PICA Programs.

Brown, R. (1973). *A first language: The early stages*. Cambridge, MA: Harvard University Press.

Brownell, R. (Ed.). (2000). *Receptive one-word picture vocabulary test*. Novato, CA: Academic Therapy Publications.

Brownell, R. (Ed.). (2010). *Expressive one-word picture vocabulary test*. (4th ed.) Novato, CA: Academic Therapy Publications.

Bruno, J. (2010). *Test of aided-communication symbol performance (TASP)*. Pittsburg, PA: DynaVox Mayer-Johnson.

Brutten, G. J., & Vanryckeghem, M. (2007). *The behavior assessment battery for school-age children who stutter*. San Diego, CA: Plural.

Bryant, B. R., Wiederholdt, J. L., & Bryant, D. P. (2004). *Gray diagnostic reading tests* (2nd ed.). Austin, TX: Pro-Ed.

Bzoch, K. R. (Ed.). (2004). *Communicative disorders related to cleft lip and palate* (5th ed.). Austin, TX: Pro-Ed.

Bzoch, K. R., League, R., & Brown, V. L. (2003). *Receptive-expressive emergent language scale* (3rd ed.). Austin, TX: Pro-Ed.

Calvert, D. R., & Silverman, S. R. (1983). *Speech and deafness* (rev. ed.). Washington DC: Alexander Graham Bell Association for the Deaf.

Carrow-Woolfolk, E. (1996). *OWLS written expression (WE) scale*. Bloomington, MN: Pearson Assessments.

Carrow-Woolfolk, E. (1999). *Comprehensive assessment of spoken language (CASL)*. Torrance, CA: Western Psychological Services.

Carrow-Woolfolk, E., & Allen, E. A. (2013). *Test of expressive language (TEXL)*. San Antonio, TX: Pro-Ed.

Chall, J. S. (1983, 1996). *Stages of reading development*. New York: McGraw-Hill.

Chomsky, N., & Halle, M. (1991). *The sound pattern of English* (2nd ed.). Cambridge, MA: MIT Press.

Coplan, J. (1993). *Early language milestone scale* (2nd ed.). Austin, TX: Pro-Ed.

CTB/McGraw-Hill. (1996). *Test of cognitive skills (TCS/2)* (2nd ed). Monterey, CA: CTB/McGraw-Hill.

Cummins, J. (1992). Language proficiency, bilingualism, and academic achievement. In P. A. Richard-Amato & M. A. Snow (Eds.), *The multicultural classroom: Readings for content-area teachers* (pp. 16–27). New York: Longman.

Dabul, B. (2000). *Apraxia battery for adults* (2nd ed.). Austin, TX: Pro-Ed.

Darley, F. L., Aronson, A. E., & Brown, J. R. (1975). *Motor speech disorders.* Philadelphia: W. B. Saunders Co.

Dikeman, K. J., & Kazandjian, M. S. (2003). *Communication and swallowing management of tracheostomized and ventilator-dependent adults* (2nd ed.). Clifton Park, NY: Delmar Learning.

Dodd, B., Hua, Z., Crosbie, S., Holm, A., & Ozanne, A. (2006). *Diagnostic evaluation of articulation and phonology (DEAP).* San Antonio, TX: Pearson.

Dunn, L. M., & Dunn, L. M. (2007). *Peabody picture vocabulary test* (4th ed.). Bloomington, MN: Pearson Assessments.

Edwards, H. T. (2003). *Applied phonetics: The sounds of American English* (3rd ed.). Clifton Park, NY: Delmar Learning.

Enderby, P. M., & Palmer R. (2008). *Frenchay dysarthria assessment* (2nd ed.) Austin, TX: Pro-Ed.

Erickson, R. L. (1969). Assessing communicate attitudes among stutterers. *Journal of Speech and Hearing Research, 12,* 711–724.

Fletcher, S.G. (1972). Time-by-count measurement of diadochokinetic syllable rate. *Journal of Speech and Hearing Disorders, 15,* 763–770.

Fluharty, N. B. (2000). *Fluharty 2: Fluharty preschool speech and language screening test.* Austin, TX: Pro-Ed.

Folstein, M. F., Folstein, S. E., & McHugh, P. R. (2001). *Mini-mental state examination.* Lutz, FL: Psychological Assessment Resource.

Fudala, J. B. (2000). *Arizona articulation proficiency scale* (3rd ed.). Los Angeles: Western Psychological Services.

Gauthier, S. V., & Madison, C. L. (1998). *Kindergarten language screening test* (2nd ed.). Austin, TX: Pro-Ed.

Gentry, J. R. (2004). *The science of spelling: The explicit specifics that make great readers and writers.* Portsmouth, NH: Heinemann.

German, D. J. (1989). *Test of adolescent/adult word finding.* Austin, TX: Pro-Ed.

Gillam, R. B., & Pearson, N. A. (2004). *Test of narrative language (TNL).* Austin, TX: Pro-Ed.

Gillam, R. B, Logan, K. J., & Pearson, N. A. (2009). *Test of childhood stuttering (TOCS).* Austin, TX: Pro-Ed.

Glennen, S. L., & DeCoste, D. C. (1997). *Handbook of augmentative and alternative communication.* Clifton Park, NY: Delmar Learning.

Goldman, R., & Fristoe, M. (2000). *Goldman-Fristoe test of articulation 2.* Circle Pines, MN: American Guidance Service.

Goldstein, B. (2000). *Cultural and linguistic diversity resource guide for speech-language pathologists.* Clifton Park, NY: Delmar Learning.

Goldsworthy, C. (2003). *Developmental reading disabilities: A language-based treatment approach.* Clifton Park, NY: Cengage Learning.

Goodglass, H., Kaplan, E., & Barresi, B. (2000). *Boston diagnostic aphasia examination* (3rd ed.). Baltimore: Williams & Wilkins.

Hall, K. D. (2001). *Pediatric dysphagia resource guide.* Clifton Park, NY: Thompson Learning.

Hammill, D. D., & Newcomer, P. L. (1997). *Test of language development—intermediate.* Austin, TX: Pro-Ed.

Hammill, D. D., Mather, N., & Roberts, R. (2001). *Illinois test of psycholinguistic abilities* (3rd. ed.). Austin, TX: Pro-Ed.

Hammill, D. D., Brown, V. L., Larsen, S. C., & Wiederholt, J. L. (2007). *Test of adolescent and adult language (TOAL-4)*. Austin, TX: Pro-Ed.

Hammill, D. D., & Larsen, S. C. (1996). *TOWL-3 test of written language* (3rd ed.). Austin, TX: Pro-Ed.

Hammill, D. D., Wiederholt, J. L., & Allen, E. A. (2006). *Test of silent contextual reading fluency (TOSCRF)*. Austin, TX: Pro-Ed.

Hasbrouck, J. E., & Tindal, G. (2006). Oral reading fluency norms: A valuable assessment tool for reading teachers. *The Reading Teacher, 59* (7), 636–644.

Haynes, W. O., & Pindzola, R. H. (2012). *Diagnosis and evaluation in speech pathology* (8th ed.). Needham Heights, MA: Allyn & Bacon.

Hegde, M. N., & Davis, D. (2005). *Clinical methods and practicum in speech-language pathology* (4th ed.). Clifton Park, NY: Delmar Learning.

Helm-Estabrooks, N. (1992). *Aphasia diagnostic profiles*. Austin, TX: Pro-Ed.

Helm-Estabrooks, N. (2001). *Cognitive linguistic quick test*. San Antonio, TX: Psychological Corporation.

Helm-Estabrooks, N., & Hotz, G. (1991). *Brief test of head injury*. Austin, TX: Pro-Ed.

Helm-Estabrooks, N., & Nicholas, N. (2003). *Narrative storycards*. Austin, TX: Pro-Ed.

Helm-Estabrooks, N., Ramsberger, G., Morgan, A. R., & Nicholas, M. (1989). *Boston assessment of severe aphasia*. Austin, TX: Pro-Ed.

Hickman, L. A. (1997). *The apraxia profile*. San Antonio, TX: Psychological Corporation.

Hodson, B. W. (2003). *Hodson computerized analysis of phonological patterns (HCAPP)* (3rd ed.). Wichita, KS: PhonoComp Software.

Hodson, B. W. (2004). *Hodson assessment of phonological patterns* (3rd ed.). Austin, TX: Pro-Ed.

Holland, A. L., Frattali, C. M., & Fromm, D. (1999). *Communication activities of daily living* (2nd ed). Austin, TX: Pro-Ed.

Hresko, W., Herron, S., & Peak, P. (1996). *Test of early written language (TEWL-2)* (2nd ed.). Austin, TX: Pro-Ed.

Hresko, W., Reid, D. K., & Hammill, D. (1999). *Test of early language development* (3rd ed.). Austin, TX: Pro-Ed.

Huer, M. B. (1988). *The nonspeech test for receptive/expressive language*. Wauconda, IL: Don Johnston Developmental Equipment, Inc.

Huisiugh, R., Bowers, L., LoGiudice, C., & Orman, J. (2003). *Test of semantic skills–intermediate (TOSS)*. East Moline, IL: Linguisystems.

Hutson-Nechkash, P. (2001). *Narrative toolbox*. Eau Claire, WI: Thinking Publications.

Jelm, J. (2001). *Verbal dyspraxia profile*. DeKalb, IL: Janelle Publications.

Johnson, M. (Ed.). (2005). *Dangerous decibels teacher resource guide*. Portland, OR: The Oregon Museum of Science and Industry.

Kaufman, N. (1995). *Kaufman speech praxis test for children (KSPT)*. Detroit, MI: Wayne State University Press.

Kertesz, A. (2006). *Western aphasia battery-revised (WAB-R)*. San Antonio, TX: Harcourt.

Khan, L., & Lewis, N. (2003). *Khan-Lewis phonological analysis (KLPA-2)* (2nd ed.). Austin, TX: Pro-Ed.

Kinzler, M. (1993). *Joliet 3-minute preschool speech and language screen*. Austin, TX: Pro-Ed.

Kinzler, M., & Johnson, C. (1993). *Joliet 3-minute speech and language screening test* (Revised). Austin, TX: Pro-Ed.

Langdon, H. W., & Cheng, L. L. (2002). *Collaborating with interpreters and translators: A guide for communication disorders professionals*. Eau Claire, WI: Thinking Publications.

LaPointe, L., & Horner, J. (1998). *Reading comprehension battery for aphasia (RCBA-2)* (2nd ed.). Austin, TX: Pro-Ed.

LaPointe, L. L., & Eisenson, J. (2008). *Examining for aphasia: Assessment of aphasia and related impairments* (4th ed.). San Antonio, TX: PRO-ED.

Larsen, S., Hammill, D., & Moats, L. (1999). *TWS-4: Test of written spelling* (4th ed.). Bloomington, MN: Pearson Assessments.

League for the Hard of Hearing. (2007). *Noise levels in our environment fact sheet*. Retrieved May 2, 2007 from http://www.lhh.org/noise/facts/evironment.html.

Leonard, R. and Kendall, K. (1997). *Dysphagia assessment and treatment planning: A team approach*. San Diego, CA: Singular.

Lindamood, P. C., & Lindamood, P. (2004). *Lindamood auditory conceptualization test (LAC-3)* (3rd ed.). Austin, TX: Pro-Ed.

Lippke, B., Dickey, S., Selmar, J., & Soder, A. (1997). *Photo articulation test* (3rd ed.). Austin, TX: Pro-Ed.

Lombardino, L. J., Lieberman, R. J. & Brown, J. C. (2005). *Assessment of literacy and language (ALL)*. San Antonio, TX: Harcourt.

Long, S. H., Fey, M. E., & Channell, R. W. (2006). *Computerized profiling for phonology (Version 9.7.0)* Computer program available as Freeeware on the internet at http://www.computerized profiling.org

Lowe, R. J. (2000). *Assessment link between phonology and articulation revised (ALPHAR)*. Mifflinville, PA: Alpha Speech and Language Resources.

Lund, N. J., & Duchan, J. F. (1993). *Assessing children's language in naturalistic contexts* (3rd ed.). Englewood Cliffs, NJ: Prentice-Hall.

MacWhinney, B. (2000). *The CHILDES project: Tools for analyzing talk (3rd ed.)*. Mahwah, NJ: Lawrence Erlbaum Associates.

Manning, W.H. (1994, November). *The SEA-Scale: Self-Efficacy Scaling for Adolescents Who Stutter*. Paper presented at the annual convention of the American Speech-Language-Hearing Association, New Orleans, LA.

Martin, N., & Brownell, R. (2005). *Test of auditory processing skills–3 (TAPS-3)*. Austin, TX: Pro-Ed.

Masterson, J., & Bernhardt, B. (2001). *Computerized articulation and phonology evaluation system (CAPES)*. San Antonio, TX: Psychological Corporation.

Masterson, J. J., Apel, K., & Wasowicz, J. (2002). *Spelling performance evaluation for language and literacy (SPELL)*. San Antonio, TX: Harcourt Assessment.

Mather, N., Hammill, D. D., Allen, E. A., & Roberts. R. (2004). *Test of silent word reading fluency (TOSWRF).* Austin, TX: Pro-Ed.

Mattes, L. J., & Schuchardt, P. R. (2000). *Stories for oral language development.* San Diego, CA: Academic Communication Associates.

Mattis, S., Jurica, P. J., & Leitten, C. L. (2001). *Dementia rating scale (DRS-2)* (2nd ed.). Lutz, FL: Psychological Assessment Resources.

McNeil, M. R., & Prescott, T. E. (1978). *Token test—revised.* Baltimore, MD: University Park Press.

Mecham, M. (2003). *Utah test of language development* (4th ed.). Austin, TX: Pro-Ed.

Miller, J. F. (2012). *Systematic analysis of language transcripts (SALT).* Madison, WI: SALT Software.

Miller, J. F., & Chapman, R. (1981). The relation between age and mean length of utterance in morphemes. *Journal of Speech and Hearing Research, 24,* 154–161.

Miller, L., Gillam, R. B., & Pena, E. D. (2001). *Dynamic assessment and intervention: Improving children's narrative abilities.* Austin, TX: Pro-Ed.

Morgan, D., & Guildford, A. (1984). *Adolescent language screening test (ALST).* Austin, TX: Pro-Ed.

Naremore, R. C., Densmore, A. E., & Harman, D. R. (2001). *Assessment and treatment of school-age language disorders: A resource manual.* San Diego, CA: Singular.

National Institute for Literacy. (2006). What is literacy?. Retrieved from http://www.nifl .gov/nifl/faqs.html/literacy

Newborg, J. (2004). *Battelle developmental inventory* (2nd ed). Itasca, IL: Riverside Publishing Co.

Newcomer, P., & Barenbaum, E. (2003). *Test of phonological awareness skills (TOPAS).* Austin, TX: Pro-Ed.

Newcomer, P. L., & Hammill, D. D. (1997). *Test of language development—primary* (3rd ed.). Austin, TX: Pro-Ed.

Owens, R.E. (1995). *Language disorders: A functional approach to assessment and intervention* (3rd ed.). Needham Heights, MA: Allyn & Bacon.

Owens, R. E. (2013). *Language disorders: A functional approach to assessment and intervention.* (6th ed.). Needham Heights, MA: Allyn & Bacon.

Pimental, P. A., & Knight, J. A. (2000). *Mini inventory of right brain injury* (2nd ed.). Austin, TX: Pro-Ed.

Poole, E. (1934). Genetic development of articulation of consonant sounds in speech. *Elementary English Review, 11,* 159–161.

Prather, E., Hedrick, D., & Kern, C. (1975). Articulation development in children aged two to four years. *Journal of Speech and Hearing Disorders, 40,* 179–191.

Purcell, R. M., & Runyan, C. M. (1980). Normative study of speech rates of children. *Journal of the Speech and Hearing Association of Virginia, 21,* 6–14.

Richard, G. J., & Hanner, M. A. (2005). *Language processing test 3: Elementary.* East Moline, IL: Linguisystems.

Riley, G. D. (1981). *Stuttering prediction instrument for young children* (rev. ed). Austin, TX: Pro-Ed.

Riley, G. D. (2008). *Stuttering severity instrument* (4th ed.). Austin, TX: Pro-Ed.

Robertson, C., & Salter, W. (1995). *The phonological awareness profile*. East Moline, IL: Linguisystems.

Robertson, C., & Salter, W. (2007). *The phonological awareness test–2* (2nd ed). East Moline, IL: Linguisystems.

Robins, D., Fein, D., & Barton, M. (2009). *Modified checklist for autism in toddlers–revised with follow-up (M-CHAT-R/F)*. Retrieved from http://www.M-CHAT.org

Roseberry-McKibbin, C. (2008). *Multicultural students with special language needs* (3rd ed.). Oceanside, CA: Academic Communication Associates.

Rosenbek, J. C., & LaPointe, L. L. (1985). The dysarthrias: Description, diagnosis, and treatment. In D. F. Johns (Ed.), *Clinical management of neurogenic communicative disorders* (2nd ed., pp. 97–152). Boston: Little, Brown and Co.

Rossetti, L. (2006). *The Rossetti infant-toddler language scale*. East Moline, IL: LinguiSystems.

Ross-Swain, D. (1996). *Ross information processing assessment* (2nd ed.). Austin, TX: Pro-Ed.

Ross-Swain, D. (1999). *Ross information processing assessment—primary*. Austin, TX: Pro-Ed.

Ross-Swain, D., & Fogle, P. (1996). *Ross information processing assessment—geriatric*. Austin, TX: Pro-Ed.

Rustad, R. A., DeGroot, T. L., Jungkunz, M. L., Freeberg, K. S., Borowick, L. G., & Wanttie, A. M. (1993). *The cognitive assessment of Minnesota*. San Antonio, TX: Harcourt.

Rutter, M., Bailey, A., Lord, C., & Berument, S. K. (2003). *Social communication questionnaire*. Los Angeles: Western Psychological Services.

Salter, W., & Robertson, C. (2001). *The phonological awareness and reading profile—intermediate*. East Moline, IL: Linguisystems.

Saxton, J., McGonigle, K. L., Swihart, A. A., & Boller, F. (1993). *Severe impairment battery*. Bury St. Edmunds, UK: Thames Valley Test Company.

Secord, W. A. (1981). *Test of minimal articulation competence*. San Antonio: Psychological Corporation.

Secord, W. A., Boyce, S. E., Donohue, J. S., Fox, R. A., & Shine, R. E. (2007). *Eliciting sounds: Techniques and strategies for clinicians* (2nd ed.). Clifton Park, NY: Delmar, Cengage Learning.

Secord, W., & Donohue, J. (2002). *Clinical assessment of articulation and phonology (CAAP)*. Greenville, SC: Super Duper.

Secord, W., Donohue, J., & Johnson, C. (2002). *Clinical assessment of articulation and phonology (CAAP)*. Greenville, SC: Super Duper.

Sell, D., Harding, A., & Grunwell, P. (1994). A screening assessment of cleft palate speech (Great Ormond Street Speech Assessment). *European Journal of Disorders of Communication, 29*, 1–15.

Semel, E., Wiig, E. H., & Secord, W. (2004). *Clinical evaluation of language fundamentals (CELF-4) screening test*. San Antonio: Pearson.

Semel, E., Wiig, E. H., & Secord, W. (2013). *Clinical evaluation of language fundamentals (CELF)* (5th ed.). New York: Psychological Corporation.

Shaywitz, S. E. (2003). *Overcoming dyslexia: A new and complete science-based program of reading problems at any level*. New York: Alfred A. Knopf.

Shipley, K. G., & Roseberry-McKibbin, C. (2006). *Interviewing and counseling in communicative disorders: Principles and procedures* (3rd ed.). Austin, TX: Pro-Ed.

Shipley, K. G., Recor, D. B., & Nakamura, S. M. (1990). *Sourcebook of apraxia remediation activities*. Oceanside, CA: Academic Communication Associates.

Shipley, K. G., Stone, T. A., & Sue, M. B. (1983). *Test for examining expressive morphology (TEEM)*. Tucson, AZ: Communication Skills Builders.

Shriberg, L. D., & Kwiatkowski, J. (1983). Computer-assisted natural process analysis (NPA): Recent issues and data. *Seminars in Speech and Language, 4*, 397–406.

Simon, C. S. (1994). *Evaluating communicative competence: A functional pragmatic procedure* (2nd ed.). Tempe, AZ: Communicos Publications.

Smit, A. B., & Hand, L. (1997). *Smit-Hand articulation and phonology evaluation (SHAPE)*. Los Angeles: Western Psychological Services.

Smit, A., Hand, L., Frelinger, J., Bernthal, J., & Byrd, A. (1990). The Iowa articulation norms project and its Nebraska replication. *Journal of Speech and Hearing Disorders, 55*, 779–798.

Stein, N. L., & Glenn, C. G. (1979). An analysis of story comprehension in elementary school children. In R. O. Freedle (Ed.), *Current topics in early childhood education* (Vol.,) (pp. 261–290). Norwood, NJ: Ablex.

Stevens, N., and Isles, D. (2011). *Phonological screening assessment*. Bicester, Oxon, U.K.: Speechmark.

Stone, W. L., Coonrod, E. E., & Ousley, O. Y. (2000). Screening tool for autism in two-year-olds (STAT). *Journal of Autism and Developmental Disorders, 30*, 6, 607–612.

Swigert, N.B. (1998). *The source for pediatric dysphagia*. East Moline, IL: LinguiSystems.

Swiburn, K., Porter, G., & Howard, D. (2004). *Comprehensive aphasia test (CAT)*. New York: Psychology Press.

Tanner, D., & Culbertson, W. (1999). *Quick assessment for aphasia*. Oceanside, CA: Academic Communication Associates.

Tanner, D., & Culbertson, W. (1999). *Quick assessment for apraxia of speech*. Oceanside, CA: Academic Communication Associates.

Tanner, D., & Culbertson, W. (1999). *Quick assessment for dysarthria*. Oceanside, CA: Academic Communication Associates.

Templin, M. (1957). *Certain language skills in children: Their development and interrelationships* (Institute of Child Welfare, Monograph, No. 26). Minneapolis: The University of Minnesota Press.

Tompkins, C. A. (1995). *Right hemisphere communication disorders: Theory and management*. Clifton Park, NY: Delmar Learning.

Torgesen, J., Wagner, R., & Rashotte, C. (1999). *Test of word reading efficiency (TOWRE)*. Austin, TX: Pro-Ed.

Torgesen, J. K., & Bryant, B. R. (2004). *Test of phonological awareness–second edition: Plus (TOPA-2+)*. Austin, TX: Pro-Ed.

Venkatagiri, H. S. (1999). Clinical measurement of rate of reading and discourse in young adults. *Journal of Fluency Disorders, 24*, 209–226.

Vinson, B. (2001). *Essentials for speech-language pathologists*. Clifton Park: NY: Delmar Learning.

Vinson, B. (2007). *Language disorders across the lifespan* (2nd ed.). Clifton Park, NY: Delmar Learning.

Wagner, R. K., Torgesen, J. K., & Rashotte, C. A. (2009). *Comprehensive test of phonological processing (CTOPP-2).* Austin: Pro-Ed.

Wallace, G., & Hammill, D. D. (2013). *Comprehensive receptive and expressive vocabulary test* (3rd ed.). San Antonio, TX: Pro-Ed.

Wechsler. D. (2001). *Wechsler individual achievement test (WIAT-11)* (2nd ed.). San Antonio, TX: Psychological Corporation.

Weiner, A. E. (1984). Vocal control therapy for stutterers. In M. Peins (Ed.), *Contemporary approaches in stuttering therapy* (pp. 217–269). Boston: Little, Brown and Co.

Wellman, B., Case, I., Mengurt, I., & Bradbury, D. (1931). *Speech sounds of young children* (University of Iowa Studies in Child Welfare No. 5). Iowa City: University of Iowa Press.

Westby, C. E. (2002). Multicultural issues in speech and language assessment. In J. B. Tomblin, H. L. Morris, & D. C. Spriestersbach (Eds.), *Diagnosis in speech–language pathology* (2nd ed., pp. 35–62). Clifton Park, NY: Delmar Learning.

Wiederholt, J. L., & Blalock, G. (2000). *Gray silent reading tests (GSRT).* Austin, TX: Pro-Ed.

Wiederholt, J. L., & Bryant, B. B. (2001). *Gray oral reading test, (4th ed.)(GORT-4).* Austin, TX: Pro-Ed.

Wiig, E. H., Nielsen, N. P., Minthon, L., & Warkentin, S. (2002). *Alzheimer's quick test: Assessment of parietal function.* San Antonio, TX: Psychological Corporation.

Williams, K. T. (2007). *Expressive vocabulary test (EVT-2)* (2nd ed.). Bloomington, MN: Pearson Assessments.

Williams, W. B., Stemach, G., Wolfe, S., & Stanger, C. (1995). *Lifespace access profile: Assistive technology planning for individuals with severe or multiple disabilities* (rev.). Irvine, CA: Lifespace Access. Assistive Technology Systems.

Wilson, B. A., & Felton, R. H. (2004). *Word identification and spelling test (WIST).* Austin, TX: Pro-Ed.

Woodcock, R. W. (1998). *Woodcock reading mastery test (rev./normative update).* Bloomington, MN: Pearson Assessments.

Woodcock, R. W., McGrew, K. S., & Mather, N. (2001). *Woodcock-Johnson III complete.* Itasca, IL: Riverside.

Yorkston, K. M., Beukelman, D. P., & Traynor, C. (1984). *Assessment of intelligibility of dysarthric speech.* Austin, TX: Pro-Ed.

Zimmerman, I., Steiner, V., & Evatt-Pond, R. (2011). *The preschool language scale* (5th ed.). San Antonio, TX: Pearson.

GLOSSARY

A

Acculturation: The change in the cultural behavior and thinking of an individual or group that occurs through contact with another group.

Acoustic reflex: An involuntary movement to sound that stiffens the ossicular chain and decreases the compliance of the tympanic membrane.

Adenoidectomy: Surgical removal of the adenoidal tissue.

Adjective: A word that modifies a noun or pronoun. It adds description or definition of kind (*red* car), which one (*that* man), or how many (*three* children).

Adverb: A word that modifies a verb, adjective, or another adverb. It adds description or definition of how (ran *quickly*), when (went *immediately*), where (walked *here*), or extent (ran *far*).

Agrammatism: A problem with grammatical accuracy commonly associated with aphasia.

Alternate form reliability: See *Reliability*.

Ambulatory: Capable of walking.

Anomia: Inability to identify or to recall names of people, places, or things. Seen with some aphasias.

Anterior: See *Distinctive feature*.

Aphasia: Loss of language abilities and function as a result of brain damage. It may affect comprehension or expression of verbal language, as well as reading, writing, and mathematics.

Apraxia: A neurologically based motor speech disorder that adversely affects the abilities to execute purposeful speech movements. Muscle weakness is not associated with apraxia.

Article: A noun modifier that denotes specificity, that is—*a, an,* or *the*.

Articulation: Use of articulators (lips, tongue, etc.) to produce speech sounds. It also describes a person's ability to make sounds, as in "her *articulation* contained several errors."

Aspiration: The action of a foreign material (e.g., food) penetrating and entering the airway below the true vocal folds.

Assimilation: The process by which something absorbs, merges, or conforms to a dominant entity. In articulation, assimilation occurs when a phoneme becomes similar to a neighboring phoneme. In cultural groups, assimilation occurs when the traits of a minority group conform to the traits of the dominant cultural group.

Asymmetry: Lack of similarity of parts of a structure; unevenness or lack of proportion. For example, drooping on one side of the face makes it *asymmetrical* with the other side.

Ataxia: Disturbance of gait and balance associated with damage to the cerebellum. It is a type of dysarthria characterized by errors in articulation, uneven stress patterns, monopitch, and reduced loudness.

Atresia: Congenital absence, pathological closure, or severe underdevelopment of a normal orifice or cavity. As used in audiology, it often refers to an abnormally small or malformed pinna (the visible outside part of the ear).

Atrophy: The wasting away of tissues or an organ due to disease or lack of use.

Audiogram: A graphic illustration of hearing sensitivity. An audiogram depicts hearing levels (in dB) at different frequencies (Hz) of sound.

Auricle: The outside visible part of the ear. Also called the *pinna*.

Autism: A serious disorder characterized by significant deficits in social communication and fixated interests and/or behaviors.

Automatic speech: Speech that is produced with little conscious effort or thought, such as counting from 1 to 10 or reciting the alphabet. Examples of automatic speech include saying "Excuse me" after bumping against something, or responding to a greeting with "Fine, how are you?" without thinking about it.

Auxiliary verb: A verb used with a main verb to convey condition, voice, or mood; a "helping verb" *be*, *do*, or *have*, such as *is* going, *did* go, or *have* gone.

B

Back: See *Distinctive feature*.

Ballism: Violent or jerky movements observed in chorea (a group of disorders characterized by rapid and usually brief involuntary movements of the limbs, face, trunk, or head).

Bifid uvula: The complete or incomplete separation of the uvula into two parts. Associated with cleft palate.

Bilateral: Pertaining to both sides, such as a *bilateral* hearing loss that involves both ears.

Blue-dye test: A dysphagia test often used with tracheostomized clients. Blue dye is placed in the oral cavity, either directly applied to a client's tongue or mixed in with food or liquid, and then monitored for its progression through the body. If blue dye appears in the lungs or at the site of the stoma, it is an indication of aspiration. Blue dye is used because there are no natural body secretions that are blue.

Bolus: Food in the mouth that is chewed and ready to be swallowed.

Brachydactyly: Shortness of the fingers.

C

Carhart notch: A dip in bone conduction hearing (seen on an audiogram) of 5 dB at 500 and 4000 Hz, 10 dB at 1000 Hz, and 15 dB at 2000 Hz. It is often observed with otosclerosis because of the inability of fluids to move freely when the footplate of the stapes is fixed firmly to the oval window.

CAS: See *Childhood apraxia of speech*.

Catenative: A specific type of verb such as *wanna* (want to), *gonna* (going to), and *hafta* (have to).

Central nervous system: Part of the nervous system that includes the brain and spinal cord.

Cerebellar ataxia: See *Ataxia*.

Cerebral vascular accident (CVA): Also called a stroke. Damage to part of the brain due to a disturbance in the blood supply.

Charting: Ongoing recording of client's actions or responses. For example, recording each instance of a correct or incorrect sound production.

Childhood apraxia of speech (CAS): A motor speech disorder characterized by difficulty coordinating the articulators for speech in absence of muscle weakness or paralysis.

Circumlocution: A roundabout way of speaking; or nonuse of a particular sound, word, or phrase. In aphasia, the client may be unable to recall the desired word and, therefore, defines or uses a related word. In stuttering, the client may fear stuttering on a particular word and use an alternative word or description.

Cluttering: A speech disorder characterized by rapid and sometimes unintelligible speech; sound, part-word, or whole-word repetitions; and often a language deficit.

Coloboma: A clefting defect of the eye that may involve the iris, choroid (the heavily pigmented tissue in the eye), or retinal structures.

Compliance: The ease with which the tympanic membrane and middle ear mechanism function; mobility of tympanic membrane.

Concurrent validity: See *Validity*.

Conductive hearing loss: Reduced hearing acuity from diminished ability to conduct sound through the outer or middle ear; often due to abnormalities of the external ear canal, eardrum, or ossicular chain.

Congenital: Describes a disease, deformity, or deficiency that is present at birth. The abnormality may be hereditary or acquired prior to birth.

Conjoining: Joined together.

Conjunction: A word that joins two or more grammatical units. Examples include you *and* me, wanted to *but* couldn't, he went *because* he wanted to, I would *if* I could.

Consonantal: See *Distinctive feature*.

Construct validity: See *Validity*.

Contact ulcer: An inflammation that develops on the laryngeal cartilage; usually results from vocal abuse but can also result from acid irritation or intubation during surgery.

Content validity: See *Validity*.

Copula: A form of the verb "to be" that links a subject noun with a predicate noun or adjective. For example, the puppy *is* young, or they *were* late.

Coronal: See *Distinctive feature*.

Covert cleft: A cleft of the lip or palate that is not overtly visible.

Craniosynostosis: Premature fusion of the cranial sutures that can adversely affect the shape and structure of the head.

Cuff: A part of a tracheostomy tube that can be inflated to close off the airway.

Cul-de-sac resonance: A hollow-sounding, somewhat hyponasal voice quality often associated with cleft palate speech.

CVA: See *Cerebral vascular accident*.

D

Dementia: Mental deterioration characterized by confusion, poor judgment, impaired memory, disorientation, and impaired intellect.

Denasality: See *Hyponasality*.

Diadochokinesis: Abilities to make rapid, repetitive movements of the articulators to produce speech. Often tested by using preselected syllables such as /pʌ/, /tʌ/, and /kʌ/.

Diastema: Widely spaced teeth.

Diplegia: Bilateral paralysis affecting parts of both sides of the body.

Disfluency: An interruption that interferes with or prevents the smooth, easy flow of speech. Examples include repetitions, prolongations, interjections, and silent pauses.

Distinctive feature: The articulatory or acoustic characteristics of a phoneme (e.g., voiced or unvoiced, consonant or vowel, tense or lax) that make it unique from all other phonemes; the specific features attributed to each sound.

> **Anterior:** Produced in the front region of the mouth, at the alveolar ridge, or forward. It includes /l/, /p/, /b/, /f/, /v/, /m/, /t/, /d/, /θ/, /ð/, /n/, /s/, and /z/.
>
> **Back:** Produced in the back of the mouth with the tongue retracted from the neutral position. It includes /k/, /g/, /ŋ/, /w/, /u/, /oʊ/, /ɑɪ/, /ɔɪ/, /ʌ/, /ʊ/, /o/, and /ɔ/.
>
> **Consonantal:** Produced with narrow constriction. It includes all consonant sounds except /h/.
>
> **Continuant:** Produced with partial obstruction of air flow. It includes /r/, /l/, /f/, /v/, /θ/, /ð/, /s/, /z/, /ʃ/, /ʒ/, and /h/.
>
> **Coronal:** Produced by raising the blade of the tongue above the neutral position, it includes /r/, /l/, /t/, /d/, /θ/, /ð/, /n/, /s/, /z/, /tʃ/, /dʒ/, /ʃ/, and /ʒ/.
>
> **High:** Produced by raising the body of the tongue above the neutral position. It includes /tʃ/, /dʒ/, /ʃ/, /ʒ/, /k/, /g/, /w/, /j/, /i/, /u/, and /ɪ/.
>
> **Low:** Produced by lowering the body of the tongue below the neutral position. It includes /h/, /ɑɪ/, /ɑʊ/, /æ/, and /ɔ/.
>
> **Nasal:** Produced by lowering the velum to allow air to pass through the oral cavity. It includes /m/, /n/, and /ŋ/.
>
> **Round:** Produced by narrowing the lips. It includes /u/, /ɔɪ/, /ʊ/, /o/, /ɔ/, and /w/.
>
> **Strident:** Produced with rapid airflow pressing against the teeth. It includes /f/, /v/, /s/, /z/, /tʃ/, /dʒ/, /ʃ/, and /ʒ/.
>
> **Tense:** Produced by maintaining muscular effort of the articulators for an extended period of time. It includes /i/, /u/, /e/, /ɑɪ/, and /ɔɪ/.
>
> **Vocalic:** Produced without significant constriction and with voicing. It includes all vowel sounds and the consonant sound /h/.
>
> **Voiced:** Produced with vocal fold vibration. It includes /r/, /l/, /b/, /v/, /m/, /d/, /ð/, /n/, /z/, /dʒ/, /ʒ/, /g/, /j/, and all vowel sounds.

Distortion: A speech error whereby the intended sound is recognizable, but is not produced correctly. Examples include "slurred" or imprecise sound productions.

Dominant language: The language in which a person is most fluent and proficient.

Dysarthria: A group of motor speech disorders associated with muscle paralysis, weakness, or incoordination. It is associated with central or peripheral nervous system damage.

Dysfluency: See *Disfluency*.

Dysphagia: A disturbance in the normal act of swallowing.

Dysphonia: An impairment of normal vocal function.

E

Earmold: A fitting designed to conduct amplified sound from the receiver of a hearing aid into the ear.

Echolalia: An involuntary, parrot-like imitation or repeating back of what is heard. It is frequently seen with some autisms and schizophrenias.

Ectrodactyly: Absence of one or more fingers or toes.

Edentulous: Absent dentition.

Ellipsis: The omission of known or shared information in a subsequent utterance when it would be redundant; construction may be incomplete, but missing parts are understood. In cluttering, it may refer to omission of sounds, syllables, or entire words.

Encephalitis: Inflammation of the brain, usually caused by a viral infection.

Eustachian tube: A tube that connects the nasopharynx and the middle ear. It equalizes pressure in the middle ear with atmospheric pressure.

Expressive abilities: The abilities to express oneself. This usually refers to language expression through speech, but it also includes gestures, sign language, use of a communication board, and other forms of expression.

F

Face validity: See *Validity*.

Failure to thrive: Inability to maintain life functions. People in this condition are bedridden and "just barely alive."

Fasciculations: Tremor-like movements of a band of muscle or nerve fibers.

Fenestrated: A tracheostomy tube that has small holes in it to allow passage of air through the airway.

Fistula: An abnormal channel, often a hole, connecting two spaces. For example, a palatal fistula may connect the oral and nasal cavities.

Fluency: The smooth, uninterrupted, effortless flow of speech; speech that is not hindered by excessive disfluencies.

G

Gerund: A verb form that ends in *-ing* and is used as a noun. For example, *stealing* is bad, or *swinging* is fun.

Glossoptosis: A downward displacement of the tongue, typically associated with neurological weakness.

Grammar: Systems, rules, or underlying principles that describe the aspects (phonology, semantics, syntax, pragmatics, morphology) of language.

Granuloma: A mass of tissue produced in response to an inflammation; pertaining to voice, a granuloma can develop at the site of a contact ulcer.

H

Hematoma: A collection of blood in an organ, space, or tissue. It is caused by a break in the wall of a blood vessel.

Hemifacial microsomia: A condition in which portions or all of the head is abnormally small.

Hemiparesis: Paralysis or weakness on one side of the body. Commonly associated with stroke.

Hemorrhage: Excessive bleeding, typically from a ruptured blood vessel.

Heterochromia iridis: More than one color of the iris of one eye (e.g., a brown patch in a blue eye), or differences in color between the two eyes (e.g., one blue eye and one brown eye).

High: See *Distinctive feature*.

Hydrocephaly: Enlargement of the head caused by excessive accumulation of cerebrospinal fluid in the cranial spaces.

Hypernasality: Excessive, undesirable nasal resonance during phonation; nasal resonance on a sound other than /m/, /n/, and /ŋ/.

Hyperplexia: Underdevelopment. For example, a *hyperplexic* mandible is underdeveloped.

Hypertelorism: Increased distance between the eyes.

Hypertonia: Excessive muscle tone or tension.

Hypogonadism: Decreased gonadal function or size, often the result of deficient hormone production.

Hyponasality: Lack of normal nasal resonance on the nasal consonants /m/, /n/, and /ŋ/, often a result of obstruction in the nasal tract.

Hypoplasia: Incomplete or underdevelopment of a tissue or organ. For example, lingual *hypoplasia* is an underdeveloped tongue.

Hypotonia: Reduced or absent muscle tone or tension.

I

Idiom: Short, figurative language expression such as *hit the roof, in the ballpark,* or *blew their cool.*

Idiosyncratic language: Language that is particular to one person or a very limited group of people, such as twins or other siblings.

Imitation: Repetition of a behavior. In speech treatment, the client repeats a verbal stimulus. Clinicians use imitation as one technique to teach newly desired behaviors.

Impedance: Resistance to a vibratory source of energy. Resistance may be acoustic, mechanical, or electric. In impedance audiometry, impedance of air pressure and air volume differences are measured to detect conductive hearing loss and middle ear pathology.

Intelligibility: The degree or level to which speech is understood by others.

Interjection: The addition of a sound or word that does not relate grammatically to other words in the utterance. For example, "I want, *you know*, to go," or "He was, *uh*, going."

Intermittency: Episodic or variable. In voice, it is the inappropriate cessation of phonation during speech. In reference to a hearing aid, it is the inappropriate interruption of the transmission of a signal through the hearing aid.

Intertester reliability: See *Reliability*.

Intonation: Changes in pitch, stress, and prosodic features that affect speech. The lack of intonation makes the speech sound monotone and "colorless."

Intratester reliability: See *Reliability*.

J

Jargon: (1) Verbal behavior of children (approximately 9–18 months) containing a variety of inflected syllables that resemble meaningful, connected speech. (2) Fluent, well–articulated speech that makes little sense; illogical speech consisting of nonsense words or words used in an inappropriate context. For example, *Get this a splash of arbuckle.*

Joint attention: More than one person is focused on the same stimulus; the sharing of visual and auditory attention to the same stimulus.

K

Klunking: An undesirable, audible sound that occurs when air is injected into the esophagus too quickly during the production of esophageal speech.

L

Labial pit: A small hole in the lip sometimes seen with cleft lip or palate.

Labyrinthitis: An inflammation of the inner ear. Symptoms are vertigo, balance problems, or vomiting.

Language proficiency: A person's ability to produce and comprehend a language.

Lesion: A specific site of injury or disease.

Lingual frenum: The fold of skin underneath the tongue that connects the tongue to the floor of the mouth.

Literal paraphasia: See *Paraphasia*.

Low: See *Distinctive feature*.

M

Macroglossia: Abnormally large tongue.

Malocclusion: Misalignment of the upper and lower teeth. A normal occlusion is the correct alignment of the upper and lower molars; deviations from this are malocclusions.

    Class I (neutroclusion): Normal anterior-posterior relationship of the upper and lower molars; individual teeth may be misaligned.

    Class II (distoclusion): The lower molars (dental arch) are posterior to the alignment of the upper molars.

    Class III (mesioclusion): The lower molars (dental arch) are anterior to the alignment of the upper molars.

Mandible: The lower jaw.

Mandibular hypoplasia: Underdevelopment of the lower jaw.

Mastoiditis: An inflammation of the mastoid process.

Mastoid process: The bony protuberance (bulge) behind and below the outer ear.

Maxilla: The upper jaw.

Mean length of utterance (MLU): The average length of each utterance taken from multiple utterances. It is usually the average number of morphemes per utterance, but it can also be used to describe the average number of words per utterance.

Ménière's disease: A disease of the inner ear characterized by progressive sensorineural hearing loss in the affected ear, recurrent dizziness, tinnitus, nausea, or vomiting.

Meningitis: An inflammation of the tissues that surround the brain and spinal cord. It is usually caused by a bacterial infection but can also result from a viral or fungal infection.

Metaphor: A figure of speech with an implied comparison between two entities. For example, *big as a house* or *meaner than a junkyard dog*.

Metathetic errors: Speech errors involving the transposition of sounds or syllables in a word or phrase. For example, *puck* for *cup*, or *warday* for *doorway*.

Microcephaly: Abnormal smallness of the head; imperfect, small development of the cranium.

Microglossia: Abnormally small tongue.

Micrognathia: Unusually small lower jaw, often associated with a recessed chin.

Microstoma: Abnormally small mouth.

Microtia: Congenital underdevelopment of the external ear.

Mixed hearing loss: A hearing loss with conductive and sensorineural components.

Morpheme: The smallest unit of language that has meaning. Free morphemes (*cat*, *dog*, *me*, etc.) can stand alone to convey meaning and cannot be reduced any further without losing meaning. Bound morphemes (*-ing*, *-s*, *-er*, etc.) cannot stand alone; they must be attached to a free morpheme to convey meaning.

Morphology: The study of how sounds and words are put together to form meaning.

Myopia: Short sightedness; inability to see distances.

N

Nares: Nostrils.

Nasal: See *Distinctive feature*.

Nasal emission: Escape of airflow through the nasal cavity. Often seen in the presence of an inadequate velopharyngeal seal between the oral and nasal cavities. It is most frequently heard during the production of voiceless sounds, especially voiceless plosives or fricatives.

Nasality: Sounds made with air moving through the nasal cavities. It is appropriate during productions of /m/, /n/, and /ŋ/; it is inappropriate with all other English sounds.

Nasogastric tube: A tube that leads from the nose to the stomach. It is used to provide liquid nutrients and medications to clients who cannot eat orally.

Nasopharynx: The section of the pharynx located above the level of the soft palate that opens into the nasal cavity.

Neologistic paraphasia: See *Paraphasia*.

Nominal: A word or phrase that acts as a noun.

O

Occult cleft: See *Submucosal cleft*.

Omission: The absence or deletion of a needed sound. For example, articulating *so* instead of *soap*.

Orthographic processing: The ability to retrieve sight words from memory.

Ossicles: The three small bones of the middle ear (incus, malleus, and stapes). Also referred to as the ossicular chain.

Otitis media: An infection of the middle ear frequently acquired by children and often associated with upper respiratory infection. There are three varieties:

Acute otitis media: A sudden onset of otitis media caused by an infection.

Chronic otitis media: The permanent condition of a ruptured tympanic membrane. It may or may not be associated with infection.

Serous otitis media: Inflammation of the middle ear, with the presence of a thick or watery fluid that fills the middle ear space.

Ototoxicity: Damage to the ear caused by a harmful poison. It is usually associated with certain drugs.

Overt cleft: A clearly visible cleft of the lip and palate.

P

Palpebral fissures: The slits of the eyes formed by the upper and lower eyelids.

Paralinguistic cues: Vocal or nonvocal cues that are superimposed (added onto) on a linguistic code to signal the speaker's attitude or emotion or to add or clarify meaning. For example, sarcasm is usually conveyed more through paralinguistic cues than through the actual words or syntax used.

Paralysis: Impairment or loss of muscle power or function due to muscular dysfunction.

Paraphasia: A problem with word or sound substitution commonly associated with aphasia. There are several types:

Neologistic paraphasia: The use of a nonmeaningful word. For example, "I want *arbuckle*."

Phonetic or literal paraphasia: The substitution of one sound for another or the addition of a sound. For example, *mandwich* for *sandwich* or *skandwich* for *sandwich*.

Verbal paraphasia: Substitution of an entire word for another. There are two types:

Random paraphasia: Substitution of a word that is not similar to the intended word. For example, *dog* for *flower*.

Semantic paraphasia: Substitution of a word that is similar to the intended word. For example, *father* for *mother*.

Paresis: Partial or incomplete paralysis; weakness.

Participle: A verb used as an adjective. For example, the *flowing* water or the *swaying* branch.

Peripheral nervous system: The collection of nerves outside the brain and spinal column that conducts impulses to and from the central nervous system. The peripheral system includes the cranial nerves, spinal nerves, and some portions of the autonomic nerves.

Peristalsis: Alternate contraction and relaxation of the walls of a tube-like structure, which helps its contents move forward (e.g., within the intestinal tract).

Perseveration: Inappropriate continuation or repetition of the same word, thought, or behavior, commonly associated with aphasia and other neurologic impairments.

Phonation: The physiological process by which air moving through the vocal tract becomes acoustic energy in the larynx; production of voiced (versus voiceless) sounds.

Phoneme: An individual sound.

Phonetic decoding: Using alphabetic strategies to decode new words.

Phonetic paraphasia: See *Paraphasia.*

Phonology: The study of the sound system of language, including speech sounds, speech patterns, and rules that apply to those sounds.

Pinna: The outside, visible part of the ear. Also called the *auricle.*

Polydactyly: Extra fingers or toes.

Polyneuritis: The inflammation of multiple nerves.

Pragmatics: The study of the rules that govern and describe how language is used situationally, in light of its context and environment.

Predictive validity: See *Validity.*

Preposition: A word used to relate a noun or pronoun to another word in a sentence. It can be used to modify a noun, adjective, or adverb. For example, *in* there, *on* the bed, *between* them.

Presbycusis: Progressive loss of hearing as a result of the aging process.

Presupposition: Taking the other person into consideration or perspective when communicating. It is the process of understanding what information the other person has or may need.

Primary language: The language a person learned first and used most often during the early stages of language development. It is often referred to as L1.

Prognathic: A marked projection of the jaw.

Prognosis: A prediction or judgment about the course, duration, and prospects for the improvement of a disorder. It may include judgments about future changes with or without professional intervention.

Prolongation: The inappropriate lengthening of a sound production. For example, prolonging the vowel in the word *gooood.*

Pronoun: A word that takes the place of a noun. Examples are *I, mine, we, myself, whose, which,* and *that.*

Prosody: Variations in rate, loudness, stress, intonation, and rhythm producing the melodic components of speech.

Proverb: A figure of speech that often contains advice or conventional wisdom. For example, *Don't put all your eggs in one basket* or *Nothing ventured—nothing gained.*

Psychosis: A severe mental or behavioral disorder characterized by a disordered personality or inability to deal with reality. It may include disorientation, delusion, and hallucination.

Ptosis: Drooping of the eyelids, usually affecting the upper eyelids.

Puree diet: A diet that consists of foods that are blended to a soft texture, like that of pudding or applesauce. It may be recommended for clients who have dysphagia.

R

Random paraphasia: See *Paraphasia.*

Receptive abilities: The ability to understand or comprehend language. It usually refers to the ability to understand verbal expression, but it also includes the ability to understand sign language, writing, Braille, and other forms of language.

Reflux: Backward flow of food or liquids that have already entered the stomach.

Regurgitate: Vomiting of food or liquids that have already entered the stomach.

Reliability: The consistency and subsequent dependability of obtained results. For example, a test administered on two occasions produced the same or similar results.

> **Alternate form reliability:** Consistency of results obtained when using different forms of the test. For example, obtaining similar results after administering Form L and Form M of the *Peabody Picture Vocabulary Test.*

> **Intertester reliability:** Consistency of results obtained when the same test is administered by two or more examiners.

> **Intratester reliability:** Consistency of results obtained when the same test is administered by the same examiner on two or more occasions.

> **Split-half or internal reliability:** Consistency of difficulty throughout a test that is not intended to be progressively more difficult. For example, the first half of a test is equally difficult to the second half.

> **Test-retest reliability:** Consistency of results of a test administered on two occasions. Administration by one examiner on different occasions is intratester and test-retest reliability. Administration by more than one examiner on different occasions is intertester and test-retest reliability.

Repetition: In disfluent speech, the abnormal additional productions of a sound, syllable, word, or phrase. For example, *I-I-I-I-I* want to go.

Resonance: Vibration of one or more structures related to the source of the sound; vibration above or below the sound source (the larynx for speech). In voice, resonance relates to the quality of the voice produced.

Respiration: The act of breathing, including drawing air into the body (inspiration) and expulsion of the air from the body (expiration).

Retinitis pigmentosa: A hereditary, deteriorating condition involving inflammation and pigmentary infiltration of the retina.

Revisions: Verbalizations in which a targeted word or phrase is changed and a different word or phrase is substituted.

Rime: the part of a syllable that remains when the initial consonant(s) are deleted. For example, the rime of *boy* is *oy*; the rime of *stop* is *op*.

Round: See *Distinctive feature.*

Rugae: Ridges of flesh on the hard palate located immediately behind the front teeth.

S

Semantic paraphasia: See *Paraphasia.*

Semantics: The study of the meaning of language, including meaning at the word, sentence, and conversational levels.

Sensorineural hearing loss: Reduced hearing acuity due to a pathological condition in the inner ear or along the nerve pathway from the inner ear to the brainstem.

Social (pragmatic) communication disorder: A disorder characterized by persistent and significant deficits in verbal and nonverbal social communication.

Splay: Spread or turn outward. For example, a hand with the fingers spread apart and turned outward from the palm is called *splayed*.

Split-half reliability: See *Reliability*.

Spoonerism: The transposition of sounds in a word, phrase, or sentence. For example, *half-warmed fish* for *half-formed wish*.

Stammer: Synonym for *stutter*.

Stoma: A surgically placed opening in the body. Following laryngectomy, the stoma is in the anterior portion of the neck.

Strabismus: A visual disorder in which both eyes do not focus on the same thing at the same time.

Strident: See *Distinctive feature*.

Stridor: An abnormal breathing noise characterized by a tense, nonmusical laryngeal sound.

Submucosal cleft: A cleft of the palate whereby the surface tissues of the hard and soft palate are joined but the underlying bone or muscle tissues are not. Also called an occult cleft.

Substitution: One sound is substituted in place of the target sound. For example *wabbit* for *rabbit*.

Symbolic play: Using one object to represent another during play activity. For example, pretending a wooden spoon is a microphone during play.

Synchondrosis: A joining of two bones by cartilaginous tissue.

Syndactyly: Persistent soft tissue between the fingers or toes; webbing.

Syntax: The order of language, especially the way words are put together in phrases or sentences to produce meaning.

T

Telecoil switch: A hearing aid switch that allows the induction coil in the hearing aid to pick up signals from a telephone. It is also used in loop induction auditory training units.

Telegraphic speech: Short utterances consisting primarily or exclusively of content words (nouns, verbs, adjectives, adverbs). Grammatical words such as *the*, *to*, or *and* are typically omitted. For example, *I want to go* may be reduced to *want go*.

Tense: See *Distinctive feature*.

Test-retest reliability: See *Reliability*.

Tonsillitis: An inflammation of the tonsils usually caused by a bacterial infection.

Tracheostomy: The construction of an artificial opening through the neck into the trachea.

Tracheotomy: The operation of cutting into the trachea.

Transposition: See *Metathetic errors*.

Traumatic brain injury: An acute assault on the brain that causes mild to severe injury. The two types of traumatic brain injury are penetrating injuries and closed head injuries. The damage is localized or generalized depending on the type and extent of the injury.

Tympanogram: A graph depicting eardrum and middle ear compliance measured during air pressure changes in the external auditory canal.

U

Unilateral: Pertaining to one side of the body, such as a *unilateral* hearing loss involving only one ear.

V

Validity: Estimate of the degree to which a test actually measures or evaluates what it is intended to measure or evaluate.

    Concurrent validity: The relationship between what a given test measures and the results of a separate test. For example, the relationship between results obtained from two language tests.

    Construct validity: The relationship between what the test measures and a known construct such as age, sex, or IQ.

    Content validity: Whether the items contained on the test are appropriate for measuring what it intends to measure.

    Face validity: Whether a test appears, at face value, to measure what it intends to measure.

    Predictive validity: The ability of a test to predict future performance or abilities.

Velopharyngeal: Pertaining to the velum (soft palate) and the posterior nasopharyngeal wall.

Ventilation: Movement of air from one place to another.

Ventilation tube: A small tube placed in the tympanic membrane, creating a hole in the ear drum. It is used for the treatment and prevention of chronic otitis media.

Verb: A word expressing action or making a statement about the subject or noun phrase of a sentence.

Verbal paraphasia: See *Paraphasia*.

Vestibular system: The inner-ear structure containing three semicircular canals. The system is important for body position, balance, and movement.

Vitiligo: Unpigmented, pale patches of skin due to loss of pigmentation.

Vocalic: See *Distinctive feature*.

Vocal nodule: A small growth on the inner edge of the vocal folds. Acute nodules are similar to bruises, but they can harden and thicken over time. Vocal nodules are most common among children and adults who misuse and abuse their voices.

Voiced: See *Distinctive feature*.

INDEX

693